An Occupational Perspective of Health

Second Edition

An Occupational Perspective of Health

Second Edition

ANN A. WILCOCK, PHD, BAPPSCOT, GRADDIPPH, FCOT

HONORARY PROFESSOR OF OCCUPATIONAL SCIENCE AND THERAPY
DEAKIN UNIVERSITY, VICTORIA, AUSTRALIA

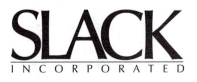

Delivering the best in health care information and education worldwide

www.slackbooks.com

ISBN-10: 1-55642-754-9
ISBN-13: 978-1-55642-754-1

An Occupational Perspective of Health, Second Edition Instructor's Manual is also available from SLACK Incorporated. Don't miss this important companion to *An Occupational Perspective of Health, Second Edition.* To obtain the Instructor's Manual, please visit http://www.efacultylounge.com

The procedures and practices described in this book should be implemented in a manner consistent with the professional standards set for the circumstances that apply in each specific situation. Every effort has been made to confirm the accuracy of the information presented and to correctly relate generally accepted practices. The authors, editor, and publisher cannot accept responsibility for errors or exclusions or for the outcome of the material presented herein. There is no expressed or implied warranty of this book or information imparted by it. Care has been taken to ensure that drug selection and dosages are in accordance with currently accepted/recommended practice. Due to continuing research, changes in government policy and regulations, and various effects of drug reactions and interactions, it is recommended that the reader carefully review all materials and literature provided for each drug, especially those that are new or not frequently used. Any review or mention of specific companies or products is not intended as an endorsement by the author or publisher.

SLACK Incorporated uses a review process to evaluate submitted material. Prior to publication, educators or clinicians provide important feedback on the content that we publish. We welcome feedback on this work.

Published by: SLACK Incorporated
                  6900 Grove Road
                  Thorofare, NJ 08086 USA
                  Telephone: 856-848-1000
                  Fax: 856-853-5991
                  www.slackbooks.com

Contact SLACK Incorporated for more information about other books in this field or about the availability of our books from distributors outside the United States.

Library of Congress Cataloging-in-Publication Data
Wilcock, Ann Allart.
   An occupational perspective of health / Ann A. Wilcock. -- 2nd ed.
      p. ; cm.
   Includes bibliographical references and index.
   ISBN-13: 978-1-55642-754-1 (alk. paper)
   ISBN-10: 1-55642-754-9 (alk. paper)
   1. Occupational therapy--Philosophy. 2. Industrial hygiene. I. Title.
   [DNLM: 1. Occupational Therapy. 2. Rehabilitation, Vocational. 3. Work--psychology. WB 555 W667o 2006]

RM735.4.W55 2006
615.8'515--dc22

                              2006008716

For permission to reprint material in another publication, contact SLACK Incorporated. Authorization to photocopy items for internal, personal, or academic use is granted by SLACK Incorporated provided that the appropriate fee is paid directly to Copyright Clearance Center. Prior to photocopying items, please contact the Copyright Clearance Center at 222 Rosewood Drive, Danvers, MA 01923 USA; phone: 978-750-8400; website: www.copyright.com; email: info@copyright.com

Printed in the United States of America.

Last digit is print number: 10   9   8   7   6   5   4   3   2   1

Dedication

This edition is dedicated to the life of 2 remarkable brothers, Eric John Richard (Dick) Heyward and Bruce Stanley Heyward of Koonya, a tiny rural community in the South East corner of the world, who epitomize to me the health-giving properties of doing, being, and becoming according to different natures and capacities.

Born to parents engaged in community service and primary production, Dick became an economist and an energetic, insightful, very respected long-established Director of UNICEF at the UN in New York. A frequent visitor to third-world countries for the World Bank, he was an early advocate of breastfeeding as an important public health measure. He died last year at 91 years of age.

Bruce, deafened as a result of aero engineering in World War II, followed the family tradition of growing high quality fruit for export to European and Eastern markets and as a local councilor. Following retirement, he built a large steel boat, took his skipper's license, and chartered groups of adventurers around the untamed waters of Southern Tasmania. After 10 years, he retired a second time to take up community service to help older and disadvantaged people and to learn to fly gliders. His greatest challenge could be as my husband supporting me as I struggle to write what I think is important—the recognition by world governments, health professions, and the general population of the complex but vital relationship of occupation to health.

Contents

Acknowledgments

My sincerest thanks go to all those who have supported and assisted me over the years and in the production of the first and second editions of this book: particularly my thanks go to my late husband, Derek, Dr. Neville Hicks, Janet Crowe, and other friends and professional colleagues, clients, and students who have contributed (in many ways) to my work and ideas.

About the Author

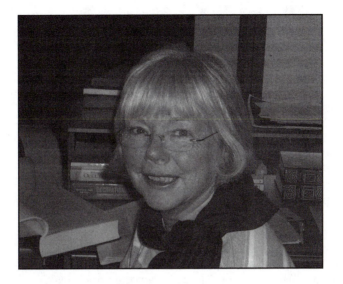

Ann A. Wilcock (née Ellison), PhD, BAppScOT, GradDipPH, FCOT, was born in the United Kingdom and was brought up in the Lake District. She graduated as an occupational therapist from the Derby School in 1961. She learned early of the need to think about the purpose of the profession because, in order to obtain some financial assistance for her training, at 16 years of age, she had to convince the Westmorland Education Authority of the merits of the profession, and the reason they should support her tertiary education in this field. No occupational therapists were employed in Westmorland at that time.

After graduating, Ann worked at Black Notley Hospital and Farnham Park Rehabilitation Centre before going to live in Australia in 1964. There, she worked in large general hospitals in a variety of fields, including mental health, orthopedics, geriatric medicine, and neurology. After many years as a practitioner, she moved into the academic sphere eventually becoming Head of the School of Occupational Therapy at the University of South Australia in 1987. Her formal academic career culminated in her appointment to establish a new and innovative program as Professor of Occupational Science and Therapy at Deakin University. Other appointments have included Visiting Professor at Brunel University, London; Adjunct Professor at Dalhousie University, Canada, and Charles Sturt University, Australia; and Doctoral Supervisor at Auckland University of Technology, New Zealand. Ann's research interests have spanned active aging; children's occupational potential; physiological influences on occupational performance; occupational balance; well-being; the effect of neurological disorder on the human need for occupation; population health; and the relationship between occupation, health, illness, occupational therapy, and public health. The highlight of her career has been in encouraging the development of occupational science as an international and interdisciplinary force. As well as introducing occupational science to Australasia, she founded the *Journal of Occupational Science* in 1993, convened the first Australasian Occupational Science Symposium, and was elected as the Inaugural President of the International Society of Occupational Scientists (ISOS). Her personal direction within the science is exploration of the relationship between people's occupational natures and health. This was firmly established as Ann undertook graduate studies in public health, and was the subject of her PhD thesis.

She is the author of 5 books; the first 2 are about stroke—*Help Yourselves: A Handbook for Hemiplegics and Their Families* in 1966 followed by *Occupational Therapy Approaches to Stroke* in 1986. The most recent *Occupation for Health: A Journey from Self-Health to Prescription* (2001) and the second volume, *A Journey from Prescription to Self-Health* (2002), were written when Ann was the commissioned historian for the British College and Association of Occupational Therapists. The first edition of this text, *An Occupational Perspective of Health*, was published by SLACK Incorporated in 1998. As well as numerous chapters and articles, Ann has delivered keynote addresses at the World Federation of Occupational Therapists Congress in Montreal in 1998, and at other conferences in Australia, New Zealand, Canada, United Kingdom, Sweden, Portugal, Japan, Thailand, Hong Kong, and the United States. She is the recipient of a range of prestigious awards, internationally:

2005	Honorary Professor of Deakin University, Victoria, Australia
2004	Honorary Fellow of Brunel University, UK
	Honorary Doctor of the University of Derby, UK
	Fellow of the British Association and College of Occupational Therapists
	Barbara Sexton Lectureship: University of Western Ontario, Canada
2000	Thelma Cardwell Lectureship: University of Toronto, Canada
1999	The Sylvia Docker Lectureship: OT Australia (National)
	The Doris Sym Memorial Lectureship: Glasgow Caledonian University, UK
	Inaugural Henry Nowic Trust "Occupation and Health" Lectureship: Charles Sturt University, Australia
1995	Wilma West Lectureship: University of Southern California, United States in recognition of outstanding contribution to the development of occupational science

Preface

This book addresses health from an occupational perspective. Drawing on history to inform the present, critical comment is offered to inform both a broad-based understanding of occupation within present-day health care and approaches that may be useful in the future. Like the first edition, it is written principally to inform those interested in improving the health of populations about the potential place of occupation-based initiatives in public health. It should be of interest to all workers in the field of public health, but public health practitioners have been constrained by a lack of understanding of occupation as a holistic concept and have devoted "occupation"-focused population health research and strategies toward specific aspects that have been identified by medicine and/or sociology as concerns. That provides only snapshots of understanding about how what people do throughout their lives to meet economic, social, and personal needs impacts on their health. The snapshots have effectively decontextualized and biased appreciation, exploration, and action of a phenomenon of great importance to health.

The first edition of the book was adopted largely by occupational therapists who, ironically, are often restricted in their fields of interest and expertise by the expectation of others. In large part, the occupational therapy profession's contribution is overlooked. In some cases, it not considered relevant in the present economically driven system in which time matters and people are left to get on with their lives in a way that possibly contributed to illness in the first place. It may also be that occupational therapists are hesitant to let go of current practice and have few opportunities to develop other forms more relevant to today's world. With the intention of informing public health experts of the potential of occupational therapists to work toward population health in the spirit of the World Health Organization's (WHO) directives, the first edition introduced the philosophical bases and the development of occupational therapy to provide insight into the profession's ideology. These are not provided separately in this edition, which continues to inform both occupational therapists and public health practitioners of their potential role in largely unexplored territory. Some aspects of both public health and occupational therapy history are, however, included as the story develops throughout the text.

The story focuses on the present reality of health experiences throughout the world and the views of the WHO as to necessary future directions for all health care. It concentrates on how occupation is integral to the experience of health or illness within populations complementing other public health and occupational therapy texts. In this edition, 4 chapters address suggested approaches to population health, expanding and encapsulating the 5 approaches outlined in the original edition. They center on the evidence that such approaches are valid and useful, the type of people or circumstance for which each may be appropriate, and the essential nature or characteristics that distinguish each from the others, although all could be used in conjunction. It would, at this stage, be inappropriate to give detailed recipes for how to go about such work. This is for occupation-focused public health professionals to develop according to the health needs they seek to address in participation with the populations involved. Despite its difference to other texts, the book is pertinent and informative to the new public health and traditional occupational therapy in providing a collection of background studies that support the professions' beliefs.

In informing both occupational therapists and workers from other professions in the population health field, the book tells of a long history that precedes current ideas about the relationship between occupation and health, providing evidence from many disciplines that suggests new ways forward. It takes a holistic view of health in line with that of the WHO, addressing the necessity for all health professions to move in the direction of preventing illness and promoting health and well-being for all people. To focus the research and discussion, important directives provided by the WHO are used as themes for each chapter.

Like other public health approaches, this occupational perspective respects and complements the medical approach to health. It acknowledges the long-held expertise and place of conventional medicine in tackling somatic and psychological problems of physical and mental disease and injury. Occupational therapy has a useful and respected role within that. This perspective also respects the medical role in preventing and treating disease principally but not exclusively with pharmaceutical knowledge founded on laboratory-based sciences and on researching the causes of disease and the effects of drug-based therapy. The view taken here is that, particularly over the last century, priority in medicine has been given to finding and using technical and pharmaceutical remedies for illness, and that less time has been given to advising people about living wisely and healthily. This has begun to change in part because of the new public health direction of the last 2 decades. Within that newer wave of thinking there is, however, limited attendance to the complexity of occupational issues in population health, and present day initiatives are aimed principally at health risks in paid employment and on physical exercise to counter obesity.

The WHO has begun to address occupational issues of health in the rhetoric of documents such as the *Ottawa Charter for Health Promotion*,[1] the *Social Determinants of Health*,[2] *Mental Health*,[3] *Global Strategy on Diet, Physical Activity and Health*,[4] and in its active aging policy.[5]

The Purpose of This Book

This book presents an occupational perspective of public (population) health that is founded on WHO definitions and policies, drawing heavily on the documents listed above and addressing important themes as a focal point of each chapter. Four suggested approaches are complementary to and supportive of conventional medical practice but address broader personal, social, economic, and environmental goals that are in line with WHO and public health in a changing world and a global economy.

The book endeavors to uncover a different way to understand health in the light of how, what, and why people spend time and effort in "doing, being, and becoming" through engagement in occupations. It explores the relationships between occupation, health, illness, health care, and the ideologies that surround them; the potential importance to public/population health of these relationships; and how these are or could be addressed by occupational therapists or public health practitioners. In doing so, it links occupational terminology with that of public health so that interdisciplinary speak becomes easier.

Throughout the text, *occupation* is used to mean "all the things that people need, want, or have to do" across the sleep-wake continuum, and a theory about people's occupational natures and their needs, wants, and obligations in this regard is outlined in the second chapter. The third chapter addresses the prerequisites of health and survival, and the fourth chapter embraces the impact of how people feel about what they do. In the fifth chapter, the growth, development, and enhancement potential of involvement is considered. The 3 aspects of occupation in Chapters 3, 4, and 5 are conceptualized within the phrase "doing, being, and becoming" and are addressed throughout the text, as well as being the hub of the 3 separate chapters.

Public health relates to health concerns and initiatives for the population at large. The terms *public health* and *population health* will therefore be used interchangeably throughout the text. While the book's primary purpose is to address the occupation-health nexus at population levels within communities across the globe, many of the issues are relevant to individual health and illness initiatives, as readers of the first edition found.

Explorations that have preceded both editions of the book have been influenced by observations and reflections of the health care system over several decades, professional and academic experience in occupational therapy, and graduate work in public health. Study in the latter over close to 2 of those decades has provided a guide to the broad range of health issues deemed important in that sphere and by the WHO. Marrying these perspectives has been a fascinating, enlightening, and stimulating experience. For each profession, particular perspectives of health and illness are somewhat different, and for each professional, there are also slight differences according to underlying beliefs, values, and experiences. Nevertheless, there is scant acknowledgment that basic ideas about what health is may not be constant between health professions or even within the general population. There is little appreciation that in order to meet professional, population, community, and individual goals, health care workers, including occupational therapists and public health practitioners, need to be able to define clearly what they, their clients, and the communities they serve mean by health and illness. Because ideas about "health and well-being" do differ, it is important to search for factors that may have been overlooked as well as those common to the experience of "health." It is also necessary to describe clearly each profession's particular views and underlying values.

The WHO Primary Health Care Report of the International Conference held at Alma Ata in 1978 also prompted the explorations.[6] That report and the 1986 *Ottawa Charter for Health Promotion*[1] inspired the continuing development of an occupational view of human nature and health that is described in early chapters and underlies the perspective presented. Those WHO documents, as well as more recent ones, stressed the need for the reorientation of all health professions toward the pursuit of health. For occupational therapists, it is reasonable that such reorientation should be founded on study of the relationship between health and occupation. For public health practitioners, it is important to recognize a holistic view of occupation as a largely ignored aspect of health and illness.

Developing a health perspective centered on occupation is particularly difficult because occupation is such an integral part of living and of already accepted, but different, perspectives on life. To rethink issues from this divergent, yet familiar, focus demands that "the ways of thinking which seem so natural and inevitable that they are not [usually] scrutinized with the eye of logical self-consciousness" be identified and analyzed, and, following scrutiny, resynthesized.[7] Throughout recent decades this has been made more difficult because of the prevailing reductionism of traditional scientific methods that are central within medical and epidemiological research.

At the start of this exploration, occupational science, or the study of people as occupational beings, was in the first stages of development. This science was initially conceived by occupational therapists in the United States.[8] Work by others in Australasia, Canada, Japan, the United Kingdom, and Scandinavia followed. It is not coincidental that the science emerged at this time throughout the world. A look at concept development in many fields other than occupational therapy illustrates a change of consciousness about the things that people do. There is, for example, renewed interest in issues related to paid employment, leisure pursuits, sports, education, and early childhood learning as determinants of health. Unfortunately, such interest has not yet reached a stage of understanding that enables adoption of occupational science as a global and far-reaching discipline that can offer insights into understanding occupation as an important issue within public health. This book attempts to provide a multidisciplinary synthesis that may assist others in recognizing common concerns and provide impetus for further developments. That may also assist leaders in the public health field to appreciate that occupational therapists with well-founded understanding of the relationship between health and what people need, want, or have to do can offer intervention and community and health-planning advice worthy of their attention.

To these ends, 5 specific issues are addressed in the second edition:

1. How health has been, is, and can be conceptualized
2. The role of occupation in human life, health, and survival
3. Occupation as a positive or negative influence on health
4. The potential contribution of occupation-focused approaches to current WHO and public/population health objectives
5. Possible occupation for health-focused action for occupational therapists and public health practitioners to take at population levels

The History of Ideas Approach

Traditional experimental researchers often see the complexities of human characteristics and the variety of occupational environments as contaminants to research design.[9] Yet to reduce people's engagement in occupation to component parts would diminish its study because it is the integrated complexities that require the most rigorous investigation.[8] It is almost impossible to explore those according to reductionist and contextually controlled studies. Gergen, a social psychologist, is one of many who criticize using traditional science methodology for studying human beings because techniques do decontextualize, are atemporal and deterministic, and can lead to inadequate and distorted findings.[10]

Open-minded consideration of different research methodologies, such as those used in anthropology, developmental and social psychology, sociology, evolutionary biology, and history, which study people contextually, view their activities diachronically and recognize individual will are more suited to building a knowledge base for a science of occupation.[8] Additionally, methods appropriate for interdisciplinary research about the "conditions which make possible the reproduction and transformation of society, the meaning of culture, and the relationship between the individual, society, and nature"[10] are valuable to consider as tools in understanding the occupational nature of people and its relationship to population health. Advocated by critical social scientists, such methods would also assist the development of transformative occupation-based programs to meet differing cultural needs. These requirements suggest that a synthesis of ideas from a wide range of disciplines is required for the broad issues being explored in this text. To meet that requirement, the exploration took the form of a history of ideas that entailed analysis of wide-ranging historical and modern documentation about how occupation has been and still is instrumental in survival and health.

Histories of ideas are really forms of critical text analysis used to consider insights into the what, why, and how of particular phenomena. Arthur Lovejoy first advanced the term in the 1920s to describe a form of research that reconsiders already known concepts from a different perspective so that new insights emerge.[11] He argued that this approach is most useful if the history is concerned with widely held concepts that cross cultural boundaries, disciplines, and thought such as justice, nature, and freedom.[7] Lovejoy named these as core ideas.[12] I ascribe that both health and occupation are core ideas so fundamental to any time and place that they are taken for granted and assumed to be largely unchangeable. An unchangeable nature proves to be far from the case because ideas about both have altered throughout history as environments and cultures evolved. Indeed, it is vital to recognize that core ideas often change from generation to generation and that they might be conceived in slightly different ways by different disciplines, socio-economic groups, or ethnically disparate populations. Ideas that emerge at any one time usually manifest themselves in more than one direction. A history of ideas aims "at interpretation and unification and seeks to correlate things" that, in our present structures and reductionist ways of thinking, may appear unconnected.[7] As material is reviewed in this text from other disciplines, cultures, known experts, and ideas and artfacts of people throughout time, that phenomenon is illustrated. It is also apparent that the concept and meaning of occupation and of health has changed with occupational technology and subsequent sociocultural evolution, ideas, and expectations.

A study of this kind is fairly unusual in the field of health and at first glance may appear to be "a strange combination of incongruences: general but detailed, straightforward but intricate, pragmatic but abstract," and because it tells a story, the rigor of the research effort is easily overlooked.[13] The story line was perhaps clearer in the first edition of this book because it was presented in chapters that explored biological characteristics of people, their occupational nature and needs, and occupational evolution before progressing to a study of health and illness with those perspectives in mind. It told a second story about occupational therapy and its relationship with those ideas. In this edition, the story line is dispersed throughout the text as different issues about health and its relationship to what people do, are, and become are raised. This has been done to make clearer the links between natural health, biological needs, long-held rules for health, current population health directives, and occupation.

The study was rigorous because almost every central notion was subjected to cross-disciplinary searches and analysis and led to a voyage of discovery through evolutionary texts, anthropology, sociology, philosophy, ethology, epidemiology, sociobiology, genetics, labor studies, psychology, ecology, neural Darwinism, and public health as well as occupational therapy texts. As progress occurred, unexpected issues emerged and fresh connections were made, eventuating in a hypothesis about occupation and health that provides the substance of the second chapter.

Because the historian of an idea is compelled to gather material from several fields of knowledge, it is inevitable that error will occur in at least some parts of the synthesis.[14] To counter this as far as is possible, secondary and tertiary sources of information, as well as primary works, were used to further illuminate the original ideas and point the novice toward new or different sources of evidence. These sources suggested both lines of inquiry and other historians' viewpoints. The story that emerged from this process, like other histories of ideas, opened up "new avenues of investigation, criticism, and reflection, not simply (a) recreat(ion of) another author's interpretation of the past."[13] Historical research, in contrast to most other forms of qualitative inquiry, depends upon the quality of a reasoned argument, which is considered of more importance than particular methodological steps or stages that are in accord with scientific conventions. The writing is, therefore, an essential aspect of the research process. It can be a method of discovery and analysis as well as "a way of 'knowing'."[15]

The process facilitated a critical viewpoint because it enabled me to look at the world through a different lens. It generated a belief in the necessity for political and social change to improve occupational experience, health, and well-being, and, unexpectedly, the need for occupational therapists to become social activists who are concerned with issues of occupational injustice and with sustaining the ecology.

The story that emerges from the research process outlines a long association between occupation and health. Humans affected their health by what they did from the start of their existence, long before specific people were designated or chosen to specialize in caring for the health of others. As the latter specializations developed, the basic association between occupation and health became increasingly overlooked. This neglect is a matter for public health practitioners. It is also a matter for occupational therapists whose foundation and subsequent development is based on the natural and often overlooked relationship between health and occupation. To give due importance to this relationship, its foundation and subsequent changes throughout millennia needs to be elucidated. It is necessary to understand the hows and whys of the relationship before beginning to move forward into the population health arena. Practice not based on a firm foundation will falter, and practitioners will be unable to respond appropriately when ongoing change forces new action and places new demands. A firm foundation fosters research that can accept the challenges of approaches that fail to deliver results and articulate and fight for approaches that can deliver improved population health.

Configuration of the Text

The book has 2 main sections with an introduction to each. The introduction to the first section advances the central business of the book: health and occupation. The second induces the themes of the 4 approaches that are offered and provides information pertinent to all 4 about an action-research approach. Two pictorial devices have emerged during the updating of the book. One is a triangle shape that occurred so often it suggested the occupation pyramid for health as a health promotion device. The second is a scroll used for special bibliographical inserts. The use of a scroll is indicative of the long and shared journey between health and occupation and that the thoughts have grown from earlier ones and will be followed by others.

The first section of the book considers why and how occupation and health are related. To do so, it addresses the concepts of health and illness, the importance of occupation in human life, and the positive or negative influences of occupation on population health. In addressing health and illness, issues concerning natural health, biological needs, public health, well-being and health promotion, and ancient and modern rules for health will be explored. An occupational theory of human nature is introduced, largely unchanged from how it was conceived and presented in the first edition. This is followed by 3 chapters that address "doing," "being," and "becoming" as different but inter-related components of occupation. Discussion centers on how these relate to the WHO prerequisites for health at personal, social, cultural, and environmental as well as population levels. The occupation health and illness nexus is investigated from the angle of how people feel about what they do or do not do and how they become different through what they do. Also considered is the WHO ideology about active aging and about health promotion and the effects of occupational deprivation, alienation, or injustice.

The second section of the book presents discussion about 4 public health occupation-focused approaches to eco-sustainable community development, justice and equity, the prevention of illness and disability, and the promotion of health and well-being. The 4 approaches can be seen to cover environmental, population, and individual issues. All can be aimed at public policy to improve health experiences globally. Developing expertise relating to this broad range of approaches does demand a critical, proactive stance within community venues and at a sociopolitical level and also demands that the potential contribution of occupation-focused programs to population health be made known.

The book has been firmly based on WHO directives toward improving the health of people throughout the world. There is a strong "occupation" focus within those directives, although the terminology reflects the disintegrated concept of people's "doings, beings, and becomings" that are enacted in the current environment. The material in the first edition of this text forms the core. It appears in chapters throughout the text when relevant to the new direction outlined. Recent research that supports or refutes the positive and negative relationships between occupation and health is added and discussed. Additionally, more evidence from historical sources is included. The pre-history and genesis of occupational therapy that formed 2 chapters in the earlier edition is linked more explicitly to social change in the Western world and integrated throughout the work in contrast to being separated out. The material presented in the last chapter of the first edition is extended into separate chapters to provide more guidance to practitioners who are about to launch into public health-based practice.

References

1. World Health Organization, Health and Welfare Canada, Canadian Public Health Association. *Ottawa Charter for Health Promotion*. Ottawa, Canada: WHO; 1986.
2. Wilkinson R, Marmot M, eds. *Social Determinants of Health: The Solid Facts*. Copenhagen, Denmark: World Health Organization Regional Office for Europe; 2003.
3. World Health Organization. *Mental Health: Strengthening Mental Health Promotion. Fact sheet N°220*. Geneva: WHO; 2005.
4. World Health Organization. *Global Strategy on Diet, Physical Activity and Health. Chronic Disease Information Sheets*. Geneva: WHO; 2005.
5. World Health Organization. *Ageing and Life Course Programme Policy Framework*. Madrid, Spain: WHO Second UN World Assembly on Ageing; 2002.
6. World Health Organization. Primary Health Care. Report of the International Conference on Primary Health Care, Alma Ata, USSR, 1978.
7. Lovejoy AO. The study of the history of ideas. In: King P, ed. *The History of Ideas*. London: Croom Helm; 1983:179-194.
8. Yerxa EJ, Clark F, Frank G, et al. An introduction to occupational science: a foundation for occupational therapy in the 21st century. *Occupational Therapy in Health Care*. 1989;6(4):1–17.
9. Yerxa EJ. A mind is a precious thing. *Australian Occupational Therapy Journal*. 1990;37(4):170–171.
10. Gergen K. *Towards Transformation in Social Knowledge*. New York: Springer-Verlag; 1982.
11. Burke P. History of ideas. In: Bullock A, Stalleybrass O, Trombley S, eds. *The Fontana Dictionary of Modern Thought*. 2nd ed. London: Fontana Press; 1988:388.
12. Boas G. *The History of Ideas. An Introduction*. New York: Charles Scribner's Sons.
13. Hamilton DB. The idea of the history and the history of ideas. *Image: Journal of Nursing Scholarship*. 1993;25(1):45–48.
14. Lovejoy AO. *Essays in the History of Ideas*. Baltimore, Md: The Johns Hopkins Press; 1948:195.
15. Richardson L. Writing: a method of inquiry. In: Denzin N, Lincoln Y, eds. *Handbook of Qualitative Research*. London: Sage; 1994:516-529.

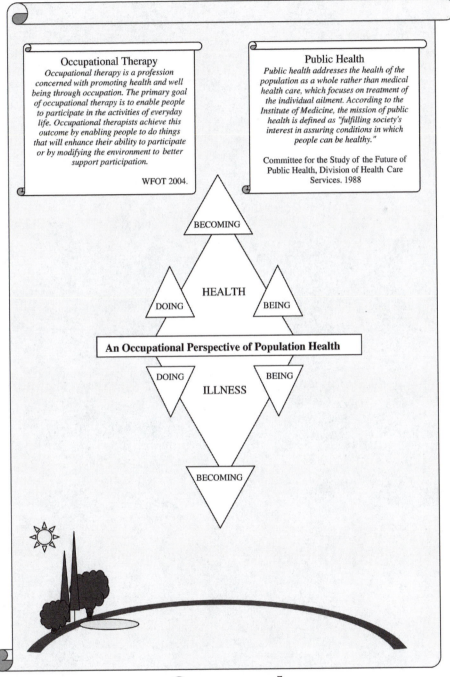

Occupational Therapy

Occupational therapy is a profession concerned with promoting health and well being through occupation. The primary goal of occupational therapy is to enable people to participate in the activities of everyday life. Occupational therapists achieve this outcome by enabling people to do things that will enhance their ability to participate or by modifying the environment to better support participation.

WFOT 2004.

Public Health

Public health addresses the health of the population as a whole rather than medical health care, which focuses on treatment of the individual ailment. According to the Institute of Medicine, the mission of public health is defined as "fulfilling society's interest in assuring conditions in which people can be healthy."

Committee for the Study of the Future of Public Health, Division of Health Care Services. 1988

BECOMING

HEALTH

DOING

BEING

An Occupational Perspective of Population Health

DOING

BEING

ILLNESS

BECOMING

SECTION I

HEALTH AND A SCIENCE OF OCCUPATION

Introduction to Section I

I get angry almost every time I read, hear, or watch the news. Yet, on the whole I would not describe myself as an angry person.
Why is this so?
Increasingly in every part of the globe, the consequences of social illness are reported. War, terrorism, rioting, ecological devastation, famine, homelessness, substance abuse, school absenteeism, unemployment, social welfare fraud, dependence on the state, an increase of food-related disorders, family breakdown, suicide, aggression, and abuse are commonly headline news. The modern world has got something very wrong, despite pockets of affluence that appear to be the focus of postmodern, economic rationalist governments. Ironically, the affluent too are subject to many of these social illnesses.
One of the causes, I believe, is a lack of understanding of social illness despite World Health Organization (WHO) attempts to bring this to the attention of governments, health practitioners, and the population at large for nearly 3 decades. Additionally, I believe that the role of occupation in terms of social health, as well as physical and mental health, is so poorly understood that it is largely ignored and not resourced adequately. Some of these complex issues will be addressed throughout this book.

Health and a Science of Occupation

Like all things in the universe, health is remarkably simple and remarkably complex. In the rapid growth of understanding of some of the complexities during the last 100 years or so, the simple and most important aspects of health have been overlooked. They are obvious and yet almost totally ignored. The first 6 chapters will try to peel back some of the millions of years of buildup to present-day neglect and to take a fresh look at one central factor in health that has been neglected: namely, the what, whys, and hows of people's doings. What humans, early homo species, and creatures of all kinds did and still do is the lynch pin of health. Animals in the wild remain able to live healthily through what they do as long as their environment is not changed too drastically. People are not so fortunate. Across the globe, natural environments and ways of life are so irreparably damaged that illness is a present reality for many and probable for most in the longer term. This negative background to people's experiences of health, in large part, can be blamed not only on what people have done or not done in the past, but also on what people do currently, and in particular, what the pursuit of wealth by advanced countries and multinational corporations has led to.

While the glories of medical science and the struggles of a young environmental movement to right those wrongs are topics that are addressed almost daily in the world's news, the fact is that the occupational needs of people and how these relate to their health or illness remain largely unexplored. This is despite the fact that from the time people began to record their observations about the causes of health or illness, rules about doing were prescribed. That remained the case until the early 20th century but is rare presently, except with regard to the taking of medication, resting, or, more recently, exercising in the interest of reducing obesity and subsequent disease. While the fascination with eating and health has been constant and evident in ancient health rules, the occupations related to the getting, preparing, and eating food have been increasingly ignored as an aspect of health. Instead they are regarded, in the main, as a social matter or one of economics. Also regarded as a social matter fairly distinct from health or illness is the way people appear to need to find enjoyment or meaning in what they do, yet this too is a basic health mechanism. Fortunately, the WHO has provided directives and guidelines. These supersede the earlier rules of health that still have much to recommend them. If taken seriously and acted upon, the new rules could lead health services toward a broader understanding of health that embraces occupational issues. While viewing public health as distinct from occupation terminology, these directives provide a way forward for those concerned with improving population health through enabling participation in health-giving occupation.

In seeking to clarify people's beliefs, values, perceptions, and ideas about the relationships between health and occupation, it is important to recall that, presently, health care is dominated by medical science in postindustrialized societies. This is based mainly on contemporary understanding of physiology, biochemistry, pathology, biostatistics, and societal acceptance of modern technological, surgical, and pharmaceutical advances. Medical science values are so integral to postindustrial culture's thinking, it is difficult for those brought up in such a society to perceive health from other than a medical science perspective. To some extent, this limits the study of health to ideas, beliefs, and approaches that are valued, advocated, and deemed important by medical science. Even the growing behavioral-health, social-health, and health-science professions, which are different and distinct from medicine, are still influenced by medical science values and perspectives. They challenge or use medical science categories and theories; accept many medical science priorities; and are concerned with strategies to diagnose or analyze, reduce, or prevent illness resulting from physical, behavioral, or social factors. Because of this emphasis, the major preoccupation in health research is to uncover the causes of illness and disease. Notwithstanding the holistic philosophy of the *Ottawa Charter for Health Promotion*,[1] which was adopted by the "new public health" movement[2] and ratified by the *Jakarta Declaration* as the way forward into the 21st century,[3] health research remains preoccupied with reducing the incidence of illness at the expense of detailed exploration of the causes of good health and well-being. Recent interest in social determinants of health, health promotion, and wellness has centered to a large extent on the prevention of illness, with many people using the terms *prevention* and *health promotion* synonymously. Preventive approaches, which dominate public health just as medicine dominates health care, generally take for granted a medical science explanation of the cause of disease and the mechanisms for prevention.

The new public health is also influenced by a postindustrial debate between the values of economic rationalism and social equality. Caught between medical science and the debate about social values, public health has largely failed to consider how basic human needs relate to health, unless the needs can be reduced to obvious physiological functioning or monetary terms. Rather like "instinct theory," the idea of human needs is unfashionable and to a large extent ignored, being associated with "naturalistic fallacy"[4] and out of step with the dominant notions of behaviorism and cultural relativism. This stance ignores many of the needs and potential of humans, which are part of their "hard-wired" neuronal structure, and, as Doyal and Gough maintain in their award-winning book *A Theory of Human Need*, even if needs are not identical with drives or a "motivational force instigated by a state of disequilibrium ... neither are they disconnected from 'human nature.'"[5] These authors state that "to argue for such disconnection would be to identify humanity with no more than human reason and to bifurcate human existence from that of the rest of the animal world."[5] It is argued in these first 6 chapters that health is related to the meeting of biological needs and potential, to learning "how nature intended human beings to live,"[6] and that the needs of any living organism are related to health from the point of view of "how a specimen" of that kind of organism "can be recognized as flourishing."[4] The simplicity and complexity of health is mirrored in the occupational nature and needs of people.

A major concept revisited in each of the first 6 chapters maintains that humans have "occupational needs" that go beyond the instinctive patterned behaviors of many other animals and that these needs are related to health. In fact, they are the species' primary health mechanism, motivating the provision of other basic requirements as well as enabling individuals to use their biological capacities and potential, meet sociocultural expectations, and thereby flourish. The integrative functions of the central nervous system, which process external and internal information, activated by engagement in occupation, are focal to survival, the maintenance of homeostasis, and facilitating health and well-being. The adaptive capacity of the human brain allows the innate drive for purposeful occupation to respond to cultural forces and values that add a social dimension to the relationship between health and doing, being, and becoming.

I explore health from an occupational perspective to uncover the innate evolutionary relationship between health and occupation. I combine an evolutionary, biological approach with a modern, culture-concept approach to determine the influence of experience, learning, and cultural evolution. This is similar to approaches taken by ethologists who seek to discover, among other ideas, the survival function of whatever behavior is under study. Konrad Lorenz, an Austrian zoologist, explained ethology as the process of examining "animal and human behavior as the function of a system owing its existence, as well as its special form, to a development process that has taken place in the history of the species, in the development of the individual and, in man, in cultural history."[7]

In line with Lorenz's perspective, I consider prehistoric occupational traits alongside "natural" health behaviors of early hominids before they were affected by millions of years of acquired health and occupational values. The assumption is that human traits resulting from biological evolution will have affected occupational evolution, just as changes in social values and occupational technology will have affected natural health behaviors. The exploration is based on archeological and anthropological research, as was much of the previous edition. It rests upon a range of hypotheses founded on the study of archeological finds and their context, the subjecting of these to scientific analysis and reconstruction, and from ethnographic studies of modern people still engaging in early lifestyles. Biological characteristics and capacities, occupational evolution, health and well-being, and the prevention of illness will be explored to uncover the ideas behind natural health and biological needs.

This exploration has added to and draws upon studies that provide the ground swell of the new academic discipline of occupational science. Recognition of the need for a science of occupation is not entirely new. In recent times, however, occupation—in the sense it is used here and in its own right rather than as therapy—has only been a focal point of

Figure 1-1A. Pioneers of occupational science: John Locke.

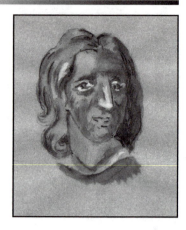

study for occupational scientists. Earlier, John Locke (1632–1704), an English philosopher and a self-styled physician (Figure 1-1A), propounded a view that only 3 sciences were necessary, one of which was closely aligned to occupational science. Locke lived in the period described as the Enlightenment at the latter part of the Renaissance when humanism emerged as a dominant philosophy, so his recognition of the need for such a science is understandable. Humanism challenged previously held views about "body and soul, flesh and spirit, mind and matter," and social concepts of identity, destiny, moral, and spiritual well-being, signalling a rebirth of interest in individual talent and interest.[8] In *An Essay Concerning Human Understanding*, Locke argued that science as the means to explore, discover, and understand the world as far as it was possible could be divided into "three sorts." In closest to current terms, these were the biological, occupational, and communication sciences:

> *First, The Nature of Things, as they are in themselves, their Relations, and their manner of Operation: Or,*
> *Secondly, that which Man himself ought to do, as a rational and voluntary Agent, for the Attainment of any Ends, especially Happiness: Or,*
> *Thirdly, The ways and means, whereby the Knowledge of both the one and the other of these, are attained and communicated.[9]*

Interestingly, these 3 sciences are central to the perspective presented in this text. Locke went on to describe them further. The second (which he called ethics) he defined as:

> *The skill of Right applying our own Powers and Actions, for the Attainment of Things good and useful. The most considerable under this Head, is Ethicks, which is the seeking out those Rules, and Measures of humane Actions, which lead to Happiness, and the Means to practice them. The end of this is not bare Speculation, and the Knowledge of Truth; but Right, and a Conduct suitable to it.[9]*

A recurring theme throughout what is considered his most important text is reference to the practical and the possible. In teasing out the issues of human understanding in this way, he anticipates 19th and early 20th century socialist reformers in Europe who recognized the value of human labor and pragmatist philosophers in the United States, such as William James, who recognized the centrality of occupation to life. Both groups were influential in the ideas of the modern occupational therapy profession in the United States of America and the United Kingdom. This was accomplished through the decisive roles played by Jane Addams in Chicago and Octavia Hill in London that led to the establishment of occupational therapy education.

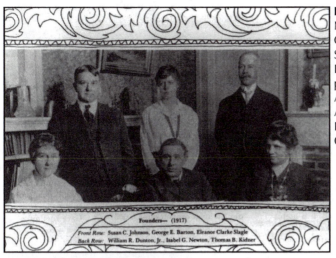

Figure 1-1B. Founders of the National Society for the Promotion of Occupational Therapy, 1917, Clifton Springs, NY. Box 123, File No. 1016. Bethesda, Md. (Reproduced with permission of the Archives of the American Occupational Therapy Association Inc, Bethesda, Md. Permission conveyed through the Copyright Clearance Center, Inc.)

Founders— (1917)
Front Row: Susan C. Johnson, George E. Barton, Eleanor Clarke Slagle
Back Row: William R. Dunton, Jr., Isabel G. Newton, Thomas B. Kidner

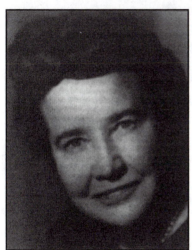

Figure 1-1C. Pioneers of occupational science: Mary Reilly. (Reproduced with permisison of American Occupational Therapy Asssociation, from American Occupational Therapy Association. *A Professional Legacy: The Eleanor Clarke Slagle Lectures.* Rockville, Md: Author; 1985:298. Permission conveyed through the Copyright Clearance Center, Inc.)

It was in 1917 that the American National Society for the Promotion of Occupational Therapy was formed. Architects George Edward Barton (Figure 1-1B) and Thomas Bessell Kidner, social worker Eleanor Clarke Slagle, physician William Rush Dunton (see Figure 1-1B), and teacher Susan Cox Johnson, who were all working in the field, came together at Clifton Springs, New York, to write the Certificate of Incorporation.[10] The objectives of the Society recognized the importance of research to back up the profession's claims.[11] They were "the advancement of occupation as a therapeutic measure; the study of the effect of occupation upon the human being; and the scientific dispensation of this knowledge."[12]

Those particular objectives, recognized as difficult to achieve because of the complex nature of occupation, have current value in terms of public health as well as pre-empting the development of occupational science some half a century later.

It was Mary Reilly (Figure 1-1C), an occupational therapy educator at the University of Southern California, who led the way to developing occupational science in the early 1960s, proposing "that man through the use of his hands, as they are energized by mind and will, can influence the state of his own health."[13] She postulated that although the First Principle, from which medical science draws its premise, explains that the nature of

Figure 1-1D. Pioneers of occupational science: Elizabeth Yerxa.

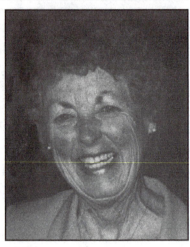

humans is to be alive, the Second Principle is for humans to grow and be productive, and she maintained that occupational therapy should derive its premise from this principle. The 2 principles "merge into a concept of function which asserts that both the existence and the unfolding of the specific powers of an organism are one and the same thing."[13] Reilly had a huge influence on the work of her graduate students,[14] as Gary Kielhofner's *A Model of Human Occupation* attests. Kielhofner, one of the best known figures of occupational therapy today, developed his model from one of Reilly's basic assumptions that "occupation is a central aspect of the human experience" and that "all human occupation arises out of an innate, spontaneous tendency of the human system—the urge to explore and master the environment."[15] Reilly also influenced her colleagues, one of whom, Elizabeth Yerxa (Figure 1-1D), was instrumental in the development of occupational science as "a unique academic discipline sufficient in scope and importance to merit its own doctoral degree."[16] She saw this basic science of occupation as a social science akin to anthropology, sociology, and psychology and as complementary to the applied science of occupational therapy.[16] Yerxa and her associates at the University of Southern California defined occupational science as "the study of the human as an occupational being, including the need for and capacity to engage in and orchestrate daily occupations in the environment over the lifespan."[17] In this text, this has been shortened to "the study of people as occupational beings."

Since the early 20th century, new age thinking in sociology, economics, technology, and medical science had so dominated thinking that occupation during that time had been considered from these perspectives rather than in its own right. However, it is interesting to note that the earlier socialist and pragmatist recognition of the importance of occupation in life occurred as a result of drastic social change from a technology of human labor based on agriculture to one based on industry and that occupational therapy originated as a result of this occupational interest. The current resurgence of interest in occupation and occupational science by occupational therapists may well be a response to a particular need to reconsider human occupational requirements afresh at times of change. Its relevance to population health is encapsulated in how the World Federation of Occupational Therapists (WFOT), the central organizational arm of the profession, describes its concerns:

> *Promoting health and well being through occupation. The primary goal of occupational therapy is to enable people to participate successfully in the activities of everyday life. Occupational therapists achieve this outcome by enabling people to do things that will*

enhance their ability to live meaningful lives or by modifying the environment to better support participation.[18]

Because occupation is a central theme of this text, it is necessary to clarify, as much as possible, what is meant by the word in this particular context. It will be used in the text as many English-speaking occupational therapists use it, in the generic sense, perhaps reflecting common usage of the word when their profession was developing in the first decades of this century. (Because of occupation's other meaning of a foreign power taking possession over another's territory, many occupational therapists from European nations do not feel comfortable with its usage and instead use "ergo" as a prefix). In dictionaries of the period, occupation was defined as "being occupied, what occupies one, means of filling up one's time, temporary or regular employment, business, calling, pursuit"[19] and "that which occupies or engages the time and attention."[20] In a contemporary dictionary, too, the aspect of occupation central to this text includes "being occupied or employed with, or engaged in something."[21] Despite more generic meaning, occupation is currently commonly used to refer to paid employment, specifically. The adjective *occupational* is particularly used in this way, as in "occupational health and safety" and "occupational diseases." The use of occupation to refer, as it does in this text, to all that people need, want, or are obliged to do; what it means to them; and its ever present potential as an agent of change is often misunderstood. Other words that have similar but less inclusive meaning, such as *activity, exercise,* or *task,* are seen as aspects of occupation that will be used appropriately from time to time.

Occupation is so much a part of everyday life that it is reasonable to make empirical statements about it. It can be said, therefore, that people engage in occupation, with individuality of purpose and to meet familial and communal goals; they think about the effects, conceptualize, and plan prior to engagement; and they are able to reflect and mentally alter future doing as a result of outcomes. Occupations demonstrate a community's and an individual's culturally sanctioned intellectual, moral, social, and physical attributes. It is only by what they do that people can demonstrate what they are or what they hope to be. Occupation also provides the mechanism for social interaction and societal development and growth, forming the foundation of community, local, and national identity because individuals not only engage in separate pursuits, they are able to plan and execute group activity to the extent of national government or to achieve international goals for individual, mutual, and community purposes.

Without occupation, time appears to pass extremely slowly, as any long distance air traveler can attest, even with the frequent meals, drinks, and movies. Occupation is a natural user of time that provides a sense of purpose, and without which humans are apt to be bored, depressed, and sometimes destructive. Even the stylite, the eremite, or the monk passes the time in a way meaningful or purposeful to him or her despite the meaning or purpose perhaps appearing obscure to others. Adolph Meyer, an American psychiatrist, eminent in the first half of the 20th century and credited with providing a philosophy to occupational therapy, proposed that how people use time is very important. He asserted that in order to maintain and balance the organism that is a person, there is a need to act in time with bodily and natural rhythms and that timely activity and rest are vital components of healthy living.[22] Exploring how and why people use time the way they do provides a rich source of data on many different sociocultural and health-related issues, and thus, this perspective of occupation has been subject to scrutiny. Time-use surveys originated early this century, with most studying large population groups for comparative purposes, to inform social planners at national and international levels. Today, many time-use studies provide important sources of empirical information for occupational scientists and therapists.[23-32]

Statements by occupational therapists suggest a view within the profession that occupation is central to the human experience. In the professional literature, occupation has been described as "a natural human phenomenon" that is taken for granted because it forms "the fabric of everyday lives,"[33] and more specifically, as purposeful "use of time, energy, interest, and attention"[34] in work, leisure, play, self-care, rest, sleep, and social interactions.[35] It includes "activities that are playful, restful, serious, and productive," that are "carried out by individuals in their own unique ways" based on societal influences; their own needs, beliefs, and preferences; "the kinds of experiences they have had; their environments; and the patterns of behavior they acquire over time."[36] Occupation, to a large extent, is dependent on political will and environmental factors. It is culturally sanctioned and seen by some as "a primary organizer of time and resources," enabling humans to survive, control, and adapt to their world; be economically self-sufficient[17]; to create their self-image and organize their lives[37]; and to experience social relationships and approval, as well as personal growth.[38] It is perceived as part of personal and social identity[39] and is an interactive process between people and their environment of "culturally valued, coherent patterns of actions" that may be either socially expected or freely chosen.[40] Not all occupational scientists include sleep within their definitions, although recognizing its importance and affiliation,[16] I have included it here. This holistic view of occupation is applicable to populations and communities at local to global levels and should not be seen as referring only to individuals. All aspects of this description will be integral to the meaning given to occupation throughout this text. Figure 1-2, which is based on work done by occupational science and therapy students at Deakin University in Australia, succinctly encapsulates the dimensions of occupation taken in this text.

References

1. World Health Organization, Health and Welfare Canada, Canadian Public Health Association. *Ottawa Charter for Health Promotion.* Ottawa, Canada: Author; 1986.
2. Ashton J, Seymour H. *The New Public Health: The Liverpool Experience.* Milton Keynes: Open University Press; 1988.
3. World Health Organization. *Jakarta Declaration on Leading Health Promotion into the 21st Century.* Geneva: Author; 1998.
4. Watts ED. Human needs. In: Kuper A, Kuper J, eds. *The Social Science Encyclopedia.* Rev ed. London: Routledge; 1989:367-368.
5. Doyal L, Gough I. *A Theory of Human Need.* London: Macmillan; 1991:353-368.
6. Coon CS. *The Hunting Peoples.* London: Jonathan Cape Ltd; 1972:393.
7. Lorenz K. *Civilized Man's Eight Deadly Sins.* Latzke M, trans. London: Methuen and Co Ltd; 1974:1.
8. Porter R. *Disease, Medicine and Society in England 1550-1860.* London: MacMillan Education; 1987:13-17.
9. Locke J. *An Essay Concerning Humane Understanding.* London: Tho, Basset; 1690:361.
10. Woodside HH. The development of occupational therapy 1910-1929. *Am J Occup Ther.* 1971;XXV(5):226-230.
11. Schartz KB. The history of occupational therapy. In: Crepeau EB, Cohn ES, Boyt Schell BA, eds. *Willard & Spackman's Occupational Therapy.* 10th ed. Philadelphia: Lippincott, Williams & Wilkins; 2003.
12. Dunton WR Jr. *Prescribing Occupational Therapy.* 2nd ed. Springfield, Ill: Charles C Thomas; 1928.
13. Reilly M. 1961 Eleanor Clarke Slagle lecture: occupational therapy can be one of the great ideas of 20th century medicine. *Am J Occup Ther.* 1962;16:1-9.
14. Van Deusen J. Mary Reilly. In: Miller BRJ, Sieg KW, Ludwig FM, Shortridge SD, Van Deusen J, eds. *Six Perspectives on Theory for the Practice of Occupational Therapy.* Rockville, Md: Aspen Publications; 1988.
15. Kielhofner G, Burke JP. A model of human occupation. Part 1, conceptual framework and content. *Am J Occup Ther.* 1980;34:572-581.
16. Larson E, Wood W, Clark F. Occupational science: building the science and practice of occupation through an academic discipline. In: Crepeau EB, Cohn ES, Boyt Schell BA, eds. *Willard & Spackman's Occupational Therapy.* 10th ed. Philadelphia: Lippincott, Williams & Wilkins; 2003.

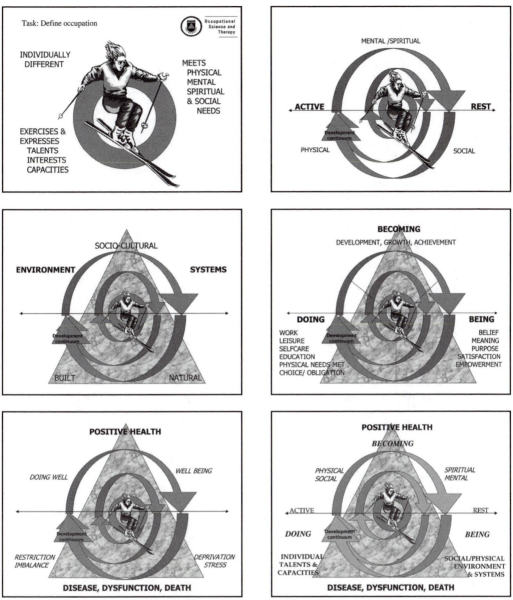

Figure 1-2. Occupational therapy students' ideas about the nature of occupation.

17. Yerxa EJ, Clark F, Frank G, et al. An introduction to occupational science: a foundation for occupational therapy in the 21st century. *Occupational Therapy in Health Care.* 1989;6(4):3.

18. World Federation of Occupational Therapists. Definition: 2004. Available at: http://www.wfot.org.au/office-files/ final%20definitionCM20042.pdf. Accessed December 2005.

19. *The Concise Oxford Dictionary of Current English.* Oxford, UK: Clarendon Press; 1911.

20. *Webster's Revised Unabridged Dictionary of the English Language.* London: G Bell and Sons Ltd; 1919.

21. *The Oxford English Dictionary.* 2nd ed. Vol XII. Oxford, UK: Clarendon Press; 1989:130,633.

22. Meyer A. The philosophy of occupational therapy. *Archives of Occupational Therapy.* 1922;1:1-10.

23. Castles I. How Australians Use Their Time. Catalog No. 4153.0. Australian Bureau of Statistics, 1992.

24. Harvey AS. Quality of life and the use of time theory and measurement. *Journal of Occupational Science: Australia.* 1993;1(2):27-30.

25. Robinson JP. *How Americans Use Time: A Social-Psychological Analysis of Everyday Behaviour.* New York: Praeger Publishers; 1977.
26. Szalai A. *The Use of Time: Daily Activities of Urban and Suburban Populations in Twelve Countries.* The Hague: Mouton; 1972.
27. Yerxa EJ, Locker SB. Quality of time used by adults with spinal cord injuries. *Am J Occup Ther.* 1990;4:318-326.
28. Pentland W, Harvey A, Powell Lawton M, McColl MA, eds. *Time Use Research in the Social Sciences.* New York: Kluwer Academic/Plenum Publishers; 1999.
29. Winkler D, Unsworth C, Sloan S. Time use following a severe traumatic brain injury. *Journal of Occupational Science.* 2005;8(1):17-24.
30. Walker C. Occupational adaptation in action: shift workers and their strategies. *Journal of Occupational Science.* 2001;12(2):69-81.
31. Weeder TC. Comparison of temporal patterns and meaningfulness of daily activities of schizophrenics and normal adults. *Occupational Therapy in Mental Health.* 1986;6:27-45.
32. Gallew HA, Mu K. An occupational look at temporal adaptation: night shift nurses. *Journal of Occupational Science.* 2004;11(1):23-30.
33. Cynkin S, Robinson AM. *Occupational Therapy and Activities Health: Toward Health Through Activities.* Boston, Mass: Little, Brown and Co; 1990.
34. Occupational therapy: its definitions and functions. *Am J Occup Ther.* 1972;26:204.
35. Stein F, Roose B. *Pocket Guide to Treatment in Occupational Therapy.* San Diego, Calif: Singular Publishing Co; 2000:201.
36. Kielhofner G, ed. *A Model of Human Occupation, Theory and Application.* Baltimore, Md: Williams and Wilkins; 1985.
37. Cara E, Macrae A. *Psychosocial Occupational Therapy: A Clinical Practice.* New York: Delmar Publishers; 1998:669.
38. Wilcock AA. *Occupational Therapy Approaches to Stroke.* Melbourne, Australia: Churchill Livingstone; 1986.
39. Turner A, Foster M, Johnson SE, eds. *Occupational Therapy and Physical Dysfunction: Principles, Skills and Practice.* 4th ed. New York: Churchill Livingstone; 1996:873.
40. Humphry R. Young children's occupations: explicating the dynamics of developmental processes. *Am J Occup Ther.* 2002;56:171-179.

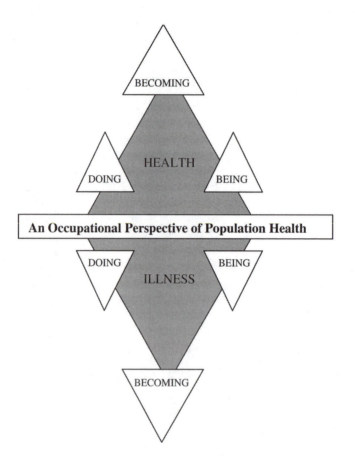

HEALTH AND ILLNESS

Theme 1:

*A state of complete physical, mental, and social well-being
not merely the absence of disease or infirmity*
WHO definition of health, 1946[1]

The chapter addresses:
* Understanding health
  * Health from a population perspective
  * Natural health and biological needs
    * Natural health
    * Biological needs as a mechanism for health
  * Rules of health
    * Ancient: humoral physiology and the *Regimen Sanitatis*
    * Modern: WHO and *Ottawa Charter for Health Promotion* (OCHP)
* Physical, mental, and social well-being
* Absence of illness

In presenting an account of the history of ideas that surround the understanding of occupation within population health, it is important to set the scene. So, the story begins with an exploration of health and illness. This chapter examines ideas that have been deemed important in promoting population health throughout time and identifies contemporary concepts in public health based on those of the WHO. It is the ideas and concepts that surface in this chapter that guide the occupational perspective presented throughout the book and form the basis of the approaches discussed in the last 4 chapters.

Health and illness are complex subjects. Their introduction in this foundation chapter will only scratch the surface of the complexity. Still, it is important to begin to explore the labyrinth of ideas that are their makeup so that a beginning appreciation of an occupational perspective of health is possible. What makes for the complexity? At the very least, ideas about what is health differ according to types of economy, cultural and spiritual philosophies, ecology, socially dominant and individual views, and the health technology available, as do the myriad of opinions about the possible causes of illness. The discussion focuses on ideas, action, and explorations about what helps to make and keep people well, what appears to cause morbidity or makes resistance to it difficult. Within the public health fraternity, the range of "personal, social, economic, and environmental factors which determine health status of individuals or populations" is known as the determinants of health.[2] The determinants are many and they frequently interact; some can be modified, but others cannot. The determinants outside the apparent control of individuals, communities, or health care providers need to be addressed by sociopolitical or environmental action, and that calls for intersectoral participation along with greater understanding of what that entails for health practitioners.

To help with understanding basic concepts about the nature of health as well as the underlying determinants, the starting point is a brief look at how health is viewed from a population or public health perspective. This is followed by an exploration of how biological needs and "natural" behaviors relate to health and illness. The basic nature of species health can be easily forgotten in the complexities of the postmodern present. That will set a baseline for the story to unfold how, as civilizations evolved, ideas, explanations, theories, and approaches formed the foundation of rules for health. As important examples of that, 2 theories are scrutinized. First are the ideas held in 6 long-lived rules for health known as the "non-naturals" that grew from humoral physiology and were widely promulgated through what was known as the *Regimen Sanitatis*. Second are the ideas held in health directives provided by the WHO in the OCHP and more recent documents based on, or ratifying, its directives. The WHO was created in the mid 20th century, its constitution providing the modern world with a definition of health as "a state of complete physical, mental, and social well-being not merely the absence of disease or infirmity."[1] This has stood the test of time and provides a pointer to both the promotion of health and the prevention of illness. Both aspects of the definition are important components of population health, and both will be addressed throughout the rest of the text.

Understanding Health

To understand the complexities of health, this section of the chapter, which is substantial, will consider 3 themes. It will first explain a global, population, or public health perspective; then it will explore natural health and biological needs; and finally, it will outline 2 sets of rules for maintaining or promoting health and reducing illness: one ancient and one modern.

HEALTH FROM A POPULATION PERSPECTIVE

Throughout this book, health is conceptualized according to the WHO definition that provides the theme of the chapter and is linked with, informed by, and centered on the OCHP, which describes health as a resource for everyday life that emphasizes social and personal resources as well as physical capabilities.[3] The OCHP is central within the doctrines and directions of public health, having been ratified at the 4th International Conference on Health Promotion in 1997 in the *Jakarta Declaration* that was adopted to lead health promotion into the 21st century.[4] The OCHP picks up on the broad intent obvious in the wording of the WHO definition and provides a listing of the prerequisites for health that includes peace, income, a stable ecosystem, sustainable resources, social justice, and equity, as well as shelter, education, and food.[3]

The OCHP resulted from the combined wisdom of 212 delegates from 38 countries when they met in Ottawa at the first WHO Health Promotion Conference in 1986. It has provided the guiding wisdom of 3 further meetings in other parts of the world: in

Adelaide (1988), in Sundsvall (1991), and in Jakarta (1997). These have explored the OCHP themes, actions, and strategies further. All remain relevant today and are accepted by the health promotion fraternity as the way forward in population health around the globe. The 3 basic strategies proposed in the OCHP are advocating for the political, environmental, economic, social, cultural, biological, and behavioral conditions essential for health; enabling people to strive for and reach their health potential; and mediating between different sociopolitical interests in the pursuit of health for all people in all walks of life wherever they live. The new public health is closely tied conceptually to the OCHP, which is a central document in world health policy.

It was recognized at the 1977 World Health Assembly that greater emphasis needed to be given to the effect of socially and economically productive factors as important aspects of health. The year 2000 was set as the target by the WHO and world governments to attain the best possible economic and social conditions and health for all the citizens of the world.[5] This was affirmed at a Primary Health Care Conference held in Alma Ata in Soviet Kazakhstan in 1978 by representatives of 134 nations in what became known as the *Declaration of Alma Ata*. This recognized that action was required across social and economic sectors as well as in health care if the inequities between the developing and the developed world were to be reduced.[6] The year 2000 was overambitious as Don Nutbeam of the WHO Collaborating Centre for Health Promotion recognized in a glossary originally prepared as a resource document for the Jakarta Conference only 3 years before the deadline. At that time he reaffirmed that:

> A comprehensive understanding of health implies that all systems and structures which govern social and economic conditions and the physical environment should take account of the implications of their activities in relation to their impact on individual and collective health and well-being.[2]

The WHO, in developing the subsequent document *Health for All in the Twenty-First Century*, consulted widely before establishing the key values in the visionary document. The values are recognition of the highest attainable standard of health as a fundamental right; continuity and strengthening of ethics in research, health policy, and service provision; the implementation of equity-oriented policies; and the incorporation of a gender perspective into health policies and strategies. While the vision continues to recognize the need to promote health and to alleviate illness and suffering for all humanity, its societal platform acknowledges both unity and diversity. It does this by validating "the uniqueness of each person and the need to respond to each individual's spiritual quest for meaning, purpose, and belonging" as part of health.[7] In terms of ethics, the policy focuses on equity and social justice in access to and utilization of quality health care, in addition to the provision by health workers of compassion; respect of others' values, needs, and individual choice; and issues of confidentiality and autonomy. It also highlights ethical issues in science and research such as those that concern the integrity of the human genome and questions relating to intergenerational matters, environmental sustainability, and equitable and effective gender perspectives. The policy calls for international collective action across diverse sectors of societies in order to achieve its goals because the determinants of positive health and well-being, like those of much illness and death, lie outside the health service domain. To stimulate the type of action required, health professionals, such as occupational therapists, need to take positive steps to make that a reality.

The WHO definition has been criticized over the decades. Some believe the focus is too broad and should be limited to that which is responsive to interventions of medical science only. Others have argued that the focus is too narrow by seeming to exclude the spiritual and ethical dimensions of health, although the latter has been addressed more recently.[8] In this text, it is taken that mental well-being refers to spiritual and ethical as well as cognitive and affective factors. A third concern is that the WHO definition implies that health cannot be achieved because it and disease are discrete and mutually exclusive entities.[9] Other medical scientists agree that it is idealistic, unattainable, largely irrelevant, and difficult to measure.[2] That is possibly accounted for by the emphasis of Western medical efforts on illness rather than health. This appears to gainsay the broader intent of the definition and, in particular, the nature and consequences of social illness.

Perhaps the least controversial aspect of the definition for many medical scientists is that health depends on the absence of illness and infirmity. Many others relate to that belief. Some 3 decades ago, for example, a French study of a largely middle class sample found that a significant number described health as an absence of illness.[10] About the same time, Audy described it as "potentially measurable by the individual's ability to rally from insults, whether chemical, physical, infectious, psychological or social."[11] Some 20 years later, Doyal and Gough describe physical health as optimizing life expectancy as well as a need "to avoid serious physical disease and illness conceptualized in biomedical terms,"[12] and Goodman defines it as "a function of the organism's ability to adjust to environmental constraints and stressors."[13] Mildred Blaxter found in a significant sample of 9000 adults that an absence of illness description was given by about 13% of the respondents when describing their own health and by about 37% of them when describing that of others.[14] In *Health and Lifestyles*, her 1990 monograph based on the results of a survey of how people in the United Kingdom describe health, a surprising 10% of respondents couldn't describe how health felt or its qualities, and even more couldn't think of anyone who was healthy.[14]

The definition of health as "more than the absence of illness" has elicited many ideas. In Herzlich's study, some respondents described it as the result of a reserve of health while others as a state of wellness or equilibrium.[10] Blaxter also found that people described health as having a reserve to combat problems and as psychosocial well-being.[14] Others in her study defined it as behavior aimed at healthy lifestyle, as being able to function, as physical fitness, as energy and vitality, and as social relationships.[14] Her survey outcomes support the belief that views of health differ over the life course, have clear gender differences, and are, for most, a multidimensional concept. Prior to World War II, Sigerist similarly recognized the multidimensional concept of health, even pre-empting the WHO definition by expressing his view that it is more than simply the absence of disease and is inclusive of body, mind, and social adjustment. He added other holistic and positive terms, such as *joyful, cheerful, well-balanced,* and *accepting of life's responsibilities.*[15] His view was possibly influenced by Johann Peter Frank who, as early as 1790, argued "that health and well-being could only be obtained where there was freedom from want and social deprivation."[16] (Sigerist wrote an introduction for Frank's work when it was translated from the German and re-published in 1941.) More recently, of many other attempts by workers in the field, Kass provides a useful but simple version that takes account of the physical, mental, and social dimensions when he describes health as a norm or a natural state of being in which the human organism works well as a whole.[17] A 2002 description given by Greiner, Fain, and Edelman has an occupational bias:

> *Functioning is integral to health. There are physical, mental and social levels of function reflected in terms of performance and social expectations. Loss of function may be a sign or symptom of a disease… a state of ill health.*[18]

The authors describe how functional health patterns include activity-exercise, roles-relationships, sleep-rest, cognition-perception, self-perception-self-concept, and coping-stress tolerance.

In the account given in this book, both aspects of the WHO definition are addressed: the negative and the positive. I find the following ideas from Bush and Zvelebil useful in this process despite the lack of mention of social or ecological health and illness, and the assumption that emanates from that of physical and mental states being the sole determinants of health:

> *The human organism, and its surviving remains, is comprehended as a dynamic, historical and adaptive system, reflecting the interaction between the biological organism and its environment during the individual's lifetime. Health is the biological and psychological condition of the individual, a state which can, at least in theory, be assessed by the incidence of insults and other abnormal symptoms.*[19]
>
> *Health is evaluated by cultural perceptions and parameters: ill-health and disease are culturally defined phenomena. In this non-biological sense, the definition of health can range from one of physical and mental well-being, with anything else being ill-health, to the other clinical presence of disease indicators or of the biological response to it with anything other considered healthy.*[19]

In the last decade, public health has been defined as "the science and art of promoting health, preventing disease, and prolonging life through the organized efforts of society."[2] While growing from a rich history of reform that marked its beginning, what is often described as the "new public health" is so called to give prominence to the different approaches and methods that have been advocated in the last 3 decades to solve health problems across populations. It takes a more comprehensive approach than previous approaches to living conditions and lifestyles, drawing heavily upon the WHO policies such as the OCHP (and its later additions) to guide global, national, and local strategies. It also focuses on ecological health, the recent concept that is concerned with economic and environmental determinants of health and includes attention to the effects of depletion of the ozone layer, global warming, uncontrolled water and air pollution, and so on.[2]

As explained in the preface to this edition, the health of populations is the primary concern of practitioners of public health, who, in line with directives from WHO, have made calls for all health professions, politicians, social planners, and others to move in this direction. Although its genesis, like occupational therapy's,[20] undoubtedly can be traced back to the species beginnings and forward through the rules for health known as the "non-naturals," it formally came into being in the mid-19th century somewhat prior to occupational therapy (Figure 1-1). While the prevention of disease has been the fundamental purpose of public health, from its origins it has remained a common misconception that sanitation and immunization are the focus of its concerns along with some other interests in fields such as occupational health and safety. The first Public Health Act was passed in Britain in 1842 following Edwin Chadwick's enquiry into the sanitary conditions of the laboring population.[21] Chadwick, along with Thomas Southwood-Smith, was a prime mover in the reform of industrial work and mining practices, as well as other conditions of living.[22]

While lifestyle and bad habits are blamed for many of today's chronic diseases,[23-25] with apparent support from numerous public health explorations such as the 20-year Framingham Cohort study,[26] they are insufficient to explain who gets sick and who stays healthy. Research concentrating on why people succumb to unhealthy lifestyles and habits is necessary but is rare. Health is so complex that studies carried out at the population level can only establish probable links. There are as yet many unknown determinants of illness and even fewer of well-being. Clearly, not all health-risk or health-enhancing factors have been established. This includes study of the determinants or outcomes of people's wide-ranging occupations: of all that they do, be, and strive to become. Ironically, occupational medicine is, perhaps, the oldest branch of public health, with texts on "mining" diseases being published as early as the 16th century,[27,28] and classical texts on occupational diseases in 1700[29] and 1831.[30] The focus of occupational medicine has historically

Figure 1-1. Origins and conceptual relationship between public health and occupational therapy.

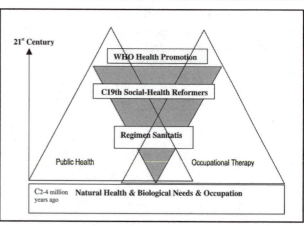

been on illness resulting from paid employment, and the prevailing public health interest reflects this limited focus, mirroring contemporary societal, political, and economic value given to that type of occupation above others.[31]

NATURAL HEALTH AND BIOLOGICAL NEEDS

In order to understand health, it is necessary to review its history, an approach taken by several notable scholars of public health, such as Rene Dubos in the mid 20th century and Thomas McKeown, a pioneer Chair of Social Health. Taking a historical viewpoint helps to uncover the characteristics of natural health and of biological needs because "clinical definitions of health cannot provide a comprehensive framework for describing the condition."[19] Basic biological health mechanisms and needs of the earliest humans would have been largely unaffected by culturally acquired knowledge, values, and behavior, so studying these should assist understanding of the basic nature of health without excessive interference of perhaps erroneous contemporary viewpoints or ways of life. To accomplish this, the health and illness experiences of the earliest peoples need to be considered. In *The Origins of Human Disease*, McKeown highlights 4 key discoveries that have contributed to the large and complex jigsaw of health[32]:

1. "Human genetic constitution is much the same today as it was 100,000 years ago." People now "face vastly changed conditions of life with the genetic equipment of hunter gatherers."

2. "In technically advanced countries the modern transformation of health, and the associated increase of population, began more than a century before effective medical intervention was possible, and must be attributed largely to advances in the standard of living."

3. Because of "the nature of infectious diseases" prevention is possible "by increasing resistance and reducing exposure."

4. "Most classes of NCDs [noncommunicable diseases] ... have environmental origins and are potentially preventable by changes in living conditions and behavior."

A brief exploration of how the natural health experience evolved to the present time discloses a broad, contextual picture of positive health, morbidity, and mortality, including some indication of its interaction with occupation. Ideas gained from that will be expanded in subsequent chapters.

Natural Health

Early Oriental theories maintain that people experienced better health when they lived naturally and harmoniously with their environment. In *The Yellow Emperor's Classic of Internal Medicine*, published in China in the 4th century BC, it was supposed that in the remote past "people lived to 100 years, and yet remained active and did not become decrepit in their activities."[33] Similarly, Lao-tzu and Chuang-tzu eulogized about a golden age, the former suggesting that when "the ancient men lived in a world of primitive simplicity ... was a time when the yin and the yang worked harmoniously, ... all creation was unharmed, and the people did not die young."[34] More recently, radical thinkers in the East picked up those ideas and observed of earlier times that when people had been free and uninhibited, working and resting according to need, there was little spread of contagious disease and life was usually long and death, natural.[35]

Similar beliefs were popular in Europe, particularly during the 18th century. Influenced by Rousseau's depiction of man as a noble savage corrupted by civilization, it had become fashionable to suppose that a state of nature was essential to the creation of health and happiness—that civilization had spoiled people physically and corrupted them mentally.[36] Such opinions were so popular that they fostered an intellectual climate that influenced both philosophers of the Age of Reason and practical sanitarians. The latter can be regarded as early workers in the field of public health who contributed to social reforms and eventual improvements in health.[37] Examples include Beddoes, a British poet-physician, who hypothesized that the blessed original state of health could only be recaptured by abiding by the simple order and purity of nature[38]; Virey, the 19th century French physician-philosopher, who asserted that humans in a state of nature are endowed with an instinct for health that permits biological adaptation and that civilized humans have lost[39]; and Jenner, who observed that people's deviation from the natural state appears to have been a prolific source of disease.[40] It is tempting to accept such romantic ideas, but it is imperative to find evidence of correctness of the claims before we do so.

A way of considering the aspects that require consideration in coming to understand the negative and positive impacts on public health of long ago is to use a current epidemiological device of identifying the interactions between host (person), environment, and potential stressors (Figure 1-2). Lucas Powell provides an example in her exploration of the prehistoric society at Moundville in the United States.[41] The host can be described in both cultural and biological terms as shown in Table 1-1. Interactions could have positive or negative effects such as diverse ecosystems include food resources and pathogens, hunting and fishing could enhance the quality of the diet but increase exposure to trauma, sedentism promotes accumulation of wastes and vermin but promotes population growth, and division of labor encourages use of particular capacities but unequal exposure to mechanical and pathological stress.

McMichael, a leader in the population health field, like McKeown, takes a historic approach to consider the nature of environmental aspects of disease suggests there are:

> ... *no guarantees of good health in the natural world. The ceaseless interplay between competing species, groups and individuals: the ubiquity of infection; the vagaries of climate, environment and food supplies; and the presence of physical hazards—these all contribute to the relentless toll of disease, dysfunction and death throughout the plant and animal kingdom.*[42]

Usefully, he describes 3 inter-related and distinctive features in the "long history of human ecology and disease." Readers can identify these features as this exploration continues. They are[42]:

* The encounters of human societies with new environmental hazards.

Figure 1-2. Three-way relationship between host, environment, and stressor.

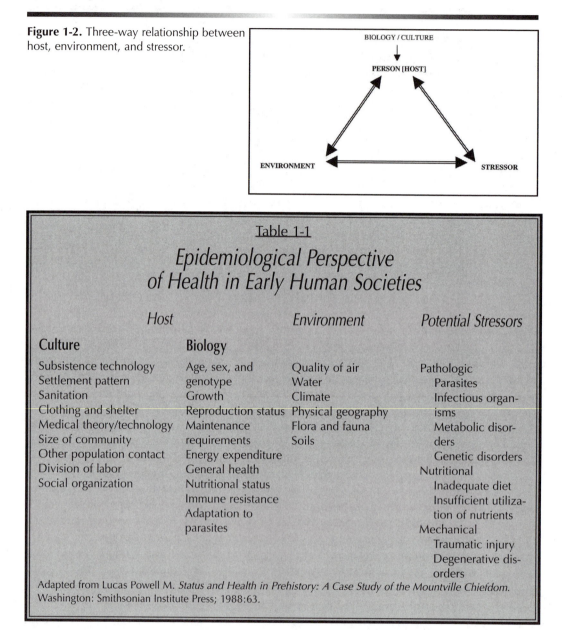

Table 1-1

Epidemiological Perspective of Health in Early Human Societies

Host		Environment	Potential Stressors
Culture	**Biology**		
Subsistence technology	Age, sex, and	Quality of air	Pathologic
Settlement pattern	genotype	Water	Parasites
Sanitation	Growth	Climate	Infectious organ-
Clothing and shelter	Reproduction status	Physical geography	isms
Medical theory/technology	Maintenance	Flora and fauna	Metabolic disor-
Size of community	requirements	Soils	ders
Other population contact	Energy expenditure		Genetic disorders
Division of labor	General health		Nutritional
Social organization	Nutritional status		Inadequate diet
	Immune resistance		Insufficient utiliza-
	Adaptation to		tion of nutrients
	parasites		Mechanical
			Traumatic injury
			Degenerative dis-
			orders

Adapted from Lucas Powell M. *Status and Health in Prehistory: A Case Study of the Mountville Chiefdom.* Washington: Smithsonian Institute Press; 1988:63.

✳ The recurring tension between biological needs and capacities and changes in living conditions.

✳ The impact of urban living and population aging on patterns of health and illness.

Participation in the majority of occupations was directly related to maintenance of the organism and survival of individuals, their communities, and the species, and challenges were in tune with the natural world. Within early human cultures, provision to meet the needs of survival and health through sustenance, self-care, shelter, safety, self-esteem, and life satisfaction was similar for the total population. All able-bodied people were involved first-hand in the gathering and preparing of food and water, with finding or devising adequate environments and shelter for safety and temperature control, and with the care and education of offspring. Few would have suffered the fate, or enjoyed the privilege, of not being able or eligible (for whatever reason) to participate in providing for themselves and others. Occupations were communal with on-the-job training and only limited division of labor. Such simple occupational structures did not obscure innate physiological needs but catered for them. The very limited numbers of people on earth posed no threat to ecosystems despite, even then, the characteristic of seeking to control or change an environment, to exploit and deplete a locality before moving on.

Unlike many other animals, people "exploit almost every link in the food chain."[43] This characteristic supported flexibility of habitat and provided motivation for hunter-gatherers to move from "one resource to another."[43] This provided a health advantage by reducing the probability of illness due to unhygienic waste disposal and assisted physical fitness by providing communities with the type of physical activity now being rediscovered as advantageous by world health authorities. A case in point is provided by first nation Australians. Their "practice of moving camp as they journeyed throughout the tribal land ensured that many of the health problems associated with permanent settlement sites could not develop."[44] Such hunter-gatherer nomads were constrained to balance physical exertion with sedentary and rest occupations because, at least until they learned to create and control fire to their advantage, they would have been diurnal, following basic circadian patterns of sleeping and waking. Additionally, contrary to popular belief, the obligatory occupations of providing for immediate needs was not as time-consuming as the modern 8-hour day.[45-48]

The nomadic lifestyle contributed to mental and social health benefits by providing adventure, preventing boredom, and facilitating bonding with fellow nomads. Communities were small enough not to require restrictive rules and regulations and probably, more so than in later occupational eras, the groups who lived together on a regular basis were stable and supportive. Survival would often have depended on the strength created by a cohesive group in combined activity. In fact, because of the constraints imposed by a nomadic way of life, the people making up each social band constituted the movable assets of the group (ie, the people, rather than material assets, were valued as central to survival). Because of this advantage, any early human or community whose "cooperation gene" was prevalent would have both an individual and a group selection advantage: "those individuals less able to participate in group activity would have been marginalized in the survival stakes."[42] This would have influenced the development of a communal rather than an individual view of the world and of health and would have been integral to social well-being. We can look again to first nation Australians to see this community/individual dual value reflected in the way in which their current health organization defines health as:

> *The social, emotional, spiritual, and cultural well-being of the whole community.*
> *Health services should strive to achieve that state where every individual can achieve*
> *their full potential as human beings (Aboriginals) and thus bring about total well-being*
> *of their community as a whole.*[49]

The type of lifestyle followed by all early homo species and humans for several million years provided a real test to whether engagement in occupations can sustain health of ecosystems, as well as the well-being of people. Many consider that the occupational pursuits of the hunter-gatherer era generally would not have disturbed the environmental balance,[43,44,50] and there have been numerous positive speculations and comments about the health status of early humans from a rich variety of sources, most of which are supported by archeological, anthropological, and other explorations. Stephenson, for example, in *The Ecological Development of Man* observes, "we know that people living a culturally primitive life (with less medical care) are generally more physically perfect than those from affluent societies,"[43] and McNeill in *Plagues and People* considers that "ancient hunters of the temperate zone were most probably healthy folk" despite short life spans compared with modern humans.[51] Such views are supported by reports from explorers in their initial contacts with people of primitive cultures, which suggest that they appeared happy, healthy, and vigorous.[52-54] More recent medical and anthropological surveys of "several South American tribes and undisplaced Pygmies of the Congo Basin" also give credence to these views.[55] Meindl, in considering the demography of human populations before agriculture, cites evidence that these peoples remain healthy and resilient unlike many whose demographic patterns have been altered by contact with modern cultures.[55]

Despite some idealized advantages of the lifestyle, early mortality and morbidity resulting from ecological forces acting on the population is believed to have been the common experience. Changes of climate, as McMichael along with Dobson suggested, would have been more of a hazard then especially as "older people suffer gradual loss of the ability to buffer temperature extremes."[56] So too would availability of food and water, and "parasites with high transmission rates and little or no induced immunity," such as worms, lice, ticks, and pathogens such as *Salmonella* and *Trypanosoma* (sleeping sickness). "Occupational" accidents, aggression, and infanticide are also suggested hazards.[55] When resources could support only limited numbers of hunter-gatherers, it appears that social strategies, such as prolonged lactation, were used to control population numbers.[57] Additionally, the abandonment of unwanted infants was probable.[58] The modern assumption that life must be preserved at all costs can sit uncomfortably with a natural ecological point of view. Those who survived and procreated were those most able to live and adapt effectively to life's demands and, in fact, could be designated as healthy. In this way, "natural selection is not thwarted, and in their breeding populations they do not build up increasing loads of disabling genes."[59]

McNeill explains how early humans and their hominid predecessors, like other animals, fit into a self-balancing, self-regulating ecological system, preying on other forms of life as they were preyed upon by large-bodied organisms, parasites, and microorganisms.[51] They were, in fact, "caught in a precarious equilibrium between the microparasitism of disease organisms and the macroparasitism of large-bodied predators." In a natural state, some microparasites provoke acute disease, killing the host; some provoke immunity reactions; others achieve a stable relationship with the host who perhaps experiences continuous, low-level malady; and yet others are carried by the host and are the cause of disease in others. It was, however, occasional disturbances such as drought, fire, and floods that set limits to population imbalance. Within this natural scenario, any change to one living creature is compensated for by genetic or behavioral change in co-organisms. "Undisturbed" biological evolution is a slow process, but when humans began to evolve culturally and to adapt to different habitats by changes in their occupation, they transformed the balance of nature, and patterns of disease altered along with this occupational transformation.

Such demographic and epidemiologic deductions do not contradict the claims that hunter-gatherers experienced general well-being, but rather, in common with modern humans, they experienced ill health and accidents; the different nature of which, coupled with lack of specialist knowledge, led to early death for many of the population. McKeown argues that "in the limited sense that they were essentially free from many diseases that are now common, our hunter gather ancestors may be said to have been healthy."[32] Possibly because of a shorter lifespan, few would have experienced the NCDs prevalent today such as heart disease, dementia, osteoarthritis, cancer, and diabetes. Indeed, studies of recent hunter-gatherers have shown a virtual absence of those disorders, raised blood pressure, or obesity. McMichael concludes that "many of those diseases are an expression of a mismatch between human biological inheritance and current way of life" as "urban sedentariness, dietary excesses and various socialized addictive behaviors (alcohol consumption and tobacco smoking) have become prominent features of modern human ecology."[42] On that note, he points to several other anomalies that are factors in current day disease and disorder resulting from a human biology attuned to the Pleistocene age (2–1 million years ago) when, for example, diets included only moderate amounts of plant oils and predominantly unsaturated fats, or the earlier Pliocene age (6–2 million years ago) when bipedal gait was superimposed on skeletal structures attuned to quadrupedal gait.[42]

These deductions support the notion that occupation, survival, health, and illness are inextricably linked. As Gandevia maintained, "in the social environment of a man or a community occupation looms large."[60] Additionally, because of their occupational nature and potential, humans were able to strive to improve survival odds and decrease the experience of ill health. Their technology, in the main, addressed the potential risk factors of a world in which people are not the fastest, strongest, largest, or best camouflaged of animals. Much has been written about "fight or flight" behavior and its appropriateness for the natural dangers facing early humans since Cannon's description in the 1920s of the single automatic pattern of response of the organism to any challenge to equilibrium.[61] However appropriate, the response would have been unpleasant to experience and provided strong motivation to develop artifacts and social structures to overcome fear-producing situations. Social cohesion and education were used by hunter-gatherers, along with tool technology, as vehicles to improve superiority over prey and predators in the long term. Survival pressures provided meaning, motivation, and opportunity for engagement in a variety of individual and community occupations that addressed the obvious health risks of the day. All this may have been largely unconscious, and it is not known whether early humans made any cognitive efforts to maintain health and prevent illness apart from shelter, sustenance, and the seeking out of substances they instinctively craved when sick, in a way similar to other animals.[62] It did lead to an eventual appreciation of "the curative values of a wide range of plant products, many of which are still in medicinal use."[43] This can be thought to have produced, in time, acceptance of the people most skilled in healing as "medicine" experts. Many records exist that point to remarkable understanding of homeopathic medicine notwithstanding a striking healing capacity subsequent to injury.[44]

Following this story, it is possible to see how subsequent changes in need, culture, and environment have influenced patterns of health and illness throughout time. As human hunter-gatherers began to dominate the food chain, populations increased; as they overcame cold through the use of clothing, shelter, and fire, they were able to expand into colder environs, leaving behind many parasites and disease organisms. In new environments, populations escalated.[51] This was aided by the circumstance that in nomadic life "the small collections of human beings were too scattered to sustain microorganisms which do not readily achieve a carrier state."[58,63]

Conditions in some parts of the world led to fixed settlement and agriculture, which had mixed consequences in terms of health and illness. This occupational change is thought to have started about 12,000 years ago in what is known as the Fertile Crescent. Jared Diamond explains that the ancestors of the greatest variety of what are now the world's most valuable domestic plants grew in that area when the local people were becoming increasingly dependent on harvesting wild crops and settling down in areas where that was possible. This led to the development of stone sickles and methods for grain storage. However, the advent of farming led to a decline in life expectancy. For example, people became smaller and more diseased with nutritional deficiencies, arthritis, and dental decay because they got less exercise and their diet was not as diverse.[42,64]

Eventually, morbidity and mortality due to starvation were reduced comparitively in many places because agriculture provided more constant access to food. Additionally, improved shelters provided better facilities to nurture and care for infants, the sick, and the aged. However, low life expectancy remained the common experience because of the increased incidence of infectious diseases.[65]

The continual development of agriculture, which prevented the re-establishment of natural ecosystems, along with the rise of villages, towns, and cities, provided ideal conditions for hyperinfestations of various potential disease organisms. Throughout the world, diseases such as diphtheria, scarlet fever, malaria, typhus, smallpox, syphilis, leprosy, and tuberculosis caused ongoing morbidity, along with various plagues that took a periodic but devastating toll. Indeed, the bubonic plague, at its peak, killed 10,000 people daily in Constantinople during the 6th and 7th centuries.[66] In the 14th century, between one-third and one half of the population of mainland Europe and the British Isles died within a few years.[67] Such epidemics and infectious diseases occurred, in part, because of more travel and contact from trade. As occupations such as oceanic exploration, trading, and conquest grew, so did the spread of disease, sometimes with disastrous consequences. For example, in 1520 smallpox arrived in Mexico along with the relief expedition for Cortez and played a major role in the outcome of the Spanish conquest[51]; a few centuries later, first nation Australians having "no racial experience with diseases such as measles, mumps, smallpox, chickenpox, and influenza" were devastated when exposed to these disorders along with white settlement.[68] Infectious diseases did not cease to be the major threat to health until the 20th century, long after agriculture had been overtaken by industrial economies in the Western world.

Increased population density that came about with the growth of industry led to another increase of infectious diseases and epidemics; those that had been checked by generations of adaptation gained new leases on life. The industrial revolution initially provided few health benefits for the vast majority of people who moved to towns and cities to find paid employment. In 1780, only 15% of the population in the United Kingdom and 5% in the United States lived in towns or cities. This had risen to 50% in the United Kingdom by 1851 and in the United States by about 1910.[69] Perhaps the most obvious result of this urban population explosion was overcrowding in environments not constructed for comfortable and sanitary living, which, aggravated by industrially polluted working conditions, led to a widespread increase in illness. Eversley suggests that people living in the 20th century could:

> ... hardly imagine the significance of pain, disfigurement, and the loss of near relations as a constant factor in every day life. Slight wounds became infected and suppurated for weeks. Fractures healed badly. Minor irritations like toothache and headache became major preoccupations, paralyzing ordinary activity ... Even where no acute injury or identifiable major disease was involved, common colds, gastric upsets from the consumption of rotten foodstuffs, and permanent septic foci such as those provided by bad teeth were common, if not universal.[70]

Many factors have brought about an improvement in this state of affairs, including public health initiatives from the mid 19th century, particularly the improvement of sanitary conditions, water supply, and housing. Other social and economic changes, such as improved nutrition, smaller families, less overcrowding, and improved education, along with major advances in medical and pharmaceutical science, have also contributed to a decrease in disease[71] and to longer life expectancy. Indeed, it is possible to appreciate Gordon's suggestion that medicine's role in making life more bearable "is probably its major achievement and for this it receives little credit."[68] Making life more bearable depends, in large part, on understanding basic human needs and helping people to meet these through sociopolitical, as well as individual, intervention. This has been the particular focus of public health in more recent years. An anticipated focus in coming years is the health and economic concerns of an aging population.

It is possible to conclude from this overview that hazards' leading to much of present day illness and morbidity occur as a result of how people live and what they do. For hunter-gatherer, it was parasites, poor nutrition, and the physical dangers of lifestyle elements such as the chase, exploration, and environmental dangers that posed the greatest threats; for farmers and again for early industrial workers, there was an increase of infectious diseases probably due to fixed habitation, a greater interaction between people as travel escalated and personal and community environments became crowded, coupled with a poor understanding of sanitation and hygiene; and for people living and working in postindustrial societies, there is a predominance of NCDs that are probably a result of changed conditions of life coupled with a genetic predisposition. As McKeown reminds us:

> We are genetically ill-equipped for the ways of life that we have made for ourselves. A school child eating potato chips while watching television, a driver steering a bus or taxi through a congested city, an adolescent smoking in front of a computer, are far removed from the conditions for which their genes had prepared them.[32]

Biological Needs as a Mechanism for Health

Closely connected to the idea of natural health is that of biological needs. In order to survive, there is a basic requirement for all animals, including humans, to meet biological needs and to avoid serious hazards.[32] This depends upon a close working link between the unconscious and the conscious: between anatomy, physiology, and action. Indeed, as Lorenz suggests, the principal purpose of both anatomical characteristics and behavior patterns is survival.[72] It is the major stimulus to engage in healthful behavior albeit largely unconsciously.

Humans have 4 very basic needs, namely:

1. Oxygen—within minutes.
2. Warmth (or excessive heat loss)—within hours.
3. Water—within days.
4. Food—within weeks.

"Unlike the other essentials food is not a given; it has to be gathered, hunted, cultivated, preserved and, at times, competed for. It is the crucial determinant of health and population growth ..."[32] The occupations that people followed for millennia were more often than not centered around the acquisition or cultivation of food. However, exploration of the environment in the search for food-rich habitats had to take into account the availability of water, the availability of shelter, and the adequate supply of oxygenated air, scarce at high altitudes. Apart from those essential requirements, humans were able to adapt to life in many different environments. Such adaptations did not necessarily meet other biological needs of almost equal importance in the most health-giving way. Indeed, because some of the needs are now obscured by millions of years of acquired values and behaviors, present-day health awareness may not reflect needs that were, and probably still are, fundamental to healthy survival.

At this point it is useful to consider homeostasis. This is described as "a tendency to stability in the normal body state's (internal environment) of the organism."[73] It "is an evolutionary strategy for preserving internal sameness by resisting and smoothing out the changes" and variations from the external environment, and is especially necessary:

> ... for the proper functioning of the central nervous system of animals on the higher rungs of the evolutionary ladder. Before intelligent life could appear, and well before

the culminating event of consciousness, the mechanism to ensure the sameness of the internal milieu had to be in place.[74]

It was Claude Bernard, a 19th century French physiologist, who developed the concept that the "milieu interior" of a living organism must maintain reasonable constancy despite external circumstances. He recognized that humans, despite their apparent indifference to the environment, are "in a close and wise relationship with it, so that its equilibrium results from a continuous and delicate compensation established as if by the most sensitive balances" and that animals able to maintain "inner sameness" have greater freedom to live in many different environments and are less vulnerable to ecological change.[75] This perhaps results in their apparent indifference to the environment. American physiologist, Walter Cannon, who suggested the term *homeostasis,* recognized it as a system working cooperatively with both the brain and body.[76] He found that at "critical times" of environmental stress "economy is secondary to stability"; that important substances such as water, sugar, or salt are eliminated in order to maintain constancy.[77] Cannon researched and described the way a fluid matrix provides a stable context for highly specialized cells, which, by themselves, can only survive in specific conditions, to enact their part in complex, flexible, and versatile activities. He postulated that homeostasis leaves humans free to do new occupations, to be adventurous, and to seek beyond survival to the "unessentials" that are part and parcel of civilization.[77]

Because the study of biological needs has been neglected of late, it is necessary to discuss the concept in order to understand their role in health. The lack of discussion may be because it is not currently a fashionable concept within the scientific community, although it is addressed from time to time. As Allport remarked about the ever-changing focus of scientific inquiry, "we never seem to solve our problems or exhaust our concepts; we only grow tired of them."[78] Alternatively, the neglect may be a result of the more recent emphasis on nurture in the long-running nature versus nurture debate. When the emphasis tended to be on nature, as in the 1930s, numerous need theories were hypothesized.[79-83] The 1960s and 1970s saw a resurgence of interest in attempts to identify what motivates human behavior from a "natural" perspective.[84-86]

The word *need*, meaning a "central motivating variable," made its debut into academic psychology in the early 1930s, eventually replacing the notion of instinct.[87] By the 1970s, need is described in the *Dictionary of Behavioral Science* as "the condition of lacking, wanting, or requiring something which if present would benefit the organism by facilitating behavior or satisfying a tension," and also as "a construct representing a force in the brain which directs and organizes the individual's perception, thinking, and action, so as to change an existing, unsatisfying situation."[88] Unlike instinct, an innate need, though undeniably goal-oriented, does not have a "repertoire of inherited, unlearned action patterns."[87] However, as Lorenz observed, although humans lack "long, self-contained chains of innate behavior patterns," they have more "genuinely instinctive impulses than any other animal."[50] In that vein, Snell bemoaned the fact that "the term instinct has gone out of fashion," but thought it "tempting to revive the term and to say we can now relate instinct to detailed brain structure."[89]

Maslow's needs theory is probably the best known and most widely used, particularly in health texts. It is founded on the premise that individuals have innate needs that act as motivating forces.[86] He identified 5 basic need levels related to one another in a prepotent hierarchy. At the first level are needs such as food that relate to the physiological function of the human organism; followed progressively by needs for safety and security; then belonging, love, and social activity; with the need for esteem and respect at the fourth level; and at the top of the hierarchy, self-actualization. His theory is that more basic needs must be largely, but not necessarily completely, satisfied before higher level needs are activated and motivating. A similar 3-level hierarchy proposed by Alderfer identifies existence, relatedness, and growth (ERG) as the need levels.[85] These theories articulate well with the 3-fold notion of doing, being, and becoming used in coming chapters to encapsulate the notion of occupation.

Both Maslow's and Alderfer's theories are compatible with notions about innate "drives" common in psychology for the greater part of the century but in disuse at present. Based on physiological discoveries, such as those pertaining to homeostasis, "drives" were seen as persistent motivations, organic in origin, that "arouse, sustain, and regulate human and animal behavior" and are distinct from external determinants of behavior, such as "social goals, interests, values, attitudes, and personality traits."[90] Dashiell, in *Fundamentals of Objective Psychology*, illustrated this view:

> *The primary drives to persistent forms of animal and human conduct are tissue conditions within the organism giving rise to stimulations exciting the organism to overt activity. A man's interest and desires may become ever so elaborate, refined, socialized, sublimated, idealistic, but the raw basis from which they are developed is found in the phenomena of living matter.*[91]

A more contemporary theory of human need by Doyal and Gough calls into question fashionable subjective and relativist approaches, arguing that health and autonomy are basic needs, the meeting of which are essential preconditions for participation in social life.[12] They recognize biological motivations or drives, but they separate discourse of universal needs founded on human reason from these. Part of their stated rationale for this separation is that physiological drives and needs can result from external sources, as in the case of someone who takes drugs needing a fix. In such cases, this is obviously not a universal need but an acquired one.

The word *need*, despite diverse common, conceptual usage, will be employed in this book to describe the mechanism by which unconscious biological requirements are communicated to neuronal systems, specifically to neuronal systems engaging with the external world or that alert the conscious state to the existence of some kind of disequilibrium. This usage conforms to the suggestion made by Anscombe that needs, which are a matter of objective fact, relate to what is required for living organisms—plants, animals, or humans—to fulfill potential and flourish.[92] Watt, in defining human needs in *The Social Science Encyclopedia*, agrees that "some human needs would seem to be very closely comparable with the needs of animals and plants" and are present to facilitate fulfilment of potential: to facilitate a good (physical) specimen.[93]

Such ideas infuse the needs debate with life, as does Ornstein and Sobel's account of how the brain makes "countless adjustments" to maintain stability between "social worlds, our mental and emotional lives, and our internal physiology."[94] To do this, each neuron produces "hundreds of chemicals" that "for the most part" are responsible for "keeping the body out of trouble, from commonplace problems like not falling over or walking into a wall to the myriad of tasks involved in maintaining the stability and health of the organism."[94] From my viewpoint, this process activates biological needs that in turn promote positive health as people meet those needs. Biological needs are, therefore, homeostatically valuable. They can be seen as inborn health agents that enable the organism as a whole to interact with the environment. They do not differentiate between physical, mental, or social issues in the way in which modern society and medical or psychological practice do, but work as part of a flow of processes within biological systems relating structures and function. They are integral to the collaboration between biological rhythms and homeostasis.

Because needs are subject to the scrutiny of, and adaptation by, the highly developed cognitive and intellectual capacities of humans, "primitive instinctive energy can be

Figure 1-3. Links between biological needs, natural health, and survival.

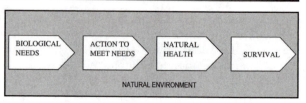

directed from its natural goal toward alternative ends that are a greater value." The cortex can override even ultradian rhythms of sleepability or wakeability. It is this process of redirection that enables the "highest achievements of humanity,"[95] and the meeting of these needs provides the essence of well-being. Indeed, the biological needs of humans are related to health from the point of view of how specimens of that kind of organism "can be recognized as flourishing."[93] People hold that in common with other living organisms. However, meeting such needs may not advance the experience of health at all times.

Survival of the species depends on individuals and populations being healthy, which in turn depends on built-in flexibility that allows for adaptation as contexts change. The latter is necessary to enable populations, communities, and individuals to flourish in different times, places, and environments. These ideas about natural health and biological needs suggest a simple linkage that is represented diagrammatically in Figure 1-3.

RULES OF HEALTH

Theories about health, the working of the human body and spirit, and rules based upon them began to be formulated as medicine developed. It is difficult to know details about any theories held before the advent of written language. However, by the time of classical medicine more than 2000 years ago, a physiological theory emerged that was to be the rationale behind much of medical and health intervention in the Western world until less than 200 years ago. This is known as humoral physiology. It has a basis in observation of mind-body occurrences, the developmental stages of people, and the natural world.

Ancient: Humoral Physiology and the Regimen Sanitatis

Best known as a mathematician of Ancient Greece, Pythagoras, in the 6th century BC, is believed to be one of the originators of a long-accepted theory of health or at least to have contributed a background of mathematical science that assisted its development. In this, the body was said to be composed of 4 elements: air, fire, water, and earth, indicative of astute observation when it is recalled that the 4 basic needs of life identified earlier are oxygen, heat, water, and food.[32] In the theory, health was contingent upon a balance between 4 humors: blood, phlegm, black bile, and yellow bile. These were thought to be the substratum of life and disease.[96] Perfect harmony, equilibrium, and balance were the guiding principles of Pythagorean theories, and numbers were thought to be the key: the number 4 was deemed central to balance and equilibrium. In addition to the 4 humors, there were 4 temperaments: the sanguine, the phlegmatic, the bilious, and the melancholy. The humors and temperaments were known as the naturals. All were interconnected, subject to the 4 seasons and 4 stages of human life; disturbance of any could be a cause of disease.[96] Each person's constitution and predisposition was underlaid with a predominant humor and temperament that determined the probabilities and type of both physical and mental illness.

There were 2 other important categories in the theory. Factors harmful to life and health were known as contranaturals, of which there were 3: diseases, their causes, and their symptoms. A group of factors regarded as necessary for life and health composed the other category known as the non-naturals. There were 6 of these related to the qualities of another 4: hot, cold, dry, and wet. The 6 non-natural factors were about activities and environments of daily life. They were characterized by a high degree of individual choice and circumstance and could be subject to either balanced use or abuse. They were:

* ✳ Air and environment.
* ✳ Motion and rest.
* ✳ Food and drink.
* ✳ Sleep and waking.
* ✳ Evacuation and repletion (including sexuality).
* ✳ Affections of the soul (including joy, anger, fear, and distress).

Interestingly, a somewhat similar humoral doctrine was prevalent in Tibet until the 20th century and this was based on 3 primal essences.[97]

Hippocrates, sometimes known as the "Father of Medicine," is attributed with putting the humoral theory together from older sources as well as his own work. Among the Hippocratic Collection of over 70 medical works is *On Regimen and Aphorisms,* which provides the core of the "Rules of Health" that are based not only on the theory of the 4 humors but also on observations of personal, lifestyle, and environmental factors. The humoral theory, which passed from Pythagoras through Hippocrates to Galen,[98] and later medical authorities including monastic-based physicians of the early medieval period, was adopted within the Arabic medical tradition from the Greek. The ideas were reintroduced with classical medicine into Europe during the late Middle Ages and continued well into the 19th century in Islamic, Jewish, and Christian practices.[20] They were encased within and disseminated widely through what is known as the *Regimen Sanitatis,* a Latin term meaning simply "rules of health."

The *Regimen Sanitatis Salernitanun* (*Regimen*) is the name given to the medico-literary phenomenon originating at the ancient University of Salerno in Southern Italy and thought to be the earliest medical school in Christian Europe. The most famous version was originally written for Robert of Normandy, son of William the Conqueror. At least 160 editions were printed prior to 1830, such publications containing many different versions, some with considerable additions and alterations or described as scientific.[99] Used throughout Europe for most of the last millennium, the *Regimen* provided a way to understand positive health as a public and a private issue, and addressed its preservation and the healing of the sick but with little reference to specific remedies for specific disorders. The *Regimen* did provide descriptions of the symptoms related to humoral excess but was mainly composed of rules for the preservation of health. Centering largely on diet, the other health rules of the non-naturals are referred to, the implication being that these were well known. Indeed, the first page of the analytical index from a 1607 English translation of the *Regimen Sanitatis Salernitanun* illustrates how the rhyming verse addressed only briefly the nonfood rules of the non-naturals (Figure 1-4). These of course were inclusive of exercise, motion (doing), and rest.[100]

The 6 rules not only provided the base for population health aimed at prevention, they also informed pathology, diagnosis, and therapeutics of medical services. The difference between what was healthy or pathologically unhealthy depended on correcting the quantity and quality of the 6 non-natural activities. Advice was provided by authentic or self-styled physicians about the management of each according to an individual's constitution and temperament in conjunction with other aspects of the humoral theory. "With or without medical guidance, patients practiced self-help," and people in all walks of life acted as their own physicians until very recently.[101]

In providing a way for everyone to understand health as both a public and a private issue, the *Regimen* was used in 3 different ways. First, it was produced beautifully in

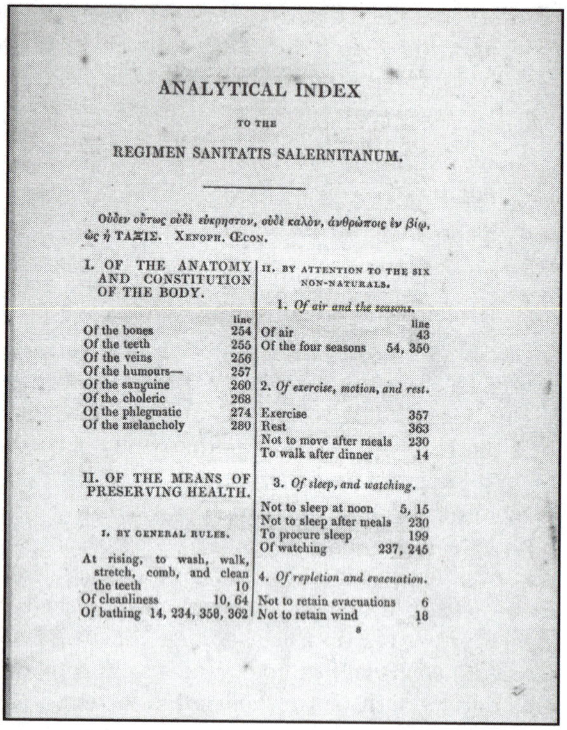

Figure 1-4. Analytical index of the *Regimen Sanitatis Salernitanun* ("of the passions" appears on the second page).

ANALYTICAL INDEX

TO THE

REGIMEN SANITATIS SALERNITANUM.

Οὐδὲν οὕτως οὐδὲ εὔχρηστον, οὐδὲ καλὸν, ἀνθρώποις ἐν βίῳ, ὡς ἡ ΤΑΞΙΣ. ΧΕΝΟΡΗ. ŒCON.

I. OF THE ANATOMY AND CONSTITUTION OF THE BODY.	II. BY ATTENTION TO THE SIX NON-NATURALS.
	1. *Of air and the seasons.*
	line
Of the bones 254	Of air 43
Of the teeth 255	Of the four seasons 54, 350
Of the veins 256	
Of the humours— 257	
Of the sanguine 260	2. *Of exercise, motion, and rest.*
Of the choleric 268	
Of the phlegmatic 274	Exercise 357
Of the melancholy 280	Rest 363
	Not to move after meals 230
	To walk after dinner 14
II. OF THE MEANS OF PRESERVING HEALTH.	3. *Of sleep, and watching.*
	Not to sleep at noon 5, 15
	Not to sleep after meals 230
I. BY GENERAL RULES.	To procure sleep 199
	Of watching 237, 245
At rising, to wash, walk, stretch, comb, and clean the teeth 10	4. *Of repletion and evacuation.*
Of cleanliness 10, 64	Not to retain evacuations 6
Of bathing 14, 234, 358, 362	Not to retain wind 18

verse format for the affluent, the authors understanding that health promotion needs to be aimed at the rich, as it does at the poor, but for different reasons. Personal regimes were individually tailored for those who had greater control over their lifestyles than the majority and could pay a physician to draw up an individualized program. The creation of these flourished across Europe for royalty, the nobility, the rich of civil life, and secular and ecclesiastical gentry, in some ways similar to the modern personal trainer programs of current days.

Second, the rules that provided the basis for *Regimen Sanitatis* were an identifiable component in major medical texts. Health care texts were also read by the nonmedical. In that way, the printed word, the state of the art technology of the time, reached the influential middle classes, the movers and shakers of their day. The 6 non-naturals provided the framework for teaching about health and the prevention of illness as medical schools became established and for centuries beyond. Trainee physicians had to learn to unite knowledge of the humoral qualities that defined the somatic constitution with the temperament of individuals. They had to link the art of medicine with the fields of science and natural philosophy and environmental and social issues. George Cheyne's 1724 *Essay of Health and Long Life* provides an example of a very respected medical textbook based on the non-naturals.[102] A firm favorite throughout the 18th century, the text made recommendations similar to WHO today that overeating, excessive drinking, late nights, restrictive clothing, and sedentary occupations should be avoided or reduced.

The scrolls provide an excerpt from the introduction to the first English translation by Thomas Paynell in 1528,[103] and from *Medicina Statica* (IV) by Italian physician Sanctorius Sanctorius (1561–1636),[104] a taste of how the rules relating to action and rest were based on empirical research (however, we might argue with the interpretation and the lack of modern objective criteria). In the excerpt on the next page, it is clear how what people did was related to the taking in and elimination of fluid according to humoral physiology.

Redynge of olde authors and stories my most honorable lorde, I fynde, that men in tyme past were of loger lyfe, and of more propsperous helthe, than they are nowe adayes...

There are 4 necessarie thynges to conserue and prolonge mans prosperite and helthe: that is abstinence from meate, abstinence from wyne, rubbyng of the body, exercise and digestion...

Yea howe greatly are we English men bounde to the maisters of the universite of Salerne [Salerne is in the realme of Naples] which vouchesafed in our behalfe to compile thus necessari, and thus holsome a boke...

So what profiteth us a boke, be hit neuer so expedient and frutefull, if we understande hit nat...

Wherefore I consydryng the frute which myght come of this boke if hit were translated in to the englishe tongue (for why euery man understandeth nat the latine). I thought hit very expedient at some tymes, for the welthe of unlerned psones to busy my selfe there in...

Thomas Paynell: 1528

Excerpts: *Medicina Statica. Of Exercise and Rest*

IV. The body perspires much more lying quietly in bed than turning from one side to another by frequent agitation.

V. Cheerful and angry persons are less wearied by long travelling than the fearful and pensive: for the former perspire more healthfully, but the other less.

VI. Those bodies which are admitted to refection, (refreshment with food and drink) after immoderate exercise, receive much prejudice; because, as they are wearied and burthened with meat, they perspire less.

VII. Exercise from the seventh hour to the twelfth after refection, does insensibly dissolve more in the space of one hour than it does in three hours at any other time.

XIII. If a person who has kept his bed long be troubled with pain in the feet, the remedy is walking; if one that is upon a journey be so troubled, the remedy is rest.

XIV. There are two kinds of exercises, one of the body, the other of the mind: that of the body evacuates the sensible excrements: that of the mind the insensible rather, and especially those of the heart and brain, where the mind is seated.

XV. An excessive rest of the mind does more obstruct perspiration than that of the body.

XVI. The exercises of the mind which most conduce to the cheering up of the spirits, are anger, sudden joy, fear, and sorrow.

XVII. Men's bodies resting in bed, and agitated with a vehement motion of the mind, for the most part become more faint, and less ponderous, than if there be a tranquility of mind, with a violent motion of the body, as it happens at tennis, or any game at ball.

(continued)

XIX. Violent exercise of mind and body renders bodies of lighter, hastens old age, and threatens untimely death: for, according to the philosopher, those persons that are exercised die sooner than such as are not.

XXI. By exercise the body perspires less, by sleep, more, and the belly is more loosened.

XXIV. Swimming immediately after violent exercise, is hurtful; for it very much obstructs perspiration.

XXV. Violent exercise in a place where the wind blows is hurtful.

XXVI. From the wind proceeds a difficulty of respiration, from the motion, acrimony.

XXVII. Riding relates more the perspirable matter of the parts of the body from the waist upwards, than downwards, but in riding, the amble is the most wholesome, the trot the most unwholesome, pace.

XXXII. The exercise of the top, consisting of moderate and violent motion, to-wit, walking and the agitation of the arms, promotes perspiration.

XXXIII. Moderate dancing, without any capering or jumping, comes near the commendation of moderate walking; for it moderately expels the concocted perspirable matter.

Sanctorius Sanctorius

In order for the greater preliterate population to know the rules of health, the *Regimen* was promulgated with verse and song, making it easier to remember. Verse and song were popular media of the day that could best disseminate messages to communities. Figure 1-5 shows Arnaldus de Villa Nova, a celebrated 13th century physician, chemist, astrologer, and divine, presenting the *Regimen* to what appears to be a broad population group. This is from an etching taken from old woodcuts in a 16th century German edition by physicians John Curio and James Crellius.[100]

The 3 very progressive methods of disseminating the *Regimen* (ie, use of personal training manuals, professional literature, and popular media) helped to promote health through what people did day by day. Although versions of the *Regimen* were usually published in verse format, they were known as *Tacuinum Sanitatis* if in table form.[105] The content of both *Regimens* and *Tacuinum* remained remarkably constant for many centuries, providing a consistent reminder of the need to promote health and prevent illness during the long period before germ theory and technologically sophisticated medicine. It was then that the long accepted messages became disregarded and largely forgotten. In the present day, rules about health are more varied than those from ancient times and, perhaps, appear to be less dogmatic. There are also many sources of modern "rules." In the spirit of this text, the modern rules for health to be considered are the directives of the WHO as presented in the OCHP.

Modern: World Health Organization and Ottawa Charter for Health Promotion

The WHO was established in 1948 as the United Nations' (UN) specialized agency for health. Its objective is the attainment of the highest possible level of health by all the people of the world and is governed through the World Health Assembly composed of

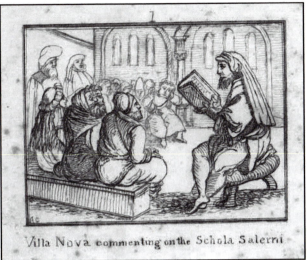

Figure 1.5. Arnaldus de Villa Nova presents the *Regimen* (from an etching taken from old woodcuts in a 16th century German edition).

Villa Nova commenting on the Schola Salerni

representatives of 192 member states. The President of the First World Health Assembly, Dr. Andrija Stampar, played a decisive role in drafting the WHO definition,[8] which has survived despite 60 years of rapid social change and has been incorporated subsequently into the International Covenant on Economic, Social, and Cultural Rights. So too has the notion of the fundamental right to and enjoyment of "the highest attainable standard of health."[106] This includes the right to adequate food, water, clothing, housing, health care, education, and security in the event of sickness, disability, old age, unemployment, or lack of livelihood beyond an individual's control. Those categories are usually regarded as social or economic issues, but the WHO recognizes the close connection with health, and it must be recalled that it defines health as social well-being as well as physical and mental well-being. While in medical dictionaries ill is defined as "not well; sick" and "a disease or disorder,"[73] in other lexicons it sits with words that cross the physical, mental, and social divide like *harmful, wretched, disastrous, hostile or malevolent, unfriendly, portending danger or disaster, unfavorable, morally bad, evil, contrary to accepted standards, improper, unsound*, and *disordered* as well as "not in good health; suffering from a disorder; sick."[107,108] Because the definition is inclusive of social as well as mental and physical health, wellness becomes everyone's concern, and the responsibility for its attainment is shared between medical and health professionals, governments and intergovernmental agencies, judiciaries, businesses, communities, families, and individuals as WHO documents outline. The OCHP applies and extends the basic concept of the WHO definition and the ideas embodied in the call for health for all people.

To achieve these ends, WHO in the OCHP called for action in 5 major directions. I am presenting these as the current "non-naturals" or the modern "rules for health." They are:

1. Building healthy public policy.
2. Creating supportive environments.
3. Strengthening community action.
4. Developing personal skills.
5. Reorienting health services beyond the provision of clinical and curative services toward the pursuit of health.

The rules are holistic in their intent as "the inextricable links between people and their environment [that] constitute the basis for a socioecological approach to health"[3] is recognized. They argue for "the conservation of natural resources throughout the world"[3]; "the need to encourage reciprocal maintenance—to take care of each other, our communities, and our natural environment"[3]; and "that the society one lives in creates conditions that allow the attainment of health by all its members."[3] It also calls for a commitment to "address the overall ecological issue of our way of living" and to "counteract the pressures toward harmful products, resource depletion, unhealthy living conditions, and environments."[3] In acknowledging that urgent consideration needs to be given to factors detrimental to the natural and social environment, the OCHP can be seen to recognize the adverse results of many current occupational structures and technology. However, it also recognizes the benefits of occupation. Although not formally acknowledged within the document by occupation-specific nomenclature, its "occupational" emphasis recognizes that what people do affects their health. Health, it is stated, "cannot be separated from other goals" because it "is created and lived by people within the settings of their everyday life; where they learn, work, play, and love."[3] The OCHP encourages communities and individuals to participate actively in life by the prescription that "to reach a state of complete physical, mental, and social well-being, an individual or group must be able to identify and to realize aspirations, to satisfy needs, and to change or cope with the environment."[3] To progress in the spirit of those directives, the *Jakarta Declaration* identified 5 priorities necessary for health promotion to go forward into the 21st century: the promotion of social responsibility for health, an increase in investments for health development, an expansion of partnerships for health promotion, an increase in empowerment of individuals and communities, and the building and safeguarding of health promotion infrastructures.[4]

The ancient and modern rules will be discussed further as this exploration expands the notion of occupation and its relationship to health in the next chapters. However, to complete this one, the 2 aspects of the WHO definition that are evident in the thrust of both ancient and modern rules will be considered.

Physical, Mental, and Social Well-Being

As early as the 5th century BC, Pericles made the connection between health and a feeling of well-being. In 2005, Web definitions include "a subject's physical and mental soundness"[109]; a "state of human existence in which a person's basic needs are adequately met and satisfied"[110]; and "a contented state of being happy and healthy and prosperous."[111] Another proclaims the importance of population well-being as a concept in economics and political science. It goes on, "a large part is standard of living, the amount of money and access to goods and services that a person has; these numbers are fairly easily measured. Others like freedom, happiness, art, environmental health, and innovation are far harder to measure."[112]

These are but a few of many descriptions because well-being has become such a popular concept that in January 2006 there were approximately 70,800,000 entries related to it on the World Wide Web. These include reports of work being carried out on this important topic, such as the Child Trends Data Bank that provides data and analyses for over 70 indicators of the well-being of children in America[113]; and *America's Children: Key National Indicators of Well-Being* from the Federal Interagency Forum on Child and Family Statistics.[114]

In the thesaurus, *well-being* stands with words like *health*, as well as *happiness* and *prosperity*.[115] Health, happiness, and prosperity have more than an intuitive fit with well-being, as the opposite appears to prove; the experiences of people living in poverty in developing countries are obvious examples. Indeed standardized mortality and morbidity statistics support the association of people wherever they live with limited resources experiencing poorer health, earlier death, and—it can be argued—less well-being.[116] For example, in the late 1980s, it was found that children of unskilled workers in Britain were twice as likely to die in their first year of life than those of professional people.[117] Numerous other studies of that time supported the notion that well-being is related to income, financial status, and employment.[118-124] In both postmodern and developing economies, those with few monetary concerns are more easily able to meet the basic requirements for health and to make the most use of health-promoting opportunities than poorer people. In addition, they experience little of the stress or worries attributed to poverty, and the high social value accorded to money in the present day increases its potential effect on health status. However, affluent people do not automatically experience well-being at all times. Prosperity is but one factor in well-being that without other physical, mental, or social elements such as energy for life's tasks, self-esteem, or social connectedness can be a negative influence. Indeed, despite acknowledged "material" associations, it appears that feelings of well-being can differ from person to person, that they can be as intangible and amorphous a concept as charm or style. Yet, despite its elusive quality, at times of absorbing interest, even when physical, social, and mental capacities are stretched to meet a challenge, people are said to be able to resist disease and seem impervious to many problems and difficulties that beset them because they are experiencing well-being. In his time-use studies, Csikszentmihalyi found that when people feel "very significantly more happy, strong, satisfied, creative, and concentrated" than at other times, they sometimes experience a sense of timelessness.[125-127] To many, that would be a good description of a state of well-being, although he calls the phenomenon "flow." Interestingly, he found it was 3 times (54%) as often at work than in their free time (17%) that a typical employed adult in the United States experienced this phenomenon.[125-127]

Many descriptors have emerged in empirical research that relate to explanations of well-being. An ongoing American project at Duke University is the development of a *Child Well-Being Index*. This provides an evidence-based measure of well-being trends over time.[128] It comprises several interrelated summary indices in 7 quality-of-life domains that have been established over 2 decades. Comparison of current results with those of 1975 and 1985 provide a sense of overall improving or deteriorating well-being for children and youths in the United States. The domains encompass physical, mental, and social criteria: health; safety and behavioral concerns; emotional and spiritual well-being; social relationships with peers and family members; place in community measured through participation in school or work; material well-being; and productive activity measured by educational attainments. At the other end of the age spectrum in the United States, a comprehensive analysis compiled by the Federal Interagency Forum on Aging-Related Statistics found that for many older Americans the indications are that well-being is increasing. However, some groups are disadvantaged disproportionately, including women, minorities, and those with limited education.[129] Across the North American border, the Canada Well-Being Measurement Act has been developed to inform that nation's citizens about the health and well-being of its people, communities, and ecosystems.[130] As well as environmental issues relating to pollution, resource depletion, and biodiversity, the act addresses social issues that relate to lack of opportunities to participate and failure to account for nonmonetary aspects of well-being. Interestingly, the act appears to accept that continual economic expansion may not lead to long-term well-being; that the fundamental goal of communities is the "well-being" of both current and future generations; and that the meaning of "well-being" is worthy of continual debate, clarification, adjustment, and measurement based on more than monetary measures.

There is similar interest in other parts of the world. Some years ago, when Pybus and Thomson asked 444 New Zealanders what, in their experience, was being well, the answers included replies like being "able to do what I want to and enjoy" and "energy and interest," as well as "being full of life" and "feeling alive and vital," with "energy for things extra."[131] Similar ideas emerged in Blaxter's British study. Women who defined health in terms of energy described it as being "properly alive," having "lots of get-up-and-go," and "being keen and interested," as well as "feeling like conquering the world."[14] In a smaller Australian survey, subjects were asked to define their concept of well-being, how it felt to them, and how often they experienced the feeling. The majority of 138 respondents were single, fit, and young women, which may well have given a particular cast to the responses. The 3 most common of those related to having a sound mind, a healthy body, and being happy. Ninety-five percent of them agreed they had felt what they would describe as well-being, with half admitting they experienced this feeling frequently. The feelings the respondents associated with well-being included happiness, peace, and confidence, and the situations or environments they most associated with that feeling concerned occupations, relationships, and surroundings. The first of those categories that was marginally the largest was a composite of responses about work, leisure, rest, religious practices, selfless activity, self-care, and achievement. They totalled 60% of the responses without taking account of any occupations carried out in conjunction with social relationships or spiritual (as opposed to religious) situations, so it could well be that most of the sample identified some form of occupational behavior, situation, or environment as one of the circumstances associated with their experience of well-being. Relationships are arguably the most often-cited factor in social-psychology research about well-being. However, in such studies, occupation in holistic, all-embracing terms is seldom factored separately, and the apparent importance of both occupations and relationships in this study gives rise to the thought that programs that link them together might be particularly effective. In other studies, well-being has been related to social supports; community cohesion; marital state; education; and religious attitudes, beliefs, and activities.[118-121,132,133] Those studies appear to be complementary to how occupation and social behavior appear to be interwoven.

Physical well-being is, perhaps, the aspect of health that has received the most attention and is the easiest to understand. Indeed, it is claimed that the research has shown that regular physical exercise is a vital aspect of well-being, not surprising when the human body is designed for exercise.[134] Blaxter found that young people, and men in particular, associate health (and presumably physical well-being) with physical fitness, with strength, energy, and athletic prowess and, in line with this, identify sports figures as their idea of health in others. Women tend to relate physical fitness and energy in terms of outward appearance and work-related activity rather than sports or particular leisure pursuits.[14] Small-scale studies carried out with students tended to confirm Blaxter's findings that young people view physical fitness and well-being as synonymous and that there are differences in how men or women perceive it, often in accord with how health and well-being are reported in the media.[135]

There is growing recognition that use of physical capacities has an effect on general well-being; for example, mental functioning benefits through increased blood supply to the brain, and aerobic power and social interactions benefit through shared activity.[136,137] Examples of such recognition are provided by a review of the relationship between physical training and mental health in which Folkins and Syme found evidence of a positive relationship between exercise, well-being, self-concept, and work ability[138]; by Chamove's study, which found that moderate physical exercise by people with psychiatric disorders decreased their depression, anxiety, and disruptive and psychotic behavior; increased self-concept and social well-being; and aided sleep and relaxation[139]; by Morgan's suggestion that nonspecific aspects of exercise such as social contact may be instrumental in improved mental health and well-being[140]; and by Oliver's report that improved play and social interaction are benefits of physical education activity along with growth, fitness, agility, and coordination.[141]

Mental well-being usually refers to the well-working and coping ability of both emotional and intellectual capacities and sometimes includes spiritual capacities. These, in combination, enable individuals to find meaning in their lives, interact effectively with others, be reflective, process and act on information, solve problems, develop skills for making decisions, clarify values and beliefs, cope with stress, and be flexible and adaptable to changes in life circumstances and demands. Mental well-being is described in these or similar terms in many popular texts addressing healthy living, such as *The Good Health Guide*,[142] *Health Through Discovery*,[143] and *Understanding Your Health*.[144] According to these conceptions, while these varied capacities may not amount to well-being in themselves and the need to use them differs between people and at different life stages, they are seen as prerequisites to the experience of well-being.[145] From Antonovsky's theory linking health with a "sense of coherence" comes the idea that one difference between who stays well and who does not is an individual's level of coping within his or her "own boundaries."[146] These boundaries, which enclose what is most important to each individual, may be narrow for some and broad for others. That is, "one need not necessarily feel that all of life is highly comprehensible, manageable, and meaningful in order to have a strong 'sense of coherence,'" but those with this sense will be better able to cope and to experience "behavioral immunology" and mental well-being.[146-149] Blaxter found that psychological fitness, which I am assuming is a term synonymous with mental well-being, was a popular concept of health across all the age groups and for both men and women when they described health for themselves rather than for others. While it tended to be used more by women and those with better education, "health is a state of mind" or "health is a mental thing more than physical" were common statements among her research participants.[14]

Psychologists have studied mental well-being over decades from various perspectives.[150-152] Strack, Argyle, and Schartz, for example, equate the concept of mental well-being with happiness,[153] and Maslow, with "full humanness."[154] The latter concept describes the highest level of personal development that enables individuals to recognize their potentials and life roles and to fully use their personal strengths without selfishness.[154] Maslow stands in a tradition of humanist psychology based on existentialism,[155] which extends from Burnham's "wholesome personality"[156] through Fromm's "productive character"[157] to Rogers' descriptions of the "fully functioning person."[158] This humanist tradition can be said to stem from the "mental hygiene movement," which was founded in America in 1909 and was influential in the growth and development of mental health services of the first half of the century, including the birth of occupational therapy. The rhetoric of this approach became "equated with productiveness, social adjustment, and contentment—'the good life' itself."[159] In turn, the "mental hygiene movement" can be seen to uphold the Renaissance tradition of human achievement and the ideals of the Age of Enlightenment. The central concept of these approaches (ie, well-being depends upon the meeting of individual potential) is an important aspect of the perspective of population health discussed in this text.

Social well-being is less researched in terms of conventional medicine despite the idea that physical and mental well-being seem to be dependent on its coexistence.[160] Throughout time, people have displayed a need to be part of cooperative social groups. Some theorists even argue that there is a correlation between the size of the neocortex and the size of social groups among primates, humans having the largest brain relative to size and the largest and most complex societies.[161] In his 1986 *Health Promotion Glossary*, Nutbeam suggests that well-being in its entirety belongs within the broad context of the social model of health.[2] In his later 1998 glossary, he provides the following definitions that relate to the concept[2]:

* Social capital: This "represents the degree of social cohesion which exists in communities. It refers to the processes between people which establish networks, norms, and social trust, and facilitate co-ordination and co-operation for mutual benefit." The stronger the bonds and networks, the greater the likelihood of mutual benefit that, in turn, creates health.

* Social networks: "Relations and links between individuals which may provide access to or mobilization of social support for health." In destabilizing circumstances, such as high unemployment or rapid urbanization, action to promote health and social well-being might focus on the re-establishment of social networks.

* Social support: "That assistance available to individuals and groups from within communities ... can provide a buffer against adverse life events and living conditions, and can provide a positive resource for enhancing the quality of life."

Empirical research supports the association of social well-being with other measures of health. Argyle's study of the psychology of happiness is a case in point. He found that relationships, such as marriage and others of a close, confiding, and supportive nature, enhance health by both preserving the immune system and encouraging good health habits.[119] He also reports that socially valued activities, including those of a religious nature, and paid employment, if satisfying, appear to have a positive correlation with both health and happiness. Going further than that, Blaxter's findings suggest "not only socioeconomic circumstances and the external environment, but also the individual's psychosocial environment carry rather more weight, as determinants of health, than healthy or unhealthy behaviors."[14] Similarly, at a 1999 conference organized in London by the Office of Health Economics, attendees were advised that social policy is more important to health than medicines.[162]

Absence of Illness

Dubos makes the claim that at least from the time of recorded history, people appear to have valued healing science more than naturally healthy living, citing the history of Hygeia and Asclepius (Figure 1-6) as symbolizing the neverending oscillation between these different points of view. The Athenian goddess Hygeia was not involved in treating the sick, but represented the natural laws that promote health of mind and body as the most important function of health care. She symbolized the belief that people would not be ill if they lived a balanced life in a pleasant environment and according to reason.[37] From the 5th century BC on, her cult progressively gave way to the god of healing, Asclepius, who before his creation as a deity lived as a physician in the 12th century BC. His followers believe that the chief role of health care is to treat disease, correct imperfections, and thereby restore health. Today, in most histories of medicine, Hygeia is mentioned briefly as subservient to Asclepius, but even in mythology, she became relegated to being either a member of his retinue or one of his daughters.[37] This cautionary tale highlights similar attitudes in the present day. The promotion of population health makes good sense in every way, but pursuit of it is not regarded as highly as the results of medical science, despite experiences of illness and the time and expense of reversing the effects of illness.

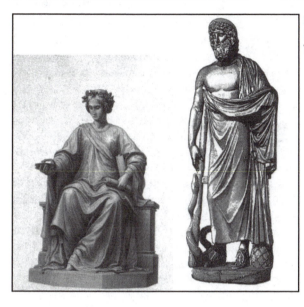

Figure 1-6. Hygeia and Asclepius. (Hygeia is reproduced with permission of The Wellcome Library.)

The Classical restorative view of health was the starting place for modern medicine and its concentration on absence of illness approaches. This was even though the rules of the non-naturals and the *Regimen* played an important role in guiding physicians about what people could do in a positive sense as well as what they should avoid doing at all. Both negative and positive approaches outlasted the spiritual focus of medicine in medieval times, the advent of humanism, the Renaissance, and the Enlightenment. They even survived, somewhat bruised, through the 19th century, particularly with the resurgence of interest in all things medieval that emerged with the pre-Raphaelite and Arts and Crafts Movements.[20] But by the end of that century, interest in hygiene and antisepsis had inspired medical advances and those of public health to suspect that societal actions as well as individual treatment might successfully eliminate much of ill health and disease. While people in third-world countries continued to endure catastrophic health conditions, for many in the postindustrial world, research and discovery changed the suspicion to belief. The Better Health Commission of Australia suggested in the mid 1980s that modern society was fostering the belief that, with the aid of modern technology, individuals could control their bodies and the environment and expect health and wellness as a right.[163] In some ways, such belief has retarded the appreciation of the holistic nature of the WHO definition of health because of what can be described as a "live now and reverse the pay later" approach within the community. They have reinforced "healing" rather than "health" ideologies and confused curative medicine with health if in no other way than by the amount of resources provided to cure illness in comparison with that provided to reduce its incidence.

The pervasiveness of "absence of illness" approaches and the current fascination with all things related to the latest technologies and cures of medical science is not surprising when apparent miracles such as organ transplants have created a myth that all illness can be overcome. Additionally, there is an illusion that modern medicine can assist people to look like and become whatever they fantasize. Miracles and illusions apart, the medical science gains over the last half century have led to an apparent unprecedented improvement in terms of life expectancy. In developed countries, there has been a substantial decline in the infant mortality rate, people are living longer, and, on the whole, experiencing lower levels of illness in childhood and early adulthood. Particularly in advanced Western societies, profound demographic changes are characterized by a rapid increase in the proportion of people living more than 70 years of age. This is despite epidemiological shifts evidenced by death resulting from a marked rise in NCDs such as diabetes, cardiovascular and respiratory disease, stress-related disorders, and mental illness such as major depression, some of which have resulted from increased consumption of high-fat foods, lack of physical activity, alcohol, cigarettes, and illegal drugs.[164]

The WHO in its policy document *Active Ageing* recognized the rapid increase in the proportion of people living longer as a global phenomenon that demands international, national, regional, and local action. It acknowledged that "failure to deal with the demographic imperative and rapid changes in disease patterns in a rational way in any part of the world will have socioeconomic and political consequences everywhere."[165] While that suggests emphasis on the ill-health consequences of the demographic changes, the policy also considers well-being. It was guided by the UN principles for older people aimed at independence, participation, care, self-fulfillment, and dignity and was developed by WHO's Ageing and Life Course Programme as a contribution to the second UN World Assembly on Ageing, held in April 2002 in Madrid, Spain. The *Active Ageing* policy will feature as an ongoing theme throughout this book because it lays the basis for many health-promoting initiatives of an occupational nature.

It is recognized more and more that aging populations could demand an increase of already stretched resources to combat the diseases that surface as time passes. That will be particularly the case if strategies are not developed and put in place to ensure people are able to maintain a healthy state throughout their lives thereby reducing the risk of illness later. In providing adequate resources to meet the 1978 WHO call for a primary health care system that is accessible to all, there tends to be a preoccupation by many government bodies that this only means everyone should have access to appropriate treatment of common diseases and injuries and that essential drugs are available. While that "absence of illness" message is an important part of the *Declaration of Alma Ata*, primary health care at the very least is also about health education for communities and individuals, adequate supplies of food and proper nutrition, safe and sufficient water supplies, basic sanitation, maternal and child health care, family planning, and immunization. It is also about addressing "the main health problems in the community, providing promotive, preventive, curative and rehabilitative services accordingly," and involves the coordinated intersectoral efforts of a range of providers in national and community development, as well as requiring and promoting "maximum community and individual self-reliance."[6]

In 1998, the WHO reported there were 1.3 billion people living in absolute poverty, mostly in developing economies.[7] The greatest burden of disease in the poorest countries remains communicable diseases such as tuberculosis and acute respiratory infections, malaria, diarrheal diseases, and HIV/AIDS. Lack of clean water and sanitation, lack of food, pollution from solid fuels, and unsafe sex remain risk factors, and poverty-related old and new infectious diseases linger as major challenges. In some parts of the world, this can be related to a rise in violence and fundamentalism; social disintegration and instability; and an increase of mental, social, and spiritual as well as physical illness.[8] Agis Tsouros, head of the Centre for Urban Health in the WHO Regional Office for Europe, wrote in the Foreword to the 2nd edition of *Social Determinants of Health: The Solid Facts* of the WHO goal "to promote awareness, informed debate and, above all, action" toward the development "of policies and programmes that explicitly address the root causes of ill-health, health inequalities and the needs of those who are affected by poverty and social disadvantage."[166] He challenges health workers who address the social determinants of health to search for "clear scientific evidence to inform and support the health policy-making process" because this field is perhaps "the most complex and challenging of all."[166] This is similarly the case for those public heath practitioners and occupational scientists, and therapists who take up the challenges of an occupational perspective of health as a largely unacknowledged but very important social (and physical and mental) determinant of health. Both the broader social determinants and occupational determinants are concerned with key aspects of[166]:

* Living and working circumstances.

* Lifestyles.

* Health implications of economic and social policies.

* Benefits of investment in health policies.

As medical science is dominant in current thinking about health, it is medical experts who, on the whole, define for the general public what health is. So it is hardly surprising that health care is aimed mainly at eradicating medically defined physical or mental ills. Occupational therapists and others working principally within medical spheres of operation are influenced, and sometimes their actions are controlled, by the dominant view held in their workplaces. This has become a deterrent to the understanding of the WHO's broader mandate for health. Like in the Classical world, we are in the midst of a conflict between the opposing views of health and healing. It is confusing because both are valuable; both are on the same side. With the increasing costs of miraculous advances, questions need to be asked about what should be the priorities across the globe according to available resources. The WHO attempts to do so, but that raises a second question about whether the most powerful forces for health in postmodern societies listen to and follow those priorities.

Hippocrates, the father of modern medicine, observed that a physician "was to be skilled in Nature and must strive to know what man is in relation to food, drink, occupation, and which effect each of these has on the other."[37] He attempted to combine the approaches of Asclepius and Hygeia, providing students of public health with a classical philosophy about the relationship between external and internal determinants of health. His tombstone in Cos is engraved:

HERE LIES HIPPOCRATES
WHO WON INNUMERABLE VICTORIES
OVER DISEASE
WITH THE WEAPONS OF HYGEIA[37]

Medicine's interest in healing, along with its popular acclaim and political influence, may account for the large number of people who do equate health with the absence of illness rather than physical, mental, and social well-being. Both aspects are considered important by the new public health that tries to act on the overarching vision of WHO.

References

1. Preamble to the Constitution of the World Health Organization as adopted by the International Health Conference, New York, 19-22 June, 1946; signed on 22 July 1946 by the representatives of 61 States. Official Records of the World Health Organization. 2:100.
2. Nutbeam D. Health promotion glossary. *Health Promotion International.* 1998;13(4):349-364.
3. World Health Organization, Health and Welfare Canada, Canadian Public Health Association. *Ottawa Charter for Health Promotion.* Ottawa, Canada: Author; 1986.
4. World Health Organization. *Jakarta Declaration on Leading Health Promotion into the 21st Century.* 4th International Conference on Health Promotion, Jakarta, Indonesia, 21-25th July, 1997.
5. World Health Organization. *Resolution WHA40.43: Technical Cooperation.* Geneva: Author; 1977.

6. World Health Organization. *The Declaration of Alma Ata.* International Conference on Primary Health Care, Alma Ata, USSR; 1998.

7. World Health Organization. *Health for All in the Twenty-First Century.* Document A51/5. Geneva: Author; 1998.

8. Yach D. *Health and Illness: The Definition of the World Health Organizatio*n. World Health Organization. Geneva: World Health Organization; 2005.

9. Wylie CM. The definition and measurement of health and disease. *Pub Health Rep.* 1970;85:100-104.

10. Herzlich C. *Health and Illness: A Social Psychological Analysis.* London: Academic Press; 1973.

11. Audy JR. Measurement and diagnosis of health. In: Shepard P, McKinley D, eds. *Environ/Mental.* Boston, Mass: Houghton Mifflin; 1971:142.

12. Doyal L, Gough I. *A Theory of Human Need.* London: Macmillan; 1991:59.

13. Goodman AH. Health adaptation, and maladaptation in past societies. In: Bush H, Zvelebil M, eds. *Health in Past Societies.* Oxford: BAR International Series 567; 1991:35.

14. Blaxter M. *Health and Lifestyles.* London: Tavistock/Routledge; 1990.

15. Sigerist HR. *Medicine and Human Welfare.* New Haven, Conn: Yale University Press; 1941.

16. Frank JP. The people's misery, mother of diseases. In: Yach D, ed. *Health and Illness: The Definition of the World Health Organization.* Available at: http://www.medizin-ethik.ch/publik/health_illness.htm. Accessed March 2005.

17. Kass LR. Regarding the end of medicine and the pursuit of health. In: Caplan AR, Engelhart HT, McCartney JJ, eds. *Concepts of Health and Disease: Interdisciplinary Perspectives.* Reading, Mass: Addison Wesley Publishing Co; 1981.

18. Greiner PA, Fain JA, Edelman CL. Health defined: objectives for promotion and prevention. In: Edelman CL, Mandle CL, eds. *Health Promotion Throughout the Lifespan.* 5th ed. St. Louis, Mo: Mosby; 2002:6.

19. Bush H, Zvelebil M, eds. *Health in Past Societies: Biocultural Interpretations of Human Skeletal Remains in Archeological Contexts.* Oxford: British Archaeological Reports International Series 567; 1991:5.

20. Wilcock AA. *Occupation for Health. Volume 1. A Journey from Self Health to Prescription.* London: British College of Occupational Therapists; 2001.

21. Girling DA, ed. *New Age Encyclopaedia: Volume 23.* Sydney: Bay Books; 1983:293.

22. Guy RDJ. *Compassion and the Art of the Possible: Dr Southwood Smith as Social Reformer and Public Health Pioneer.* (1993 Octavia Hill Memorial Lecture). Cambridgeshire: Octavia Hill Society and Birthplace Trust; 1996.

23. Department of Health and Human Services. *The Health Consequences of Smoking: Cancer.* Rockville, Md: 1982.

24. Department of Health and Human Services. *The Health Consequences of Smoking: Cardiovascular Disease.* Rockville, Md: 1983.

25. Department of Health and Human Services. *The Health Consequences of Smoking: Chronic Obstructive Lung Disease.* Rockville, Md: 1984.

26. Gordon T, Sorlie P, Kannel WB. Section 27, Coronary Heart Disease Atherothrombotic Brain Infarction. Intermittent Claudication. A Multivariate Analysis of Some Factors Related to Their Incidence: Framingham Study, 16 Year Follow Up. US Department of Health, Education and Welfare, Public Health Service. NIH Pub. No. 1740-0320, 1971.

27. Bauer G. Agricola. In: *De re Metallica 1556.* Hoover HC, Hoover HL, trans. New York: Dover Publications; 1950.

28. Paracelsus. *Four Treatises of Theophrastus von Hohenheim Called Paracelsu*s. In: Sigerist HE, ed. Temkin CL, Rosen G, Zilboorg G, Sigerist HE, trans. Baltimore, Md: Johns Hopkins Press; 1941.

29. Ramazzini B. *Disease of Occupations.* New York: Collier-MacMillan; 1980.

30. Thackrah CT. *The Effects of the Principle Arts, Trades, and Professions, and of Civic States and Habits of Living, On Health and Longevity.* London: Longman, Rees, Orme, Browne and Green; 1831.

31. Parmeggiani L, ed. *ILO Encyclopedia of Occupational Health and Safet*y. 2 Vols. 3rd rev ed. Geneva, Switzerland: International Labour Organization; 1983.

32. McKeown T. *The Origins of Disease.* Oxford: Basil Blackwell; 1988:1-2.

33. Ilza Veith, Huang Ti, Nei Ching Su Wen. *The Yellow Emperor's Classic of Internal Medicin*e. Baltimore, Md: Williams and Wilkins; 1949:253.

34. Lao-tzu. Tao Te Ching (The Way) Circe 500 BC: Chuang-tzu. In: Dubos R, ed. *Mirage of Health: Utopias, Progress and Biological Change.* New York: Harper and Row; 1959:10.

35. Pao Ching-yen. In: Needham J, ed. *Science and Civilisation in China. Vol 2. History of Scientific Thought.* New York: Cambridge University Press; 1956.

36. Rousseau JJ. Discourse on the origin and foundations of inequity amongst men. In: Mason JH, ed. *The Indispensable Rousseau.* London: Quartet Books; 1979.

37. Dubos R, ed. *Mirage of Health: Utopias, Progress and Biological Change.* New York: Harper and Row; 1959.
38. Beddoes T. *Hygeia, or Essays Moral and Medical on the Causes Affecting the Personal State of Our Middling and Affluent Classes.* 3 vols. Bristol: R Phillips; 1802.
39. Virey, JJ. *L'hygiene Philosophique.* Paris, France: Crochard; 1828.
40. Jenner E. *An Inquiry Into the Causes and Effects of the Variolae Vaccine: A Disease Discovered in Some of the Western Counties of England, and Known as the Cow Pox.* Birmingham, Ala: Classics of Medicine Library; 1978.
41. Lucas Powell M. *Status and Health in Prehistory: A Case Study of the Mountville Chiefdom.* Washington: Smithsonian Institute Press; 1988.
42. McMichael T. *Human Frontiers, Environments and Disease: Past Patterns, Uncertain Futures.* Cambridge: Cambridge University Press; 2001:xiii.
43. Stephenson W. *The Ecological Development of Man.* Sydney, Australia: Angus and Robertson; 1972:26,94,136,217.
44. King-Boyes MJE. *Patterns of Aboriginal Culture: Then and Now.* Sydney, Australia: McGraw-Hill Book Co; 1977:154-155.
45. Leakey R, Lewin R. *People of the Lake: Man: His Origins, Nature, and Future.* New York: Penguin Books; 1978:32-33,88,120.
46. Leakey R. *The Making of Mankind.* London: Michael Joseph Ltd; 1981:226-229,242.
47. Falk D. *As It Happened: Some Liked It Hot.* Television documentary. SBS.
48. Jones S, Martin R, Pilbeam D, eds. *The Cambridge Encyclopedia of Human Evolution.* New York: Cambridge University Press; 1992:369-372.
49. Agius T. Aboriginal health in Aboriginal hands. In: Fuller J, Barclay J, Zollo J, eds. *Multicultural Health Care in South Australia. Conference Proceedings.* Adelaide: Painters Prints; 1993:23.
50. Lorenz K. *Civilized Man's Eight Deadly Sins.* Latzke M, trans. London: Methuen and Co; 1987.
51. McNeill WH. *Plagues and People.* London: Penguin Books; 1979:39.
52. Tunnes N. 1656. Cited in: Dubos R, ed. *Mirage of Health: Utopias, Progress and Biological Change.* New York: Harper and Row; 1959:11.
53. Fortuine R. The health of the Eskimos as portrayed in the earliest written accounts. *Bulletin of the History of Medicine.* 1971;45:97-114.
54. Wharton WJL, ed. *Captain Cook's Journal During His First Voyage Around the World Made in HM Bark Endeavour, 1768-1771.* London: Eliot Stock; 1893:323.
55. Meindl RS. Human populations before agriculture. In: Jones S, Martin R, Pilbeam D, eds. *The Cambridge Encyclopedia of Human Evolution.* New York: Cambridge University Press; 1992.
56. Dobson A. People and disease. In: Jones S, Martin R, Pilbeam D, eds. *The Cambridge Encyclopedia of Human Evolution.* New York: Cambridge University Press; 1992:411-412.
57. Landers J. Reconstructing ancient populations. In: Jones S, Martin R, Pilbeam D, eds. *The Cambridge Encyclopedia of Human Evolution.* New York: Cambridge University Press; 1992:404-405.
58. Douglas M. Population control in primitive peoples. *Br J Sociol.* 1966;17:263-273.
59. Coon CS. *The Hunting Peoples.* London: Jonathan Cape Ltd; 1972:390.
60. Gandevia B. *Occupation and Disease in Australia Since 1788.* Sydney: Australasian Medical Publishing Co Ltd; 1971:157.
61. Cannon WB. *Bodily Changes in Pain, Hunger, Fear and Rage.* Boston, Mass: CT Branford; 1929.
62. Sigerist HE. *A History of Medicine. Vol 1. Primitive and Archaic Medicine.* New York: Oxford University Press; 1955:254-255.
63. Birdsell JB. On population structure in generalized hunting and collecting populations. *Evolution.* 1958;12:189-205.
64. Diamond J. The Animal Attraction. Fact Sheet 2. Australian Broadcasting Corporation; 2001. Available at: http://www.abc.net.au/animals/program2/factsheet2.htm. Accessed October 2005.
65. Hetzel BS, McMichael T. *L S Factor: Lifestyle and Health.* Ringwood, Victoria: Penguin; 1987:186-187.
66. Procopius. *Persian Wars 23:1. History of the Wars.* 5 Vols. Dewing HB, trans. Cambridge, Mass: Harvard University Press; 1914.
67. Mumford L. *The Condition of Man.* London: Heinemann; 1963:148,380.
68. Gordon D. *Health, Sickness and Society: Theoretical Concepts in Social and Preventive Medicine.* St. Lucia, Queensland: University of Queensland Press; 1976:5,157,164,311,337,378.
69. Jones B. *Sleepers, Wake! Technology and the Future of Work.* Melbourne, Australia: Oxford University Press; 1982:16.
70. Eversley DEC. Epidemiology as social history. In: Creighton CA, ed. *History of Epidemics in Britain.* 2nd ed. London: Cassell; 1965:1-35.

71. Doll R. *Preventive Medicine: The Objectives in "The Value of Preventive Medicine."* Ciba Foundation *Symposium 10.* London: Pitman; 1985.

72. Lorenz K. *The Waning of Humaneness.* Boston, Mass: Little, Brown and Co; 1987:21.

73. Friel JB, ed. *Dorland's Illustrated Medical Dictionary.* 25th ed. Philadelphia: WB Saunders; 1974:720.

74. Lieberman P. Evolution of the speech apparatus. In: Jones S, Martin R, Pilbeam D, eds. *The Cambridge Encyclopedia of Human Evolution.* New York: Cambridge University Press; 1992:136-137.

75. Bernard C. Lectures on the phenomena of life common to animals and vegetables (1878-1879). In: Langley LL, ed. *Homeostasis, Origins of the Concept.* Stroudsberg, Pa: Hutchinson and Ross, Inc; 1973:129-147.

76. Cannon W. *Physiological Regulation of Normal States: Some Tentative Postulations Concerning Biological Homeostatics.* Paris, France: Charles Richet; 1926:91-93.

77. Cannon W. *The Wisdom of the Body.* New York: WW Norton and Co Inc; 1939:317,323.

78. Allport GW. The open system in personality theory. *Journal of Abnormal and Social Psychology.* 1960;61:301-311.

79. McDougall W. *The Energies of Men.* London: Methuen; 1932.

80. McDougall W. *Social Psychology.* 23rd rev ed. London: Methuen; 1936.

81. Lewin K. *A Dynamic Theory of Personality.* New York: McGraw-Hill Book Co, Inc; 1935.

82. Murray HA. *Explorations in Personality.* New York: McGraw-Hill Book Co, Inc; 1938.

83. Hull C. *Principles of Behavior.* New York: Appleton-Century-Crofts; 1943.

84. Madsen KB. *Theories of Motivation.* 4th ed. Kent, Ohio: Kent State University Press; 1968.

85. Alderfer CP. *Existence, Relatedness and Growth: Human Needs in Organizational Settings.* New York: Free Press; 1972.

86. Maslow AH. *Motivation and Personality.* 2nd ed. New York: Harper and Row; 1970.

87. Eysenck HS, Arnold W, Meili R. *Encyclopedia of Psychology.* New York: Continuum Books, The Seabury Press; 1979:705-706.

88. Wolman B, ed. *Dictionary of Behavioral Science.* New York: Van Nostand, Reinold Co; 1973:250.

89. Snell GD. *Search for a Rational Ethic.* New York: Springer Verlag; 1988:147.

90. Young PT. Drives. In: Sills DL, ed. *International Encyclopedia of the Social Sciences.* New York: The Macmillan Co and The Free Press; 1968:275-276.

91. Dashiell JF. *Fundamentals of Objective Psychology.* Boston, Mass: Houghton Mifflin; 1928:233-234.

92. Anscombe GEM. Modern moral philosophy. *Philosophy.* 1958;33(124):1-19.

93. Watt ED. Human needs. In: Kuper A, Kuper J, eds. *The Social Science Encyclopedia.* London: Routledge; 1985:367,368.

94. Ornstein R, Sobel D. *The Healing Brain: A Radical New Approach to Health Care.* London, England: Macmillan; 1988:11-12.

95. Knight R, Knight M. *A Modern Introduction to Psychology.* London: University Tutorial Press Ltd; 1957:56-57,177.

96. Sigerist HE. *A History of Medicine, Volume 11: Early Greek, Hindu, and Persian Medicine.* New York: Oxford University Press; 1961.

97. Biedermann H. *Medicina Magica.* Birmingham, Ala: Classics of Medicine Library; 1986:20.

98. Berger M. *Hildegard of Bingen: On Natural Philosophy and Medicine: Selections from Cause and Cure.* Cambridge: D.S. Brewer; 1999.

99. Croke A. *Regimen Sanitatis Salernitanum: A Poem on the Preservation of Health in Rhyming Latin Verse.* Oxford: D.A. Talboys; 1830:42.

100. The Englishman's Doctor. In: Croke A. *Regimen Sanitatis Salernitanum with the Englishman's Doctor: An Ancient Translation.* Oxford: D.A. Talboys; 1830:144.

101. Siraisi NG. *Medieval and Early Renaissance Medicine: An Introduction to Knowledge and Practice.* Chicago, Ill: University of Chicago Press; 1990:127.

102. Cheyne G. *Essay of Health and Long Life.* London: Strahan; 1724:77.

103. Paynell. T. *Introduction to Regimen Sanitatis Salerni.* England: McGraw-Hill Book Co, Inc; 1528.

104. Sanctorius Sanctorius. Medicina statica. In: Sinclair J, ed. *Code of Health and Longevity.* Edinburgh: Arch Constable and Co; 1806:175-176.

105. "Tacuinum Sanitatis in Medicina". Italy:c1390. Based on Abulcasis de Baldach's "Tagwim al-sihha" (ie Tabular Summary of Health) c1060. In: Biedermann H. Medicina Magica. Birmingham, Alabama: Classics of Medicine Library; 1986:23

106. World Health Organization. *Constitution of the World Health Organization.* International Health Conference, New York, NY, 1946:1.

107. Landau SI, ed. *Funk & Wagnalls Standard Desk Dictionary.* Vol 1: A-M. USA: Harper & Row, Publishers, Inc; 1984:319.

108. Coulson J, Carr CT, Hutchinson L, Eagle D, eds. *The Standard English Desk Dictionary.* Sydney: Bay Books; 1976:419.

109. Google. Definitions of Well-being on the Web. Available at: http://www.dcri.duke.edu/patient/glossary.jsp. Accessed October 2005.
110. Google. Definitions of Well-being on the Web. Available at: http://www.undp.org/rbec/nhdr/1996/georgia/glossary.htm. Accessed October 2005.
111. Google. Definitions of Well-being on the Web. Available at: http://wordnet.princeton.edu/perl/webwn. Accessed October 2005.
112. Google. Definitions of Well-being on the Web. Available at: http://en.wikipedia.org/wiki/Well-being. Accessed October 2005.
113. Vandivere S, Pitzer L, Halle TG, Hair EC. Indicators of Early School Success and Child Well-being. Publication #2004-25. In: Cross Currents. 2004 Issue 3; October. Available at: http://www.childtrendsdatabank.org/. Accessed October 2005.
114. Federal Interagency Forum on Child and Family Statistics. America's Children: Key National Indicators of Well-Being. Available at: http://www.childstats.gov/. Accessed October 2005.
115. American Heritage Dictionary. *Roget's New Thesaurus.* Boston, Mass: Houghton Mifflin Co; 1980.
116. *Enough to Make You Sick: How Income and Environment Affect Health.* Australian National Health Strategy Research Paper, No 1, Sept 1992.
117. Whitehead M. *The Health Divide.* New York: Penguin; 1988:229.
118. Cohen P, Struening EL, Genevie LE, Kaplan SR, Muhlin GL, Peck HB. Community stressors, mediating conditions and wellbeing in urban neighborhoods. *Journal of Community Psychology.* 1982;10:377-390.
119. Argyle M. *The Psychology of Happiness.* New York: Methuen and Co; 1987.
120. Koenig H, Kvale J, Ferrel C. Religion and well-being in later life. *Gerontologist.* 1988;28(1):19-27.
121. Burckardt C, Woods S, Schultz A, Ziebarth D. Quality of life of adults with chronic illness: a psychometric study. *Res Nurs Health.* 1989;12:347-354.
122. Ullah P. The association between income, financial strain and psychological well-being among unemployed youths. *The British Psychological Society.* 1990;63:319-330.
123. Isaksson K. A longitudinal study of the relationship between frequent job change and psychological well-being. *J Occup Psychol.* 1990;63:297-308.
124. Warr P. The measurement of well-being and other aspects of mental health. *J Occup Psychol.* 1990;63(4):193-210.
125. Csikszentmihalyi M. *Flow: The Psychology of Optimal Experience.* New York: Harper and Row; 1990.
126. Csikszentmihalyi M. Activity and happiness: toward a science of occupation. *Journal of Occupational Science: Australia.* 1993;1(1):38-42.
127. Csikszentmihalyi M, LeFevre J. Optimal experience in work and leisure. *J Pers Soc Psychol.* 1989;56(58):5-22.
128. Land KC. *Child Well-Being Index.* Durham, NC: Duke University Department of Sociology. Available at: http://www.soc.duke.edu/~cwi. Accessed October, 2005.
129. Federal Interagency Forum on Aging-Related Statistics. Older Americans 2004: Key Indicators of Well-Being, The Second Comprehensive Analysis of the Lives of Older Americans. Available at: http://www.ageingstats.gov/chartbook2004/pr2004.html. Accessed October, 2005.
130. Canada Well-Being Measurement Act (Proposed by Motion M-385) Last Update: May 26, 2003. Available at: http://www.flora.org/sustain/7GB/preview5.shtml. Accessed October 2005
131. Pybus MW, Thomson MC. Health awareness and health actions of parents. In: Boddy J, ed. *Health: Perspectives and Practices.* Palmerston North, New Zealand: The Dunmore Press; 1985.
132. McConatha JT, McConatha D. An instrument to measure self-responsibility for wellness in older adults. *Educational Gerontology.* 1985;11:295-308.
133. Homel R, Burns A. Environmental quality and the well-being of children. *Social Indicators Research.* 1989;21:133-158.
134. Carnell D. Editorial: cycling and health promotion. *BMJ.* 2000;320:888.
135. Wilcock AA. Unpublished research carried out as part of student learning about the relationship between occupation and health. University of South Australia, 1991-1995.
136. Sydney KH, Shephard RJ. Activity patterns of elderly men and women. *Journal of Gerontology.* 1977;32(1):25-32.
137. Kirchman MM. The preventive role of activity: myth or reality—a review of the literature. *Physical and Occupational Therapy in Geriatrics.* 1983;2(4):39-47.
138. Folkins CH, Syme WE. Physical fitness training and mental health. *Am Psychol.* 1981;36:373-389.
139. Chamove A. Exercise improves behaviour: a rationale for occupational therapy. *Br J Occup Ther.* 1986;49:83-86.
140. Morgan WP. Psychological effects of exercise. *Behavioral Medicine Update.* 1982;4:25-30.
141. Oliver J. Physical activity and the psychological development of the handicapped. In: Kane J, ed. *Psychological Aspects of Physical Education and Sport.* London: Routledge; 1972:187-204.

142. The Open University in association with the Health Education Council and the Scottish Health Education Unit. *The Good Health Guide.* London: Pan Books; 1980.

143. Dintiman GB, Greenberg JS. *Health Through Discovery.* 4th ed. New York: Random House; 1989.

144. Payne WA, Hahn DB. Mauer EB. *Understanding Your Health.* New York: McGraw-Hill; 2004.

145. Kanner AD, Coyne JC, Schaefer C, Lazarus RS. Comparison of two modes of stress management: daily hassles and uplifts versus life events. *J Behav Med.* 1981;4:1-39.

146. Antonovsky A. The sense of coherence as a determinant of health. In: Matarazzo JD, Weiss SM, Herd JA, Miller NE, Weiss SM, eds. *Behavioral Health. A Handbook of Health Enhancement and Disease Prevention.* New York: John Wiley and Sons; 1990:117,119.

147. White RW. Sense of interpersonal competence: two case studies and some reflections on origins. In: White RW, ed. *The Study of Lives.* Chicago, Ill: Aldine; 1963.

148. Bandura A. Self efficacy: toward a unifying theory of behavioral change. *Psychol Rev.* 1977;84:191-215.

149. Kobasa SC, Maddi SR, Courington S. Personality and constitution as mediators in the stress-illness relationship. *J Health Soc Behav.* 1981;22:368-378.

150. Bradburn NM. *The Structure of Psychological Well-Being.* Chicago, Ill: Aldine; 1969.

151. Andrews FM, Withey SB. *Social Indicators of Well-Being.* New York: Plenum Press; 1976.

152. Diener E. Subjective well-being. *Psychol Bull.* 1984;95:542-575.

153. Strack F, Argyle M, Schartz N, eds. *Subjective Well-Being: An Interdisciplinary Perspective.* Oxford, UK: Pergamon Press; 1991.

154. Maslow A. *The Farther Reaches of Human Nature.* New York: Viking Press; 1971.

155. Bullock A. *The Humanist Tradition in the West.* London: Norton; 1985.

156. Burnham WH. *The Wholesome Personality.* New York: Appleton-Century; 1932.

157. Fromm E. *Man for Himself.* New York: Holt, Rinehart and Winston; 1947.

158. Rogers C. *On Becoming a Person.* Boston, Mass: Houghton Mifflin; 1961.

159. Ingleby D. Mental health. In: Kuper A, Kuper J, eds. *The Social Science Encyclopedia.* London: Routledge; 1985.

160. Kirkpatrick R, Trew K. Lifestyle and psychological well-being among unemployed men in Northern Ireland. *J Occup Psychol.* 1985;58:207-216.

161. Dunbar R. Why gossip is good for you. *New Scientist.* 1992;136(1848):28-31.

162. Richards T. News extra: social policy more important for health than medicines, conference told. *BMJ.* 1999;319:1592.

163. Better Health Commission. *Looking Forward to Better Health.* Vols 1-3. Canberra: Australian Government Publishing Service; 1986.

164. Katz AH, Hermalin JA, Hess RE, eds. *Prevention and Health: Direction for Policy and Practice.* New York: The Haworth Press; 1987.

165. World Health Organization's Ageing and Life Course Programme. *Active Ageing: A Policy Framework.* Madrid, Spain: Second United Nations World Assembly on Ageing; 2002:54.

166. Tsouros AD. Foreword. In: Wilkinson R, Marmot M, eds. *Social Determinants of Health: The Solid Facts.* Copenhagen, Denmark: World Health Organization Regional Office for Europe; 2003.

Suggested Readings

Blaxter M. *Health and Lifestyles.* London: Tavistock/Routledge; 1990.

Dubos R, ed. *Mirage of Health: Utopias, Progress and Biological Change.* New York: Harper and Row; 1959.

McMichael T. *Human Frontiers, Environments and Disease: Past Patterns, Uncertain Futures.* Cambridge: Cambridge University Press; 2001.

World Health Organization. *The Declaration of Alma Ata.* International Conference on Primary Health Care, Alma Ata, USSR; 1978.

World Health Organization, Health and Welfare Canada, Canadian Public Health Association. *Ottawa Charter for Health Promotion.* Ottawa, Canada: Author; 1986

World Health Organization. *Health for All in the Twenty-First Century.* Document A51/5. Geneva: Author; 1998.

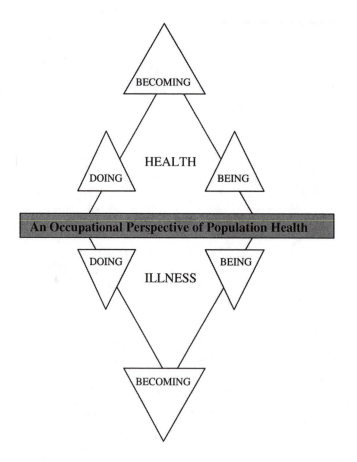

AN OCCUPATIONAL THEORY
OF HUMAN NATURE

Theme 2:
*"Changing patterns of life, work and leisure have a significant impact on health.
Work and leisure should be a source of health for people."*
WHO, *Ottawa Charter for Health Promotion*, 1986

The chapter addresses:
* Theories of human nature
* An occupational theory of human nature
  * Human evolution and occupation
  * A particular mix of physical characteristics that create the occupational human
  * Changing patterns of occupation have a significant impact on health
* 3-way link: occupation, health, and survival

In this chapter, the focus of the perspective of health taken here is introduced as a theory of human nature. This theory is based on the idea that defines the emerging discipline of occupational science—that humans are occupational beings.[1] The main direction of the theory is set out in this chapter, but the details are explored in Chapters 3 through 6. The discussion leads to the proposition that there is a 3-way link between occupation, health, and survival, in that occupation provides the mechanism for people to fulfill basic human needs essential for survival and health; to adapt to environmental changes; and to develop and exercise genetic capacities in order to maintain health and to experience physical, mental, and social well-being.

Theories of Human Nature

A theory, in the sense it is used here, is a system of ideas held to explain a group of facts or phenomena. It includes a "related set of principles" that "tie two or more concepts together, usually in a correlational or causal way," such as those in the paragraph above relating to occupation, health, and survival.[2] According to Lewin's 3 stages of theory development—the speculative, the descriptive, and the constructive—this theory is bridging the second and third stages of development: researching, testing, and trialing have already begun as evidenced by the wide-ranging material relating to occupation and health published in the *Journal of Occupational Science* since its genesis in 1993 and in the direction taken in many recent occupational therapy publications.[3-7] Since the theory was presented in the first edition, no research has become apparent that contradicts it; indeed, the opposite is the case. It is strengthened by the directives of the WHO and particularly by the ratification of the OCHP in Jakarta[8] and the policies on *Active Ageing*,[9] *Mental Health Promotion*,[10] and *Physical Activity*.[11] Throughout this text, as in the previous one, the concepts, relationships, and principles are measured against a broad range of ideas and against known research.[12]

That the theory is concerned with human nature is ambitious, but it is addressed in this way to emphasize the extent of the complexity and of the influence engagement in occupation has had upon cultural evolution, upon our present circumstances, and upon the health of individuals and communities. Some 40 years ago, in an exploration of *Occupation and Disease in Australia Since 1788*, Gandevia postulated:

> *Man's occupations are, of course, in part a function of his physical environment … are not independent of the total structure of society, its religion … its politics and legislations, its economic status, its attitudes to social problems … its approach to science and research … all these factors, and others, interact to influence the concepts and practices of every occupation. Thus the relationship of every occupation to health and disease is far from fixed and immutable over any period of time: it changes.*[13]

While the focus of Gandevia's work was mainly concerned with paid employment, he resisted using the term *occupational diseases* in the title because he felt it too restricting and technical, making it possible to ignore the relationship of occupation to "society's ever-changing attitudes and values."[13] This text holds a much wider view of occupation, as was explained in the introduction to this section of the book, but what Gandevia advanced is equally applicable to it. So too is his belief that physicians are "often baffled by it" and that any definition should be dictated "by society, not by doctors: by social concepts, not by science."[13]

It is such a complex issue that it is worthy of a theory. Diverse theories about human nature provide the context for beliefs about the meaning and purpose of life, about visions of the future, and about what humans should or should not do.[14] Well-articulated examples of differing theories of human nature range as widely as those proposed by Plato, Freud, or Sartre, as well as those embraced in creeds as diverse as Christianity or Taoism. "The notion of human nature involves the belief that all human individuals share some common features" and characteristics that are innate.[15] This is a concept central to humanist and critical theorists in that it provides the grounds for aiming toward growth models of health and for critical analysis of social or health environments that inhibit human potential; many Marxist theorists also accept it. Marx made valuable contributions to a social and occupational view of human nature, which unfortunately was dismissed in the official ideology of socialist countries and by Marxist structuralism.[16] Apart from theorists, each person thinks and acts according to a personal view of human nature but seldom attempts to articulate or to test this view, preferring instead to profess allegiance to a socioculturally accepted view.

An Occupational Theory of Human Nature

This occupational theory of human nature provides the idea around which the relationship between health and occupation is unravelled. The theory, being based upon few arbitrary elements derived from multiple and ongoing observations, meets the criteria of empirical accuracy and predictive capacity required by contemporary canons of science, such as Stephen Hawking, who suggests:

> *A theory is a good theory if it satisfies two requirements; it must accurately describe a large class of observations on the basis of a model that contains only a few arbitrary elements, and it must make definite predictions about the results of future observations.*[17]

It can definitely predict that, in the future, people will continue to engage in occupation, although the form of the occupation will change according to sociocultural evolution.

The occupational theory set out also meets Stevenson's guidelines for a theory of human nature. In *Seven Theories of Human Nature*, he sets his requirements as[14]:

* A background theory of the nature of the universe.

* A basic theory of the nature of man.

* A diagnosis of what is wrong with man.

* A prescription for putting it right.

In outline and meeting these 4 criteria, the theory is set within generally accepted scientific theories of the evolution of the universe and the species that inhabit it. Its basic concept of the nature of humans is that people are occupational beings as a result of their biological evolution and enculturation. That is, the need to engage in occupation forms an integral part of innate biological systems aimed at survival and health, that the varying potential of individuals for different occupations is a result of their genetically inherited capacities, and that the expression and execution of occupation is learned and modified by the ecosystem and sociocultural environments in which they live. "As natural selection acts on phenotypes, not genotypes, and as phenotypes always include an environmental component, it is of course fallacious to oppose genes and environment."[18] This concept is in accord with Csikszentmihalyi's view that human action is shaped by genetic, cultural, and self teleonomies[19,20] and is supported by Snell's proposal that the making of "humans" is about 50% genetics and 50% culture.[21] The theory provides a simple diagnosis and prescription—namely, that humans have not seriously considered the implications or requirements of their occupational nature; that this has caused deleterious effects to individual, community, population, and ecological health; and that addressing this lack of awareness has the potential to result in major and beneficial changes to social, political, economic, ecological, and health policies and outcomes (Figure 2-1). Having outlined the theory, it will now be discussed in some detail.

HUMAN EVOLUTION AND OCCUPATION

"Evolution provides the historical explanation for the diversity of life on earth. Insights from evolutionary biology are critical to ensuring the health and well-being of humans and all other forms on earth."[22] The background of this occupational theory of human nature is based on the following brief account of biological and cultural evolutionary theory. Current scientific thought generally accepts that living matter evolved naturally from nonliving matter in the form of single-celled creatures. Over a period of perhaps a billion years, some electrons, protons, and neutrons combined to form atoms, which formed molecules. Some of these became "more or less well-organized aggregates," one class of which is organic matter.[23] In turn, some original microorganisms went through a "comparable hierarchical evolution" to primitive plant forms to invertebrates to vertebrates, and, in the past 60 million years, to mammals.[23]

Modern science, with cross-pollination from within the fields of chemistry, geology, paleontology, and, astrophysics, plays a key role in the continuing complex discussion of life's origins nearly 4 billion years ago. It is less concerned with why life emerged from

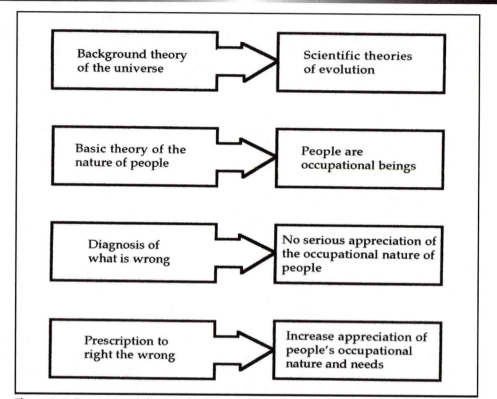

Figure 2-1. Occupational theory of human nature outlined according to Stevenson's requirements for theories of human nature.

the air, water, and rock of the barren face of the Earth than with where, when, and how. Recently, astrobiologist Robert Hazen explained many rival theories of genesis in his *2005 Genesis: The Scientific Quest for Life's Origins*,[24] pointing out, for example, how some recent theories have suggested that microbes living in rock miles below the Earth's surface might have some answers. Other theorists have been excited by the discovery of life near hydrothermal vents deep in the ocean, leading them to propose that life may have begun there. Hazen suggests:

> *Crucial features of our own cells suggest an ancient cooperative merging of early, more primitive cells. If experiments establish easy synthetic pathways to both a simple metabolic cycle and to an RNA-like genetic polymer, then such a symbiosis may provide the most attractive origin scenario of all.*[24]

Against a background of geologist and naturalist speculation, interest and theories that were out of step with dominant Christian beliefs, Darwin's *Origin of the Species by Means of Natural Selection* (1859)[25] and *The Descent of Man and Selection in Relation to Sex* (1871)[26] are recognized as the works that brought theories of evolution to public debate and inquiry in the Occident. Darwin's evidence did not come from human beings, and only his conclusion suggested that his theory would shed light on the origin of man. Nonetheless, his theories were received with moral shock, fear, and derision in the lay community, although accepted rapidly in biological science.

Dawkins suggests that although it is difficult to explain "how even a simple universe began," Darwin's theory of evolution by natural selection demonstrates a way in which "simplicity could change into complexity" and how collections of stable molecules could eventually, through "high longevity/fecundity/copying-fidelity," evolve into complex living beings.[27] Darwin's theory is based on the empirical observations and postulate that there is a tendency for parental traits to be passed to their offspring; that despite this, there are considerable and noticeable variations between individuals; and that species are capable of a rate of generation that cannot be supported by available natural resources. That is, more are born than can survive, requiring a struggle for existence. This leads to survival by natural selection of those with "certain inherited variants which increase the chances of their carriers surviving and reproducing."[28] Spencer termed this *survival of the fittest*, an often-quoted phrase that is frequently misconstrued to mean survival of those physically fit and strong, rather than those with "expected reproductive success," because it is taken literally and out of context.[29] Natural selection results in the accumulation of favored variants that will affect gradual adaptive change in every generation and, over extended periods, produce new forms of life. Diversity and individual uniqueness is the consistent message of evolutionary studies from Darwin's time to the present.[28] Individual uniqueness, particularly in relation to biological characteristics and capacities influencing engagement in occupation, has been a focal concern of occupational therapists, but not of political, social, or health planners or even public health practitioners for whom population and community needs are the major focus.

Humans are fitted for almost any environment and are dispersed across the globe in communities because their biological capacities enable flexible, adaptable, and wide-ranging occupations. Cultural and occupational evolution such as tool use, agriculture, and modern medicine have broken through natural population restraints that maintained population size of species more or less constant over long periods of time and as a result have reached a point where people dominate ecological systems, many believe, to the extent of natural resources not being sufficient to maintain predicted population growth.[28,30,31]

Working at almost the same time as Darwin, the Austrian monk Gregor Mendel studied and experimented with plant species, which led to his formulation of biological laws of heredity. Virtually ignored at the time, his work was rediscovered in 1900 by 3 scientists working separately—De Vries, Correns, and Tschermak—all within a 3-month period. Mendel's work provided the answer to the "causes of the variations on which natural selection acts."[30] Darwin's theory, modified in light of Mendelian genetics,[32] is now known as neo-Darwinism[33] or synthetic evolution.[34]

In recent times, "the discovery of the structure and function of DNA (deoxyribonucleic acid) has made clear the nature of the hereditary variations upon which natural selection operates."[35] In 1953, the elucidation of the structure of genetic DNA by James Watson and Francis Crick described how a long molecule of alternating sugar and phosphate units twisted to form a double helix (Figure 2-2) opens when chromosomes replicate. Each sugar unit is attached to a base of adenine, thymine, guanine, or cytosine that pair with those opposite. The first 2 bases always pair, as do guanine and cytosine. When chromosomes replicate, new bases are added on by pairing. These form 2 new identical molecules. An occasional mistake during replication is known as a mutation.[36]

It is now acknowledged in the scientific community that humans are mammals with much in common with other animals, and, like other species, have "a certain genetic constitution that causally explains not only the anatomical features ... but also our distinctive ... behavior."[14] As Bronowski explains so succinctly:

> The evolution of the brain, of the hand, of the eyes, of the feet, the teeth, the whole human frame, made a special gift of man ... faster in evolution, and richer and more flexible in behavior ... he has what no other animal possesses, a jigsaw of faculties which alone ... make him creative.[37]

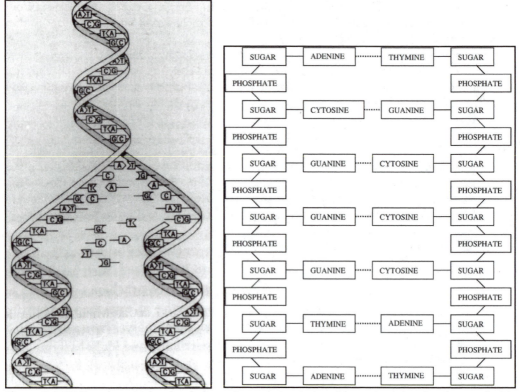

Figure 2-2. DNA: a long molecule of alternating sugar and phosphate units twisted to form a double helix. (Adapted from *The Illustrated Origin of the Species* by Charles Darwin. Abridged & Introduced by Richard Leakey. London: Rainbird Publishing Group Ltd; 1979.)

Bronowski's description of human difference is a useful bridge between Darwinist theories of evolution and the occupational nature of humans, which will be introduced here and explored more fully in the next 3 chapters.

The central concepts of the argument rely on 3 related sets of principles:

1. All people (unless prevented by congenital or acquired dysfunction, such as brain damage) engage in complex and self-initiated occupations because of their species' common combination of biological features, such as consciousness, cognitive capacity, and language. Although it is higher cortical adaptations such as these that have generated and made possible the complex occupational behavior that sets humans apart from other animals, anatomical and physiological characteristics of the body, such as bipedalism, upright posture, and hand dexterity, are vital instruments in the execution of occupation. Because of the integrated function of each, the mind and body are not seen as separate entities, but "simply one and the same."[38] Lorenz contends that this is the only possible view "tenable for the evolutionary epistemologist" and that "the razor-edge demarcation" seen as existing between them by some disciplines is only for the purpose of understanding them.[38] Certainly, because Descartes in the 17th century separated the body from the mind epistemologically, generations of scientists, up to the present day, have fed the assumption that mind and body can and should be considered separately. (Consider, for example, how the treatment of people with mental disorders is separated from those with physical disorder.) This separation has hindered the growth

and understanding of humans as occupational beings who, because of mind-body unity, are able to engage in occupation that is inclusive of both.

2. Engagement in occupation is indispensable to survival, as well as being an integral part of complex health maintenance mechanisms. The latter point will be explored further in Chapters 3 through 6. This hypothesis is in line with another of Lorenz's suggestions—that the principal purpose of both anatomical characteristics and behavior patterns is survival[38]—and with Ornstein's and Sobel's proposition that "the major role of the brain is to mind the body and maintain health."[39] My theory of occupation combines these views, maintaining that a primary function of people's anatomical characteristics, particularly the brain, is to facilitate healthy survival and that occupation is a primary mechanism for this function. To this end, the whole of the brain is involved in survival, health, and engagement in occupation. This notion is complementary to a predominant view that genomic reproduction is the principal goal of evolution, contending that, as reproduction can only occur during a particular stage of the life cycle, to reach reproductive age, individuals have to survive and resist disease and death and that positive health enhances survival and reproductive success. After reproduction, offspring require nurturing and education so that they too can eventually reproduce. Engagement in occupation is not only required for survival to the point of reproduction, but also for a long time after to provide support for the immature of the species. Views held about "kin selection" or "gene selection," which develop the concept of Darwinian "fitness" to include reproductive success of individuals who share genes,[30] account, at least in part, for social and altruistic behaviors and occupations. Given the short life expectancy of humans until fairly recently, support beyond that provided by biological parents was often necessary because human young have lengthy childhoods.

3. The theory recognizes as important that, in large part, genetic traits or capacities are inherited and that there is considerable variation between individuals because of genetic recombination, which "theoretically ... can create nearly an infinite number of different organisms simply by reshuffling the immense amount of genetic differences between the DNA of any two parents."[34] The differences between humans and the importance of exercising people's particular range of capacities are raised in later chapters as important issues in terms of promoting health and well-being and in preventing illness.

Integral to the 3 principles are ideas about the biological and sociocultural bases of behavior; the haphazard nature of evolution; the similarities and differences between species, brain size, and capacities; and the impact of occupational humans upon cultural and ecological change. Those who claim that human behavior depends on culture rather than genetics may criticize acceptance of a biological basis for occupational behavior. However, modern sociobiologists and ethologists contend that:

> Within [a] gene-environmental action model, culture can be seen as the man-made part of the environment, preselected by the specifically human genome. ... Culture can have no empirical referent outside of the human organisms that invent and transmit it, and, therefore, its evolution is inevitably intertwined with the biological evolution of our species.[18]

Such contention provides "a factual background for a middle view"[21] that is in accord with the theory of human nature proposed here. It "demonstrates the importance of evolutionary origins in the behavior of the species,"[40] but also maintains that, because of their biology, what people do is, in large part, socioculturally determined as sociologists claim. An example of that is provided by Lorenz's explanation that species have evolved in "unforeseeable ways" not "predetermined and directed toward some purpose."[38] This notion is fundamental to freedom of choice and self-responsibility. So, too, is homeostasis fundamental to people's occupational nature because the need for "sameness" maintains constancy in mental processes as well as in body physiology. To make sense of the world, psychological mechanisms seek "sameness" in what is received and perceived. This is facilitated by an "internal milieu, [which] seems to be more constant for the cells of the brain than for other parts of the body."[41] William James claimed in *The Principles of Psychology* that the capacity to recognize sameness is a prerequisite for the existence of a sense of self and "the very keel and backbone of our thinking" as it is central to recognition, of giving meaning, and of appreciating contrast and difference.[42] Without it, every time engagement in occupation occurred, it would appear as a new experience, take longer, be in the nature of trial and error, and no ongoing learning could occur. The evolution and the health experienced of the species would indeed be different.

Because people are goal-directed and committed by their nature to engage in occupation with purpose, it is difficult to appreciate that evolution may not have an ultimate purpose. The notion of predestination has led many theories of human nature, such as Marxism, to maintain that advances in cultural evolution must progress to the enhancement of human nature. In fact, the occupational nature of humans may not be progressive in terms of the ultimate "good" for the species. It may lead to less desirable outcomes for health and well-being, with occupational technology, for example, having the potential to destroy the earth's environment and the species.

All animals appear to have some special attributes that are paramount to their survival and that influence their regular occupations. This varies between and within species. For some, it is speed; for others, it is the ability to camouflage; and yet for others, it is highly developed visual or auditory capacities. Many animals possess qualities and characteristics once thought unique to humans, which is not surprising because all mammalian brains have neuronal circuitry and systems that enable them to receive, attend to, interpret, communicate with, and act upon information from the environment. In fact, "there is no strong evidence of unique brain-behavior relationships in any species within the class Mammalia."[43]

Indeed, the need to "do" is not species specific because all living things carry out survival activities. Birds build nests, decorate bowers to attract mates, and dive from great heights for fish or small prey. Domesticated dogs can learn that certain activities will be rewarded with food or praise, and will run or play with a ball for no apparent reason except for fun, which coincidentally, maintains their level of physical fitness and acuity. What animals do and how much freedom they have in the choice of occupations depends on the size, structure, and capacities of their nervous systems, as well as on environmental opportunities and constraints. Bronowski observed that while "every human action goes back in some part" to animal origins, an important distinction remains.[37] He questioned: "What are the physical gifts that man must share with the animals, and what are the gifts that make him different?"[37]

That question suggests that in order to gain some appreciation of the complex nature of doing in relation to health, it is useful to consider the most distinctive of human characteristics that create their capacity and need to do. Evolutionary scientists, archaeologists, and anthropologists have identified the human capacity to walk upright, oppose the thumb and use hands dexterously, view their world stereoscopically, and use of language as prime examples. Campbell suggests that these particular capacities have "overwhelming significance" and when "added together separate all humans from all other animals."[30] Each of these will now be considered.

A PARTICULAR MIX OF PHYSICAL CHARACTERISTICS THAT CREATE THE OCCUPATIONAL HUMAN

The brain is the starting place because it is this organ that coordinates and controls what people do. However, it cannot be studied in isolation because, as Edelman explains, "the shape of an animal's body is as important to the functioning and evolution of its brain as the shape and functioning of the brain are to the behavior of that body."[40] In evolutionary terms, "the shape of cells, tissues, organs, and finally the whole animal is the largest single basis for behavior."[40]

> *Our brain is not so much different from other brains, it is bigger. We are not a whole new experiment in the evolutionary process, but a superprimate. A quantitative change in the evolving human brain, however, has produced a qualitative change of extraordinary significance.*[30]

The human brain is "the largest primate brain that has ever existed."[44] It is 6.3 times larger than expected for mammals of the same body size.[45] Deacon suggests that the structure, configuration, and architecture are typical of other primates despite unique anatomy and functions for special human adaptations, such as "symbolic communication, speech, tool usage, and culture," and that "comparative size of brain may not be as important as its internal organization."[44]

Except for the neocortex, all cerebral regions have a rudimentary equivalent in reptilian brains.[46] Indeed, the brains of all animals have the same starting point. As they adapted to different habitats, climates, and subsistence demands, a "rather haphazard and seemingly disorganized set of structures" evolved in "archaeological" layers in the brain.[39] Each layer maintained stability and health of the organism as conditions changed, and each layer added a new dimension to what animals were capable of doing. Herbert Spencer (1820–1903), an evolutionist social philosopher, was the first to argue that "the brain evolved in a series of steps, each of which brought animals the capacity to engage in a constellation of new behaviors," and John Hughlings-Jackson (1835-1911), an English neurologist who based his work on Spencer's theory, recognized that the cortex has a special role in purposive behavior, which is supported by subcortical areas concerned with more elementary forms of the same behavior.[43]

The brainstem is the oldest part of the brain, which developed before the advent of mammals. It controls the simplest life support systems such as breathing, heart rate, and general alerting to predators or prey. The limbic system evolved to ensure stability of the organism on land, which called for structures to maintain internal temperatures, fluid levels, and emotional reactions, such as those concerned with self-protection. The cerebellum was probably the first area to specialize in sensorimotor coordination and is integral to efficiency of skilled movement. The cerebral cortex is the most recent layer. It is here that the processes occur that make humans most different from other animals, such as their capacity to analyze, organize, understand, produce, judge, plan, activate, sense, formulate, and execute complex doing.[43] Some of these processes, such as "the perceptual systems of seeing, hearing, and language comprehension," are more structured than others, such as "thinking and imagining, learning, and judging," so although "we can perceive the world only in certain modes, we can think about the finished products of perception, embellish them, and manipulate them in many different ways."[30] Such cortical functions give humans the "capacity to adapt culturally ... enabling [them] to insulate themselves from the environment and to exploit the environment."[30] That capacity has, unfortunately, led to people "struggling to come to terms with humankind's place in the biosphere."[30] This is especially so in the developed world where "culture has fostered the illusion of humans being apart from nature, rather than being part of nature" in an elitist and controlling way that has been far from egalitarian or participatory.[47]

Early hominids with the capacity to effectively meet their survival needs (such as with more food) because of their reasoning ability and social interaction skills must have had increased chances of survival, so "selection pressure would thus have favoured more complex, hence, larger brains."[47] Because brains are metabolically expensive as they increased in size, other organs, such as the colon, diminished to compensate (different food and food preparation enabled this). Additionally, much of brain growth and maturation was deferred until after birth because pelvic size could not accommodate a larger and maturer organ. This led to occupational adaptations concerned with care of offspring. Despite a remarkable similarity in what all people are able to do because of the brain's basic structure and function, subtle variations between them lead to amazing differences in terms of interest, competence, and satisfaction. The "brains of individuals vary in features just as the faces of individuals vary."[43]

Growing understanding about the relation of brain structure to behavior demonstrates "... enormously intricate brain systems at ... molecular levels, cellular levels, organismic levels (the whole creature), and transorganismic levels (ie, communication of some sort or other)," all of which interconnect.[48] In the cerebral cortex alone, it has been estimated that there are between 20 and 100 billion neurons and about 1 million billion connections, all of which are capable of many combinations so that "the sheer number and density of neuronal networks in the brain" reaches "hyperastronomical" figures and "the brain might be said to be in touch more with itself than with anything else."[48] Indeed, "the kinds of unique individuality in our brain networks make that of fingerprints or facial features appear gross and simple by comparison."[48] Many neurons, each of which is "unusual in three respects: its shape, its electrical and chemical function, and its connectivity," have specific potential.[40] In fact, just as Hughlings-Jackson had supposed, "very specific patterns of behavior are determined by very specific brain areas" with "each behavioral system probably [having] its own underlying neurophysiological mechanisms."[21] Different brain areas have different cell formations that have been described in functional and cytoarchitectonic maps.[49,50] "Mapping is an important principle in complex brains," and the fibers that connect maps with each other "are the most numerous of all those in the brain."[40]

Mapped areas of the brain that have been identified with specific functions relate to the capacity to do many things, although the "complexity of the brain's structure makes it incredibly difficult to relate its components to individual capacities."[43] Even capacities themselves have incredibly complex systems. In recent years, localization theories have been substantiated with the proviso that any area with a specific function does not work in isolation. In fact, the complexities of the interactive nature of specific areas of the brain have been demonstrated by many studies of brain activity, such as the "zenon 133" in which a 2-dimensional measure of regional blood flow (following inhalation of radioactive gases) was taken during the doing of tasks as compared to a resting state. It was found that the frontal lobes were relatively active bilaterally even at rest and that just doing simple movements of the fingers involved activity of many different areas.[51,52] Such complexity has been confirmed by 3-dimensional positron emission topography, which has been used to image the neuronal activity of both hemispheres and deeper brain structures during use (Figure 2-3). [44,53-55]

In the evolution of the human brain many pathways and connections remain from earlier developmental stages. Few structures have been discarded, although there may be alterations in size and function. Current evidence suggests that new brain functions are the result of "systematic reorganization, elaboration, or reduction of existing structures or

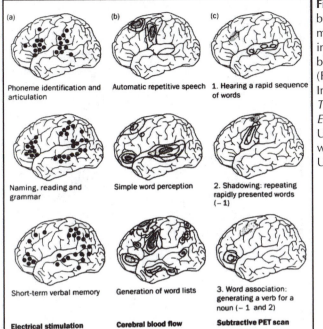

(a) Phoneme identification and articulation

(b) Automatic repetitive speech

(c) 1. Hearing a rapid sequence of words

Naming, reading and grammar

Simple word perception

2. Shadowing: repeating rapidly presented words (− 1)

Short-term verbal memory

Generation of word lists

3. Word association: generating a verb for a noun (− 1 and 2)

Electrical stimulation   **Cerebral blood flow**   **Subtractive PET scan**

Figure 2-3. The interactive nature of brain function demonstrated by various means during communication processing tasks: a) by electrical stimulation, b) by zenon 133, and c) by PET scans. (From Deacon TW. The human brain. In: Jones S, Martin R, Pilbeam D, eds. *The Cambridge Encyclopedia of Human Evolution.* New York: Cambridge University Press; 1992:121. Reprinted with the permission of Cambridge University Press.)

shifts in proportions of existing connections."[44] In answer to Bronowski's earlier question, the gifts that make humans different are not only the capacities highlighted in this section of the chapter, but also particular adaptations that evolved with increased brain size and, more specifically, the association areas of the cortex (Figure 2-4). They are responsible, in large part, for complex communication and emotional tone, language, thinking, humor, forward planning, problem-solving, analysis, judgment, and adaptation, and Lorenz has noted that:

> *Among humans ... perceptions of depth and direction, a central nervous representation of space, Gestalt perception and the capacity for abstraction, insight and learning, voluntary movement, curiosity ... exploratory behavior [and] imitation ... are more strongly developed than any of them is among an animal species, even if they represent for those animals a fulfillment of the most vital, life-furthering functions.*[38]

These highly developed capacities, along with consciousness (to be discussed in the next chapter) and particular physical characteristics, such as bipedalism, are the special survival mechanisms of humans, in that they endow unprecedented flexibility, enabling them to adapt to and meet the challenges of many different environments and dangers. The "intelligence and skills of our forebears do not only manifest themselves in the evolutionary transformations of the brain; they can also be seen in the results of their activity."[56] It is:

> *Expansion of a standard primate brain [that has provided people with] behavioral possibilities undreamed of in other even closely related species. This brain ... gives us the human potential for making tools, talking, planning, dreaming of the future, and creating an entirely new environment for ourselves.*[30]

The ongoing and progressive doings that have enabled the species to survive have stimulated and excited some people and deprived or stressed others according to what was done. That factor has health implications. Differences tend to grow or diminish

Figure 2-4. Size differences of association areas of the brain between humans and other mammals. (From Deacon TW. Primate brains and senses. In: Jones S, Martin R, Pilbeam D. *The Cambridge Encyclopedia of Human Evolution.* New York: Cambridge University Press; 1992:110. Reprinted with the permission of Cambridge University Press.)

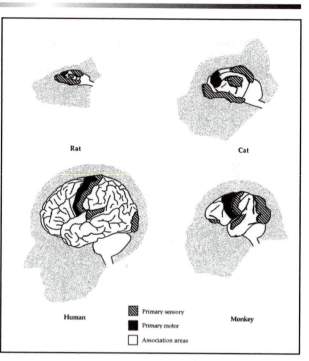

according to environmental demands, enculturation, and individual opportunity: "it is the unique blend of biology and culture that makes the species Homo sapiens a truly unique kind of animal."[57] The external variables increase individual difference, in part, because of structural change, which results from the neuronal demands of activity, "No two mixes of the inner and outer factors are just alike,"[21] and the inner factors alone are remarkably complex.

Dexterity and the anatomical advantage of hands capable of many types of prehension, and particularly of opposition of thumb to fingers, enable them to be used as tools. The capacity for manipulative skill was facilitated by a refinement of specialized brain centers within the primary sensory and motor areas of the cortex. These coordinated with other brain centers, such as the basal ganglia and the cerebellum.[49,50] As Sir Charles Bell observed in his 1833 Bridgewater Treatise on the hand, which related the hand's structure and function to environment:

> ... (the) difference in the length of the fingers (and the thumb) serves a thousand purposes, adapting the hand and fingers, as in holding a rod, a switch, a sword, a hammer, a pen or pencil, engraving tool, in all which a secure hold and freedom of motion are admirably combined.[58]

Such a hand structure, along with the capacity to walk upright, thus freeing the hands to do a variety of activities, is one of the special human attributes important to the unique ability of the species to do many things. Jelinek suggests this attribute was preadaptive to tool use, and it is probable that this preadaptive period was characterized to some extent by play.[56] Psychologist Jerome Bruner, for example, argues that "play ... can produce the flexibility that makes tool using possible," citing the laboratory studies of Birch and of Schiller, which indicate that play with materials is necessary prior to using it for "instrumental ends."[59-61]

Although Jane Goodall and others have demonstrated how chimpanzees in the wild use grasses to extract termites from their nest with great care and skill,[62,63] making and using tools is essentially a human characteristic, so much so that Benjamin Franklin is reputed to have observed, "man is a toolmaking animal."[64] Indeed, the Homo genus is said to have begun with the ancestors who are credited as being the first manufacturers of stone tools. Known appropriately as *Homo habilis* (handy man), the earliest of the remains found have been dated at over 2 million years. Although it is believed their tools were meager, statistical studies of them have shown that "their makers ... had a concept of symmetry ... and ... planned technique."[56] The doing of a variety of occupations was facilitated by a hand structure similar to our own, with a thumb positioned for opposition, essential for tool handling and manufacture, facilitated by a wrist joint that pronated and supinated.[65] "The early making of and use of stone and wooden tools placed a heightened premium on fine and gross motor coordination, and hence the elaboration of the motor cortex."[47] The appearance of *Homo erectus*, a routine toolmaker with longer legs and a larger brain, is currently dated at about 1.8 million years.

The use of upper limbs and hands has developed into a very specialized adaptation so that the unique movements, the sense of touch, the balance function, the reaching out, the gesturing, and fine manipulative capacities can be used separately or combined in infinitely varied ways, such as the preparation of food, typing, or holding a child while breastfeeding. This enables the doing of culturally derived occupations unique to humans to be carried out. Indeed, the capacity to use hands to do a multitude of activities is "one of the dominant aspects of our biological and cultural adaptation"[66] that is integral to matters of both survival and health. An ancient reference from Cicero[67] links the structure and function of the hand to the theme of this chapter: the WHO prerequisites of health.

> By the manipulation of the fingers the hand is enabled to paint, to model, to carve, and to draw forth the notes of the lyre and of the flute. And besides these arts of recreation there are those of utility, I mean agriculture and building, the weaving and stitching of garments and the various modes of working bronze and iron; hence we realize that it was by applying the hand of the artificer to the discoveries of thought and observations of the senses that all our conveniences were attained. ... (De nat. deor. II,150)
>
> *Cicero*

Bipedal gait and upright posture appear to be one of the most ancient of the species' particular features "associated with the ecological adaptations of early hominids."[68] Evidence, such as fragments of a 4-million-year-old thigh bone found in Ethiopia and the discovery in Laetoli of a trail of footprints left by 3 hominids in volcanic ash more than 3.5 million years ago, leads to anthropological opinion that hominids stood like humans before they could think like humans. Lewin suggests that the explanation of bipedalism, which currently enjoys the most scientific support, is that upright walking was a biological adaptive response to accessing traditional foods in a changing environment; that a more energy-efficient mode of walking was required because food sources became dispersed with climatic and subsequent environmental changes.[69] Doing is central to this explanation because it is to another that is favored. The second one is based on the fact that human young, who take a long time to mature, are dependent on their parents to carry them, unlike other primate offspring who are able to cling to their parents' long body hair. Erect standing and bipedal locomotion enabled mothers to move about while using arms and hands to support their children.[56] However, these are only 2 of several

Figure 2-5. Some theories of the origin of bipedal locomotion. (From Fleagle JG. Primate locomotion and posture. In: Jones S, Martin R, Pilbeam D, eds. *The Cambridge Encyclopedia of Human Evolution.* New York: Cambridge University Press; 1992:79. Reprinted with the permission of Cambridge University Press.)

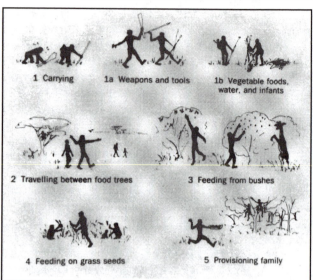

Figure 2-6. Pilocene adaptations of early hominids according to Lovejoy, drawn as a feedback system. (*Humankind Emerging.* 5th ed. Campbell BG. Copyright 1988. Reprinted by permission of Addison-Wesley Educational Publishers Inc.)

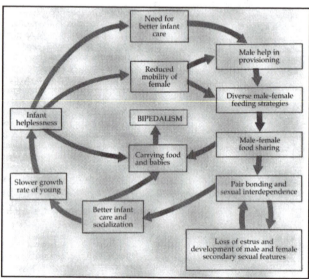

plausible explanations, all of which may have influenced bipedal evolution (Figures 2-5 and 2-6).

Although other animals have the ability to walk upright, humans have developed bipedalism into an adaptation as specialized as flight in a hovering hawk, while also developing versatility.[70-72] People can run, jump, dance, climb, swim, and cope with almost any terrain, and the health advantages of running, walking, dancing, and swimming, particularly with regard to the cardiovascular system, are well researched and applauded, even if not all epidemiologists agree about which form of activity is most valuable. Bipedal locomotion may be slower than quadrupedal, but people have thrived because of the occupational advantages of having the forelimbs free. "The tangled triple influence of bipedalism, brain development, and the manipulation of objects cannot [easily] be separated."[30] They work in cooperation with vision.

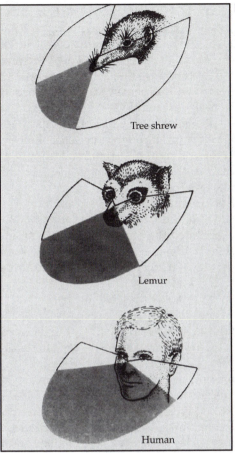

Figure 2-7. Stereoscopic vision in primates. (*Humankind Emerging.* 5th ed. Campbell BG. Copyright 1988. Reprinted by permission of Addison-Wesley Educational Publishers Inc.)

Tree shrew

Lemur

Human

Stereoscopic vision helps people to focus on objects that are close and to see these in 3-dimensional form as well as enjoying the benefits of long sight (Figure 2-7). Because of the height advantage provided by an upright posture, as well as eyes positioned at the front rather than the side of the head, people are able to see for relatively long distances. This capacity has made it possible for people to manipulate and appreciate the structure of materials, to become toolmakers, and, with practice, to produce objects of great variety and complexity that, in turn, have assisted human adaptation to different environments. Coupled with visual perception, humans are able to identify objects by color, hue, brightness, and form, in different orientations, and with sufficient clarity to pick out objects from their backgrounds whether they are still or moving. This range of visual capacity has been instrumental in the variety of occupations that people can do, giving them an evolutionary advantage over other animals despite them, perhaps, having better visual faculties of a particular kind.

People know about their world through their senses, and to many, vision is the most important. This is not surprising because there are estimates that between 75% and 90% of the information stored in the brain is derived from visual sources. "Since the world is constantly changing, the brain is flooded with information," even though "the eye [only] takes in a trillionth of the energy which reaches it."[39] In fact, the visual system and the brain select, simplify, and organize so that what humans see "is not so much a replication of the real world as a calculated and very selective abstraction of it."[73] This capacity prevents people from being overwhelmed by extraneous information and helps them make sense of what they see and choose what it is necessary to attend to so that appropriate, or even fast, action can occur as necessary for survival and safety. For example, instead of seeing each color, shape, texture, and form of parts of a room as separate, people perceive the room as a whole coherent structure in which they can move and act, or a glimpse of part of an animal or another human who may threaten will be perceived and understood as a whole. For people to be able to do this, "the brain constantly needs stimulation to develop, grow, and maintain its organization."[39] This means vision, like other capacities, is dependent, to a large extent, upon use and upon learning through experience. Indeed, sensory systems are often especially tuned in to the activities and communication systems of the same species, as a matter of survival, health, and well-being.[74,75] It is "the limitations of [human] senses [that] set the boundaries of ... conscious existence."[76]

Complex language is held by many experts to be unique to people.[77-80] Deacon puts a case that "language abilities may be the 'special intelligence' of humans," that the "brain has been shaped by evolutionary processes that elaborated the capacities needed for language, and not just by a general demand for greater intelligence," and that "when all such species-specific biases are taken into account, 'general intelligence' will be found to be less variable among species than once thought."[44]

Whether this is the case or not, the traditional view holds that, like other characteristics, it evolved through a series of adaptive changes[81] and "may rest on neural mechanisms that are present in reduced form in other living species and that were elaborated quite early during hominid evolution."[82] Although early language was, undoubtedly, based on gesture, body signals, grunts, growls, cries, or even perhaps markers on trees for directional information in the hunt for food, speech is thought by some to have developed at the same time as people became tool users. This is because, among the more obvious social advantages, speech would have facilitated complex thinking abilities necessary for the manufacture of tools and the transfer of toolmaking skills as they occurred. Such claims are supported by the fact that the brain of *Homo habilis* was larger than other hominid species of the same period. Additionally, a habilis skull, estimated to be 2 million years old, was found to possess a Broca's speech area, although not as prominent a feature as that of modern humans.[83] Earlier ancestors' remains have not revealed this feature and it is thought that their language might have depended on the limbic system. In infancy, children rely on "the workings of the limbic system to call attention to their needs ... They find temper tantrums, whimpering, or crying a much easier way ... to express [emotions] than to explain."[30] This is despite being able to use simple speech to communicate effectively about less emotional issues. Some experts believe that human speech evolved in a similar fashion.[30]

Edelman argues that humans had the capacity to "produce and act on concepts" and to ascribe meaning prior to language acquisition.[40] Then, changes occurred in the base of the skull as a result of bipedalism at about the same time as the speech areas named after Broca and Wernicke emerged in the brain. Together these "provided a morphological basis for the evolution of ... the supralaryngeal tract"[40] probably not completed until the emergence of modern *Homo sapiens* when it appears that complex speech patterns were first manifest.[82] Part of that evolutionary development was dependent on neural mechanisms involved in speech motor control and in syntax,[82] as well as adaptation of the vocal cords, tongue, palate, and teeth that facilitated better control of air flow over the vocal cords, "which in turn allowed for the production of coarticulated sounds, the phonemes."[40]

Many evolutionary scientists favor a link between doing and the evolution of language. Some emphasize the role of gesture and suggest that, as tool usage occupied hands, they became less available for communication, leading to increased use of facial gesticulation and sound.[84,85] This theory is supported by observations that hand gestures still accompany speech, and when there are difficulties in verbal communication, such as people conversing in different languages, hand and facial gestures increase. Bruner hypothesizes that language is "virtually an outgrowth of the mastery of skilled action and perceptual discrimination," basing this claim on observations of ontogenetic development.[59] From this beginning, he asserts language is progressively freed from its original dependence on action and experience.[59] Others name hunter-gatherer activities or complex social relationships as the driving forces in the evolution of language, with de Laguna suggesting that the most likely explanation lies in the need for help associated with a sociotechnical way of life.[86] A combination of causes is probable.

Spoken language is the foundation of sociocultural occupations because complex technology and social structures would be impossible without language. While no archaic material record or proof of this remains, reminiscing, singing, and the telling of stories, myths, and legends is central in handing down to the next generation occupational "know how," culturally sanctioned behaviors, taboos, and spiritual beliefs and doings, all of which are intimately related to survival, health, and well-being. McMichael suggests that the advent of early language used to enhance social cohesion "must have accelerated the later stages of evolution of the brain."[47]

CHANGING PATTERNS OF OCCUPATION HAS A SIGNIFICANT IMPACT ON HEALTH

The differences in degree of capacity, which frees people from the instinctive and functional constraints of most animals, are central to the particular occupational nature of humans, giving them their apparently strong drive to engage in daily, new, or adventurous occupations and to undertake unwelcome or unenjoyable activities according to sociocultural expectations. Indeed, popular writers such as Desmond Morris and Lyall Watson contend that most people enjoy a challenge and are neophilic in that they "actively pursue the new and different."[73,87] Bruner suggests it is only human adults who "introduce" their offspring to challenging and sometimes frightening new experiences,[59] while among both birds and other mammals the presence of mothers is required to reduce fear of novel stimuli to enable their offspring to explore.[88] If Bruner's suggestion is true, perhaps such learning experiences are a necessary precursor for people to take risks to create environments in which they feel comfortable and to brave exploration of the unknown.

It appears that humans go beyond survival needs in their pursuit of occupation.[89] The range of capacities available to humans certainly allows them to pursue many options that may not appear to have an obvious relationship to survival. Deliberation about this point has determined that this extended ability is an integral part of healthy survival mechanisms. Engagement in wide-ranging occupations enables people to hone their skills, their capacities, and their flexibility so that they are competent to deal with novel situations as they occur, as well as providing exercise to maintain the "well working of the organism as a whole."[90] This freedom and flexibility has, along with genetic and biological variability, resulted in people from different regions of the world appearing "different," although reports of recent studies suggest this is not the case biologically according to DNA evidence.[91] A large part of the difference can be attributed to the occupations in which their forebears have engaged over time, the skills and levels of interest that have been passed on, and the value given to them by the culture in which they live. As anthropologist Richard Leakey observes:

The most pronounced differences are the way in which people do things: their dress, their architecture, their myths, their songs, their ideals and so on ... The earth is populated by one people living many different styles of life because of a unique cultural capacity. And the mind that expresses this unique capacity is the one that also universally seeks beyond itself for explanations of man himself and the nature of the world around him.[83]

Indeed, from birth, children, through their predominant occupation of play, seek beyond themselves for explanations of the world and their place within it. As they do this, they develop their innate capacities through learning from others, practicing skills, and using their minds and bodies to enable them to survive, to interact, and to choose future roles. In going beyond obvious survival needs in their pursuit of occupation, people evolve and adapt as occupational beings according to their environment, cultural values, innate capacities, and interests. The brain's capacity to adapt to social environs different from those in which humans evolved has led to "culture itself" creating "norms of human behavior that, in a certain sense, can step in as substitutes for innate behavior programs."[38]

The ability of humans to adapt socioculturally enables infants at a very early age to assimilate and retain information from the environment before a conscious appreciation of meaning or significance is possible. This early absorption of observed behaviors enables ontogenetic development to be in step with sociocultural expectations. In fact, the complexity of the human brain as the species' survival mechanism means that human babies are not able to reach a stage where they can take care of themselves before birth and they require social support for many years to assume "full humanness." As part of this process, attitudes, as well as occupational behaviors, are absorbed and adopted, and it is those formed before intellectual capacities are sufficiently advanced to allow for adequate understanding or refuting that have the strongest, albeit unconscious, hold on individuals. This mechanism was central to early humans' healthy survival because it allowed essential learning to occur from birth and stimulated the development of capacities. Their view of the strength of such learned attitudes and behaviors led founding behavioral psychologists Watson[92] and Skinner[93] to argue that only physiological reflexes are inherited, Watson going so far as to claim:

Give me a dozen healthy infants, well-formed, and my own specific world to bring them up in and I'll guarantee to take any one at random and train him to become any kind of specialist I might select—doctor, lawyer, artist, merchant-chief, and yes even beggar-man and thief regardless of his talents, penchants, abilities, vocations, and race of his ancestors.[92]

Sociologists might not accept Watson's exaggerated language, but a similar understanding by them has led to one of sociology's fundamental postulates: human actions are limited or determined by past and present environments, and humans are the products and the victims of their society.[94] Sociologists, in contrast to sociobiologists, also reason that "human beings are made, not born" because "even if someone argues that human endowments such as soul and rationality are innate, these gifts are not sufficient to ensure that an infant will become a truly functional human being, capable of ethical and cultural responsibility," and that "the infant has to be learned ... in short, we enact, rehearse, work, and play our way into the human condition."[95] However, this implies that people have the genetic and biological capacity to learn, which is also part of being human. This occupational theory of human nature holds that, because of their particular mix of biological characteristics and capacities, humans are receptive to the process of enculturation and socialization to the extent that they can indeed be considered products of their particular culture.

It is also held in this theory that societies are the products of humans acting on their environment. As people engage in occupation, the physical and social environments are altered. Often, the more sophisticated the occupation, the greater the change to the environment, which in turn causes further change to and development of people. Marx suggests that "by thus acting on the external world and changing it, [man] at the same time changes his own nature,"[96] and Braverman, in the same vein, proposes that people are the special product of purposeful action.[97] He argues that occupation that "transcends mere instinctual activity is the force which created humankind and the force by which humankind created the world as we know it."[97] Neff agrees that the most revolutionary force in human history is technological change associated with the way people "wrest their living from nature."[98] He argues that social institutions are merely mirrors of technological levels. This idea, apparently well accepted in archaeological circles, as well as Marxist sociology, supports the theory that humans are occupational beings, that occupation has the potential to change the world or the species, and that it provides the mechanism to enable people to survive and to adapt to biological, sociological, and environmental demands. This view points to the need to consider humans' occupational nature from an ecological as well as a sociological or health perspective.

The many models of cultural evolution based on occupational technology are sometimes said not to address sufficiently the influences of other variables, such as local environments, ecology and climate, war and conquest, spiritual beliefs and social struggles, or the complexities of the interactions between them.[98] From my standpoint, there is some truth in the criticisms because such views have been limited to economic preoccupation with "work" or "labor" perspectives. That neglects a holistic view of occupation that, of necessity, integrates many factors. Other criticisms have been leveled at the notion of cultural evolution itself, particularly as postulated by Victorian anthropologists such as Tylor[99] and Morgan,[100] in that it seems to imply progress in advanced technological societies are somehow "better" or "higher up the evolutionary ladder" than older cultures with less technical economies.[98] The notion of cultural superiority is called into question by the argument that cultures can vary independently of race and that no one culture is superior to another.[101] Similarly, the occupational nature of humans is not seen to be more evolved in technologically advanced societies in contrast to hunter-gatherer or agrarian societies but, rather, expressed differently according to each culture's history and technological development.

Diagnosis and prescription are the final 2 points of Stevenson's notion of theories of human nature to be considered: any such theory has to include a diagnosis of "what is wrong with humans" and a prescription of how to "right the wrongs" from its particular perspective.

As to diagnosis, although the occupational behavior of early humans was in tune with self-sustaining "natural" health and ecological balance, the current direction of occupational behavior is out of step with humans' natural heritage and behaviors and the ecology. This echoes a sentiment expressed by Alexis Carrel, in 1935, that modern civilization "does not suit us," being "born from the whims of scientific discoveries, from the appetites of men, their illusions, their theories, and their desires" but "without any knowledge of our real nature."[102] He argued for a science of human individuals that views them as "an indivisible whole of extreme complexity."[102] It could be suggested that, in the present day, knowledge of human nature remains rudimentary and that Carrel's science is still necessary despite an avalanche of research in various disciplines in recent decades. The knowledge is certainly fragmentary, and, without a real appreciation of the human need to engage in occupation, it is incomplete.

As for a prescription of how to "right the wrongs," addressing the lack of awareness of people's occupational natures has the potential to influence social, political, economic, and health policies so that they are more in tune with them and with self-sustaining "natural" health and ecological balance. More concrete solutions do not seem advisable because prescriptive theories of human nature, even if they focus on occupational factors such as "Marxist Communism," do not allow sufficient flexibility to allow solutions to be responsive to contextual and evolutionary change.

Gaining an increased understanding of an occupational perspective of human nature is worthy of further extensive inquiry because it appears appropriate to many of the problems the world faces today and in the future: namely, how to maintain health and ensure human survival in an economic and self-sustaining way, that meets the biological, sociocultural, and occupational needs of people, as well as redressing ecological degradation. Because of the nature of the approach taken, the exploration that follows can only touch on these wide-ranging issues, although it is acknowledged that each requires study in its own right.

SUMMARY

Archaeologists and anthropologists recognize strong links between what humans do, biological evolution, and survival of the species. Roland Fletcher goes as far as to categorize particular forms of doing to define what being human means.[103] Along with bipedalism and toolmaking, he lists "the capacity to control fire, to interact socially with their dead, and to represent the universe in art" as marks of humanness in evolutionary terms.[103] Forms of occupation provide the framework for daily life for all people unless prevented by disorder, external constraint, or particular forms of socialization or political expectation. It is central to life and living, health, and development and has been so throughout the evolution of the species. Human evolution through what people do has helped to shape human biology, just as human biology has shaped their doing. This reciprocal and critical interaction has long-term health, illness, and survival consequences.

Three-Way Link: Occupation, Health, and Survival

Unless asked to consider such factors, or some process or part of the mechanism goes amiss, people are not usually conscious of survival and health-maintaining functions of what they do as part of their lives. These functions, rather like the autonomic nervous system, are built into the organism to just go on working. Because of this, people are able to use their capacities for their own purposes, to explain the purpose of life in abstract rather than biological ways, and to attribute meaning to activity based on sociocultural influences. It follows that, in present circumstances, many individuals are not able to distinguish their biological needs, which ultimately impact on their health, from wants or preferences.[104] This is held to be partly because the complexity of sociocultural evolution makes differentiation difficult, so that "even phylogenetically evolved programs of ... behavior are adjusted to the presence of a culture," which alters the significance of biological needs.[38]

At the center of this occupational theory of human nature is the proposal that the brain of the human species has "healthy survival" as its primary role. It is a brain that continually activates people's particular mix of characteristics and capacities through engagement in occupation. It is an occupational brain and a healing brain. Our occupational nature is the result of evolution/phylogeny, genetics, ontogeny, ecological and

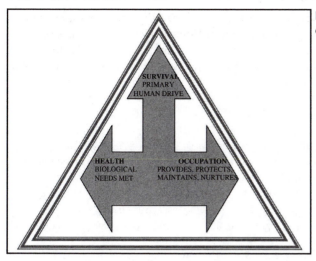

Figure 2-8. Three-way link between occupation, health, and survival.

sociocultural environments, and opportunity, all of which are centered or integrated in the brain. Engagement in occupation forms a 3-way link with health and survival, which is illustrated in Figure 2-8.

Survival is recognized as the primary drive of humans, as of all other animals. Survival of individuals is the outcome of the use of capacities through occupations that provide for essential needs of the organism, including supportive social, ecological, and material environments. The WHO terms these the *prerequisites of health*, and they will provide the focus of the next chapter. The extent and quality of survival for individuals, communities, and populations depends on their health and physical, mental, and social well-being; health is the outcome of each organism having all essential sustenance and safety needs met and of having physical, mental, and social capacities maintained, developed, exercised, and in balance. This is achieved through what people do. Engagement in occupation depends, in turn, on a level of health and its specific components, which are able to provide the energy, drive, and functional attributes necessary for engagement.

Additionally, the survival of healthy species depends on a human's capacity to live in harmony within an environment that can continue to provide basic requirements, ensure the continued acquisition of these requirements, and provide safety and education for the next generation.

The integrative functions of the central nervous system, which process external and internal information, activated by engagement in occupation, are focal to survival, the maintenance of homeostasis, and facilitating health and well-being. The next 4 chapters will consider this theory according to the ideas that emerged in the first chapter: biological needs, natural health, ancient and modern rules for health, occupational evolution in terms of the prerequisites of health and well-being as defined by the WHO, and occupation-related characteristics and capacities, health and well-being, and the prevention of illness, associated with doing, being, and becoming.

References

1. Yerxa EJ, Clark F, Frank G, et al. An introduction to occupational science. A foundation for occupational therapy in the 21st century. *Occupational Therapy in Health Care.* 1989;6(4):1-17.
2. Duldt BW, Giffin K. *Theoretical Perspectives for Nursing.* Boston, Mass: Little, Brown and Co; 1985:47.

3. Law M, Baum CM, Baptiste S, eds. *Occupation-Based Practice: Fostering Performance and Participation.* Thorofare, NJ: SLACK Incorporated; 2002.

4. Letts L, Rigby P, Stewart D, eds. *Using Environments to Enable Occupational Performance.* Thorofare, NJ: SLACK Incorporated; 2003.

5. Christiansen CH, Townsend EA, eds. *Introduction to Occupation: The Art and Science of Living.* Upper Saddle River, NJ: Prentice Hall; 2004.

6. Molineux M, ed. *Occupation for Occupational Therapists.* Oxford, UK: Blackwell Publishing; 2004.

7. Whiteford G, Wright-St. Clair V, eds. *Occupation and Practice in Context.* Sydney, Australia: Elsevier/Churchill Livingstone; 2005.

8. World Health Organization. *Jakarta Declaration on Leading Health Promotion into the 21st Century.* 4th International Conference on Health Promotion, Jakarta, Indonesia, 21-25th July, 1997.

9. World Health Organization's Ageing and Life Course Programme. *Active Ageing: A Policy Framework.* Madrid, Spain: Second United Nations World Assembly on Ageing; 2002:54.

10. World Health Organization. *Mental Health: Strengthening Mental Health Promotion.* Fact sheet N°220. Revised November 2001; Accessed 2005.

11. World Health Organization. *Global Strategy on Diet, Physical Activity and Health. Chronic Disease Information Sheets.* World Health Organization Documents and Publications: Accessed December 2005.

12. Lewin K. *Principles of Topological Psychology.* New York: McGraw Hill; 1947.

13. Gandevia B. *Occupation and Disease in Australia Since 1788.* Sydney, Australia: Australasian Medical Publishing Company Ltd; 1971:158.

14. Stevenson L. *Seven Theories of Human Nature.* 2nd ed. Oxford, UK: Oxford University Press; 1987:9,137.

15. Markovic M. Human nature. In: Bottomore T, ed. *A Dictionary of Marxist Thought.* 2nd ed. Oxford, UK: Blackwell Publishers; 1991:209.

16. Althusser L. *For Marx.* London: Allen Lane; 1969.

17. Hawking SW. *A Brief History of Time.* Toronto: Bantam Books; 1988:10.

18. Van den Berghe PL. Sociobiology. In: Kuper A, Kuper J, eds. *The Social Science Encyclopedia.* Rev ed. London: Routledge; 1989:797.

19. Csikszentmihalyi M, Csikszentmihalyi IS. *Optimal Experience: Psychological Studies of Flow in Consciousness.* New York: Cambridge University Press; 1988.

20. Csikszentmihalyi M, Massimini F. On the psychological selection of bicultural information. *New Ideas in Psychology.* 1985;3(2):115-138.

21. Snell GD. *Search for a Rational Ethic.* New York: Springer-Verlag; 1988:140.

22. Resources for Ecology, Evolutionary Biology, Systematics and Conservation Biology. Accessed January 2005.

23. Stavrianos LS. *The World to 1500: A Global History.* 4th ed. Upper Saddle River, NJ: Prentice Hall; 1988:4.

24. Hazen RM. *Genesis: The Scientific Quest for Life's Origins.* Washington, DC: Joseph Henry Press; 2005:243.

25. Darwin C. *Origin of the Species by Means of Natural Selection.* Cambridge, Mass: Harvard University Press; 1964.

26. Darwin C. *The Descent of Man and Selection in Relation to Sex.* New York: Appleton; 1930.

27. Dawkins R. The replicators. In: Dixon B, ed. *From Creation to Chaos: Classic Writings in Science.* Oxford, UK: Basil Blackwood Ltd; 1989:39-44.

28. Jones S. The nature of evolution. In: Jones S, Martin R, Pilbeam D, eds. *The Cambridge Encyclopedia of Human Evolution.* New York: Cambridge University Press; 1992:9.

29. Spencer H. *Principles of Biology.* Vol 1. New York: Appleton; 1864:444.

30. Campbell BG. *Humankind Emerging.* 5th ed. New York: Harper Collins Publishers; 1988:60-69,90-91,366.

31. Suzuki D. *The Sacred Balance.* Vancouver/Toronto: Greystone Books; 2002.

32. Stern C, Sherwood ER, eds. *The Origin of Genetics.* San Francisco, Calif: WH Freeman; 1966.

33. Medawar P. Darwinism. In: Bullock A, Stalleybrass O, Trombly S, eds. *The Fontana Dictionary of Modern Thought.* 2nd ed. London: Fontana Press; 1988.

34. McHenry HM. Evolution. In: Kuper A, Kuper J, eds. *The Social Science Encyclopedia.* Rev ed. London: Routledge; 1989:280.

35. Dyson F. The argument from design. Disturbing the universe 1979. In: Dixon B, ed. *From Creation to Chaos: Classic Writings in Science.* Oxford, UK: Basil Blackwood Ltd; 1989:49.

36. Leakey RE. Introduction. In: Darwin C, ed. *The Illustrated Origin of the Species.* Abridged. London: The Rainbird Publishing Co; 1979:26.

37. Bronowski J. *The Ascent of Man.* London: British Broadcasting Corp; 1973:31.

38. Lorenz K. *The Waning of Humaneness.* Boston, Mass: Little, Brown and Co; 1987:5,21,57-58,93,124.

39. Ornstein R, Sobel D. *The Healing Brain: A Radical New Approach to Health Care.* London: MacMillan; 1988:11,12,36,105,106,218.

40. Edelman G. *Bright Air, Brilliant Fire: On the Matter of the Mind.* London: Penguin Books; 1992:7,16-19,40,48,51,126.
41. Campbell J. *Winston Churchill's Afternoon Nap.* London: Palladin Grafton Books; 1986:54.
42. James W. *The Principles of Psychology.* Vol 1. New York: Dover Publications; 1890:239.
43. Kolb B, Whishaw IQ. *Fundamentals of Human Neuropsychology.* 3rd ed. San Francisco, Calif: WH Freeman; 1990:4,106,123.
44. Deacon TW. The human brain. In: Jones S, Martin R, Pilbeam D, eds. *The Cambridge Encyclopedia of Human Evolution.* New York: Cambridge University Press; 1992:115,119,121,123.
45. Jerison HJ. *Evolution of the Brain and Intelligence.* New York: Academic Press; 1973.
46. Rose S. *The Conscious Brain.* Rev ed. London: Penguin Books; 1976.
47. McMichael T. *Human Frontiers, Environments and Disease: Past Patterns, Uncertain Futures.* Cambridge, UK: Cambridge University Press; 2001;20,49.
48. Sperry R. *Some Effects of Disconnecting the Cerebral Hemispheres. Les Prix Nobel.* Stockholm, Sweden: Almqvist & Wikesell; 1981:209-219.
49. Penfield W, Boldrey E. Somatic motor and sensory representation in the cerebral cortex as studied by electrical stimulation. *Brain.* 1958;60:389-443.
50. Brodmann K. *Vergleichended lokalisations lehre der Grosshirnrinde in prinzipien dargestellt auf grund des zellenbaues.* Liepzig: JA Barth; 1909.
51. Lassen NA, Ingvar DH, Skinhoj E. Brain function and blood flow. *Scientific American.* 1978;239:62-71.
52. Roland PE. Applications of brain blood flow imaging in behavioral neurophysiology: cortical field activation hypothesis. In: Sokoloff L, ed. *Brain Imaging and Brain Function.* New York: Raven Press; 1985:87-104.
53. Kety SS. Disorders of the human brain. *Scientific American.* 1979;241:202-214.
54. Mazziotta JC, Phelps ME. Human neuropsychological imaging studies of local brain metabolism: strategies and results. In: Sokoloff L, ed. *Brain Imaging and Brain Function.* New York: Raven Press; 1985.
55. Restak R. *The Brain.* New York: Bantam Books; 1984.
56. Jelinek J. *Primitive Hunters.* London: Hamlyn; 1989.
57. Leakey R, Lewin R. *People of the Lake: Man: His Origins, Nature, and Future.* New York: Penguin Books; 1978:38-39.
58. Bell SC. *The Hand: Its Mechanism and Vital Endowments as Evincing Design.* Brentwood: The Pilgrims Press; 1979:108.
59. Bruner J. Nature and uses of immaturity. *Am Psychol.* 1972;August:687-708.
60. Birch HG. The relation of previous experience to insightful problem solving. *Journal of Comparative and Physiological Psychology.* 1945;38:367-383.
61. Schiller PH. Innate constituents of complex responses in primates. *Psychological View.* 1952;49:177-191.
62. Goodall J. *The Chimpanzees of Gombe.* Cambridge, Mass: Harvard/Belknap; 1986.
63. Brewer SM, McGrew WC. Chimpanzee use of a tool-set to get honey. *Folia Primatologica.* 1990;54:100-104.
64. Hill GB, ed. *Boswell's Life of Johnson.* Oxford: Clarendon Press; 1887:3,245.
65. Almquist EE. Evolution of the distal radioulnar joint. *Clinical Orthopedics.* 1992;Feb(275):5-13.
66. Tinkaus E. Evolution of human manipulation. In: Jones S, Martin R, Pilbeam D, eds. *The Cambridge Encyclopedia of Human Evolution.* New York: Cambridge University Press; 1992:349.
67. Van Den Hoven B. *Work in Ancient and Medieval Thought: Ancient Philosophers, Medieval Monks and Theologians and their Concept of Work, Occupations and Technology.* Amsterdam: J.C. Gieben; 1996:55.
68. Fleagle JG. Primate locomotion and posture. In: Jones S, Martin R, Pilbeam D, eds. *The Cambridge Encyclopedia of Human Evolution.* New York: Cambridge University Press; 1992:79.
69. Lewin R. *In the Age of Mankind: A Smithsonian Book of Human Evolution.* Washington, DC: Smithsonian Books; 1988:174,179-180.
70. Watanabe H. Running, creeping and climbing: a new ecological and evolutionary perspective on human locomotion. *Mankind.* 1971;8(1):1-13.
71. Alexander RMcN. Walking and running. *American Scientist.* 1984;72:348-354.
72. Alexander RMcN. Characteristics and advantages of human bipedalism. In: Rayner JMV, Wootton R, eds. *Biomechanics in Evolution.* New York: Cambridge University Press; 1991.
73. Watson L. *Neophilia: The Tradition of the New.* Great Britain: Hodder and Stoughton Ltd; 1989:67.
74. Hopkins CD. Sensory mechanisms in animal communication. In: Dewsbury DA, Slater PJB, eds. *Animal Behavior, Vol. 2: Communication.* New York: Freeman; 1983.
75. Leger DW. *Biological Foundations for Behavior: An Integrative Approach.* New York: Harper Collins Publishers; 1992:374.
76. Coren S, Porac C, Ward LM. *Sensation and Perception.* 2nd ed. Orlando, Fla: Academic Press; 1984.
77. Chomsky N. *Language and Mind.* New York: Harcourt Brace Jovanovich; 1972.
78. Lenneberg EH. *Biological Foundations of Language.* New York: Wiley; 1967.

79. John-Steiner V, Panofsky CP. Human specificity in language: socio-genetic processes in verbal communication. In: Greenberg G, ed. *Cognition, Language and Consciousness: Integrative Levels*. Hillsdale, NJ: Erlbaum; 1987.

80. Chomsky N. *The Origin of Language: Its Nature Origin and Use*. New York: Praeger; 1986.

81. Lieberman P. *The Biology and Evolution of Language*. Cambridge, Mass: Harvard University Press; 1984.

82. Lieberman P. Human speech and language. In: Jones S, Martin R, Pilbeam D, eds. *The Cambridge Encyclopedia of Human Evolution*. New York: Cambridge University Press; 1992:136,137.

83. Leakey R. *The Making of Mankind*. London: Michael Joseph Ltd; 1981:101-103,139,248.

84. Hewes GW. Language origin theories. In: Rumbaugh DM, ed. *Language Learning by a Chimpanzee*. New York: Academic Press; 1977.

85. Kimura D. Neuromotor mechanisms in the evolution of human communications. In: Steklis HD, Raleigh MJ, eds. *Neurobiology of Social Communication in Primates: An Evolutionary Perspective*. New York: Academic Press; 1979.

86. de Laguna GA. *Speech: Its Function and Development*. Bloomington, Ind: Indiana University Press; 1963.

87. Morris D. *The Human Zoo*. London: Jonathan Cape; 1969.

88. King DL. A review and interpretation of some aspects of the infant-mother relationship in mammals and birds. *Psychol Bull*. 1966;65:143-155.

89. Morris D. *The Human Animal*. BBC TV Production, England, 1994.

90. Kass LR. Regarding the end of medicine and the pursuit of health. In: Caplan AL, Englehardt HT, McCartney JJ, eds. *Concepts of Health and Disease: Interdisciplinary Perspectives*. Reading, Mass: Addison-Wesley Publishing Co; 1981.

91. Australian Broadcasting Corporation. News Bulletin. January 2006.

92. Watson JB. *Behaviourism*. New York: WW Norton; 1970:104.

93. Skinner BF. *Science and Human Behaviour*. New York: Macmillan; 1953.

94. Shils E. Sociology. In: Kuper A, Kuper J, eds. *The Social Science Encyclopedia*. Rev ed. London: Routledge; 1989:799-810.

95. Driver T. *The Magic of Ritual*. San Francisco, Calif: Harper Collins Publishers; 1991:16.

96. Marx K. *Capital*. Vol 1. Hamburg, Germany: Otto Meissner; 1867:179-180.

97. Braverman H. *Labor and Monopoly Capital: The Degradation of Work in the Twentieth Century*. New York: Monthly Review Press; 1974.

98. Neff WS. *Work and Human Behavior*. 3rd ed. New York: Aldine Publishing Co; 1985:20.

99. Tylor EB. *Anthropology: An Introduction to the Study of Man and Civilization*. Ann Arbor, Mich: University of Michigan Press; 1960.

100. Morgan LH. *Ancient Society*. Cambridge, Mass: Belknap; 1964.

101. Hatch E. Culture. In: Kuper A, Kuper J, eds. *The Social Science Encyclopedia*. Rev ed. London: Routledge; 1989:179.

102. Carrel A. *Man the Unknown*. London: Burns and Oates; 1935:14.

103. Fletcher R. The evolution of human behaviour. In: Buranhult G, ed. *The First Humans: Human Origins and History to 10,000 BC*. St. Lucia, Australia: University of Queensland Press; 1993:17.

104. Fitzgerald R, ed. *Human Needs and Politics*. Sydney, Australia: Permagon; 1977.

Suggested Reading

Christiansen CH, Townsend EA, eds. *Introduction to Occupation: The Art and Science of Living*. Upper Saddle River, NJ: Prentice Hall; 2004.

Darwin C. *Origin of the Species by Means of Natural Selection*. Cambridge, Mass: Harvard University Press; 1964.

Hawking SW. *A Brief History of Time*. Toronto: Bantam Books; 1988.

Lorenz K. *The Waning of Humaneness*. Boston, Mass: Little, Brown and Co; 1987.

Snell GD. *Search for a Rational Ethic*. New York: Springer-Verlag; 1988.

Stevenson L. *Seven Theories of Human Nature*. 2nd ed. Oxford, UK: Oxford University Press; 1987.

Watson L. *Neophilia: The Tradition of the New*. Great Britain: Hodder and Stoughton Ltd; 1989.

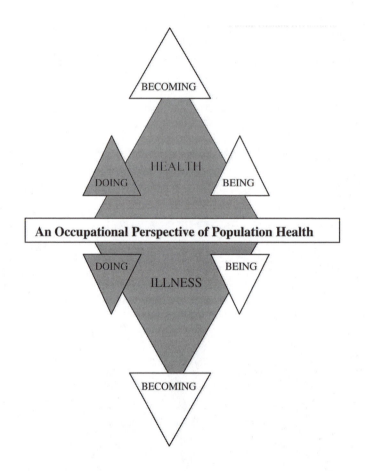

OCCUPATION: DOING, HEALTH, AND ILLNESS

Theme 3:

The prerequisites for health: "peace, shelter, education, food, income, a stable eco-system, sustainable resources, social justice and equity."
WHO, *Ottawa Charter for Health Promotion*, 1986

The chapter addresses:
* "Doing" as a determinant of population health
  * The doing-rest continuum
  * Natural health, biological needs, and the doings of early humans
    * Food and income
    * Shelter
    * Education
    * Peace
    * A stable ecosystem and sustainable resources
    * Social justice and equity
* Rules for health
  * An ancient "doing" approach
  * Modern: WHO directives for doing well physically, mentally, and socially
* Determinants of doing as a factor in well-being or illness

This chapter is the first of 3 in which occupation's basic relationship to health is examined. Despite the fact that occupation needs to be considered holistically, these chapters divide it according to the concepts of doing, being, and becoming. The division is purely arbitrary for clarity of exploration. It builds on the theory outlined in Chapter 2 and sets the scene for considering occupation that embraces a combination of the 3 concepts as an agent of public health.

Drawing on history to inform the present, this chapter challenges both occupational therapists and public health practitioners to consider the nature and place of doing within health care at present. The role of people's doings in etiology is most often overlooked, and the potential contribution of how people's doings may augment other treatments is hardly ever considered in present day, economically time-driven, medically based health care systems. Yet, in many cases, in hospitals and other medical care facilities, "range of doing" could be more important than "range of movement." In others, range of movement may be imperative to doing well in the world. For those with ongoing mental health problems living in hostels, the nature and extent of what residents do could be imperative in the control of problem behaviors. Challenging the timelines set by service providers to allow imperative life changes to be set in motion may be an important and necessary intervention to prevent further illness or to promote well-being. Those and many other health initiatives concerned with doing would be valuable. It is probable, however, that most opportunities to change unhealthy doing lie outside the world of medical care. This implies that new areas of practice need to be developed and opportunities or resources to provide new services required.

Following the structure established in the first chapter, the content of this one provides substance toward major changes in direction, intervention, and research. After introducing the concept of doing as an aspect of health, it considers how those who lived before the advantages of modern technology and medicine met the WHO prerequisites for health naturally. Then, by reflecting on the ancient rules of the non-naturals, attention is focused on how trying to understand natural mechanisms and biological needs has been instrumental in the provision of health regimes throughout millennia. While it may be tempting to overlook such "out of date material," to do so is to ignore more than 1000 years of empirical research and the foundations on which everything else is based. The ancient rules provide the context to consider the "doing" orientation within the modern rules for both well-being and the reduction of illness provided in the WHO directives. Provision of the modern rules may excite speculation about who carries them out. In turn, that could lead to deliberations about how human doings are addressed within public health research and intervention and how they could be extended within occupational therapy. But to start such exploration, it is important to define "doing" as a determinant of population health.

Doing as a Determinant of Population Health

Doing is so important in people's lives that it is impossible to envisage them without it. This is highlighted within Western cultures by the way people frequently identify themselves and each other by what they do. For example, in some parts of the world, family names reflect long past occupations of their members, some obvious like Smith and Barber and others less obvious such as Heyward. In Old English, this name describes a person who acts as a steward of an enclosure like a tithe barn, agricultural land, or a forest. Common forms of introduction, too, name the things that people do, such as, "May I introduce Bruce? He was a farmer, became a boat builder, and a charter boat skipper after retirement, and now flies gliders for a hobby." A stock question when talking with children is to ask, "What have you been doing?" or "What are you planning to do when you grow up?" It is as if what people do, in some way, defines them. Taking a long-term perspective of doing within people's lives suggests that there is some truth in that supposition.

It becomes clear that people have an innate need to do because survival, as well as health, depends on it. To find and prepare food to fuel life, people have to do; they have to do other things to be safe in their environment, to keep their temperature at a comfortable level, and to keep their bodies protected from the elements. They have to think about and plan what they will do and most have to adapt and change their doing according to environmental factors or the consequences of what they do. Doing with others is important to develop communities that can work together in supportive ways for the common good and that form local and national identity and culture. Archaeological anthropologists suggest "humans are different, not so much for what we do ... but rather the fact that we can do more or less what we want. That is what having a highly developed culture really means."[1]

In the present day, though, doing is usually separated according to culturally accepted divisions such as education, work, leisure, parenting, and rest even within a profession like occupational therapy that proclaims its holistic nature. How communities and individuals regard such segments of doing is often not only dependent on cultural viewpoints but also on political imperatives. Indeed, doing by governments, and their attitudes toward different aspects, drives the doing of individual lives as well as interacting with the doings of distant communities on the global stage. Yet, the need to do has, on the whole, been overlooked in scientific inquiry, in medicine, and in most theories of human nature because it appears so mundane, although it forms the essence of time-use studies that apply census material. Instead, it provides the unacknowledged taken-for-granted background because doing cannot be ignored; it is the foundation of living.

Such oversight has not been the case in scholarly as opposed to medical or scientific inquiry, perhaps because of classical Greek interest in what was called *praxis*. Defined as "doing" or "of action," praxis was the chosen word for almost any kind of activity likely to be performed by a citizen, as opposed to a slave, with emphasis on "all kinds of business and political activity."[2] In the 19th century, Marx described praxis as "the free, universal, creative, and self-creative activity" through which people create, shape, and change themselves and the human world,[3] although he was inconsistent about whether praxis included labor or not.[4] When it was included, his use of the word was similar to how occupation is used in this text. Praxis still appears in some modern dictionaries, retaining the earlier meaning of doing, acting, action, and "accepted practice or custom"[5] as "distinguished from theory."[6] Common usage, however, is rare in the present day. It is applied as a descriptor in some types of action-research, such as critical praxis research or critical feminist praxis.[7,8] It is also used as part of the nomenclature of a discipline, *praxiology* being the name given to a science of efficient action. At the opposite end of that skill continuum is apraxia or dyspraxia, meaning no or difficult action.[9] Resulting from congenital or acquired disorders of the brain, these medical descriptors provide something of an acknowledgment that doing is central to life and health.

However, economics is so closely intertwined with doing that it is considered from that perspective more often than it is thought of in health terms. Within public health in postindustrial societies, for example, concentration on doing has been aimed mainly at eradicating risks in paid employment—the aspect of doing that is closely tied with economic wealth of businesses and nations. A new focus in the present day recognizes that an increase of the doing of physical activity is urgently required to reduce childhood obesity, which is reaching pandemic proportions in postindustrial societies.[10] Such initiatives are vitally important, but both fail to appreciate or act upon occupation in a holistic way that is a necessary way forward. For example, a significant study with a sample of 2761 older Americans undertaken at Harvard over a period of 13 years found that doing social and productive occupations "that involve little or no enhancement of fitness" carried as much weight in terms of lowering the risk of all causes of death as doing exercise.[11]

In the present day, despite the popularity of the idiom "doing well," too few of the world's population are doing well. There is, for example, imbalance in the experience of doing between people of developed and developing countries, between the haves and the have-nots from various perspectives, between the rich and the poor, between the employed and the unemployed, between the old and the young, between the literate and the illiterate, between genders, and between those institutionalized or incarcerated and

Table 3-1

Comparison of Explanation of Terms With the International Classification of Functioning, Disability, and Health

	ICF Explanations	Text Explanations	
Activity	A person's capacity to execute occupations (with or without assistive devices or assistance); what a person could do in an environment with no barriers to performance	Synonymous with or an aspect of occupation	**Occupation** Participation in any activity of a doing, being, and becoming nature to meet health, personal, societal, and survival needs and wants
Participation	A person's actual performance of occupations in his or her current environment, including problems the person experiences due to environmental barriers	Involvement in any of life's occupations that may be self- as well as family- or sociopolitically initiated	
Environmental factors	Physical, social, and attitudinal environment within which people live their lives, which can act as barriers to or facilitators of participation	The same: all aspects of the external world including the natural and human-made physical world; other people in different relationships and roles; attitudes and values; social systems and services; and policies, rules, and laws	
Personal factors	Aspects of the person not related to his or her health condition, including gender, race, age, lifestyle, habits, coping style, education, social background, previous experiences, psychological assets, behavior patterns, etc	The same	

those who are free to pursue their doings unimpeded. Opportunities or experience of doing may, of itself, lead to lack of well-being for large numbers of people just as the right kind of doing can be considered a prerequisite of health.

The WHO recognizes the health impact of not doing well and has addressed the issue in many of its strategy documents that will be discussed later. It has also defined, to some extent, the notion of occupation as a combination of "activity" and "participation." In the *International Classification of Functioning, Disability, and Health* (ICF), for example, an indication is provided of how the WHO has explained some aspects of the doing.[12] These are provided in Table 3-1 and compared with how they are used here.

Apart from social determinants of occupation that emanate from environmental factors, many personal factors influence doing. A number of these relating to internal mechanisms, physical attributes, and biological needs have already been noted as influential. These are known as "regulatory motivators" because they are physiological in nature. They prompt "doing" to meet some of the prerequisites of health such as hunger and shelter. Other regulatory motivators might be fatigue, pain, or level of arousal.[13] Maslow's hierarchical theory of needs has already suggested other reasons why people feel driven to engage in doing to meet those and the other WHO prerequisites—peace, education, income, stable ecosystem, sustainable resources, social justice, and equity.[14] He described those as "Deficiency or D Needs." He described other forms of doing higher up on his hierarchy as "Being or B Needs," the subjects of later chapters.

A source of evidence about what people do comes from national statistics, at least in the developed world. It is relevant for those planning to work in this area to consider these as a source of vital information because they not only relate to those populations, but also to what might occur to other populations in less developed cultures in the not too distant future. More and more cease to live traditional lifestyles and turn to industry for the good or the bad. Over a lifetime, paid employment accounts for a smaller proportion of time than perhaps would be expected given the emphasis on it within public health and the way Western countries have, until fairly recently, looked to market economy to provide insight into people's needs. In recent years, and probably as a partial result of the women's movement, more appreciation is given to other forms of work such as parenting, volunteering, caregiving, and homemaking. Pentland and Harvey comment on those facts and also note "that activities and occupations vary much more among subpopulations in a given country than they do in total across countries."[15] On average, in developed countries, people spend more time sleeping than doing anything else.

THE DOING-REST CONTINUUM

The continuum of doing and resting is an important one, both in terms of the quality and quantity of occupation and of health and well-being. It was recognized as a continuum in the ancient rules of health, yet sleep is not included in some modern theories about occupation because its apparent lack of active qualities appears to gainsay the essence of doing.[16] That is a simplistic perception. Preparing for sleep is an important part of daily activities, almost reaching ritualistic proportions for some people. It encompasses preparations of body, mind, and environment; for example, in undressing, in relaxing, in ensuring appropriate ventilation, or putting out the lights.[16] Sleep, itself, is a requirement of all mammals; is integral to doing effectively, to self-care, to physical, mental, and social health; and is a complex active process. Emerging from sleep usually has a ritualistic quality that reverses relaxation and prepares mind and body for the daily doings ahead. If sleep has been disturbed, the day ahead can be also be disturbed or difficult.[17]

All sleep stages have a homeostatic function even though the system does not operate on feedback principles but on intrinsic timing mechanisms.[18] These mechanisms differ slightly for each individual and change throughout the lifespan. In evolutionary terms, the oldest form of sleep known as nonrapid eye movement sleep, or slow wave sleep (SWS), shows different patterns of EEGs for several different stages. SWS is responsible for replenishing the body and maintaining physiological and metabolic fitness. SWS increases after a day of strenuous physical occupation, and it is only during SWS that growth hormone, essential for restoring damaged tissue, is released.[19] Following sleep deprivation, SWS takes priority in "catching up." For example, studies such as those conducted by Shapiro and others on ultramarathon runners demonstrated an increase in

SWS, as well as total sleeping time, over 4 nights following the run.[20] This effect appears most developed among people who are physically fit,[21] suggesting a close relationship between sleep patterns and regular occupations. Additional "servicing" is required for the maintenance of structures specializing in mental and social functions. This is provided by rapid eye movement (REM) sleep when circuits are tested and neurotransmitters are replenished by being rested selectively.[18] During this stage, the brain is very active and "actually consumes more oxygen than it does during intense physical or mental activity when one is awake."[22] Speculations about other functions of REM sleep include the integration of knowledge acquired during the day, consolidation of information, assistance in dealing with emotionally charged material, and the laying down of long-term memory.[18,23,24] Patients in forensic care, for example, some of whom committed crimes while mentally ill, have found that resting and sleeping allowed them to dream of other life possibilities and to find new meaning.[25,26] (Some claim that SWS also assists memory formation and recall.[27]) Fox speculates from animal experiments that "current information, blocked from the hippocampus and the limbic circuit during waking, is allowed in there during sleep to be 'matched' against those wired-in survival behaviors."[28] If the information is deemed relevant, it is processed "for at least 3 years in some form or other" during dreams before being "stamped in" to long-term memory and eventually stored in the neocortex.[28] This process enables the neocortex to assess experience toward future goal-directed action. REM sleep may serve a similar purpose in humans, but Fox suggests that dreaming has been freed, to some extent, from phylogenetic and species-specific experience, allowing the "matching" to relate to prenatal and childhood experience.[28]

Duration of sleep is a need that differs from person to person. "Gating mechanisms" facilitate passage between sleep and awake states.[29] REM sleep, which usually occurs 4 to 5 times a night, is seen as the easiest exit point from sleep and possibly evolved in part as a "sentinel device, a monitor in case of danger."[18] At rhythmical times during wakefulness, there are "sleepability gates" when it is easier to sleep. The most obvious of these is the biological slump occurring in the afternoon, which is taken as siesta time in many traditional cultures. Biphasic activity peaks are part of our biological heritage, are evident in behaviors of other primates, and are probably an adaptation resulting from the need to reduce occupation during the hottest part of the day. Ultradian rhythms of arousal and nonarousal concerned with placement of sleep are easily overruled for doing obligatory or freely chosen occupations.[30] Differences in brainwaves throughout sleep and awake states appear to relate to when the organism is best fitted for different types of occupation or rest. These are flexible and can be overridden, as happens in 8-hour working days or 24-hour working shifts, which enable humans to behave as nocturnal rather than diurnal animals. The sleep systems, therefore, facilitate occupational flexibility, as well as servicing all systems so they can be used as required for whatever is being done.

NATURAL HEALTH, BIOLOGICAL NEEDS, AND THE DOINGS OF EARLY HUMANS

In the first chapter, it was shown how doing provided the means of maintaining health in a natural way and that the opposite can also be the case. What people do can lead to illness and death, and a greater understanding of the fine line between well-being or illness as a result of doing is imperative, particularly because doing is the inbuilt human mechanism to fulfil the requirements seen by the WHO as a prerequisite of health. The lifestyles of early humans will be revisited to trace more extensively what they did in order to survive in reasonable health. Debate about the daily doings of our early ancestors is speculative, based on skeletal remains, the environment in which they were found, and fossils and tools found adjacent. Despite the speculative nature, it remains important to study the experiences of our early ancestors according to the WHO criteria of the prerequisites of health: that is, according to food and income, shelter, education, peace, a stable ecosystem and sustainable resources, and social justice and equity.[31-33]

Food and Income

Food and income are recognized as prerequisites of health. Food is a biological need that is essential to life itself. In most instances it equated to income for early Homo species, so that we find successive economies are described according to their means of procuring food: hunter-gathering, agriculture, and industry. The acquisition of daily food requirements is paramount to what has been done throughout time. Food has to be earned through what people did or do according to their degree of skill or luck and is dependent upon the community and environment in which they live. Recall the discussion in the first chapter that suggested early hunter-gatherers usually experienced general well-being. Premature death for many was due to accidents possibly related to the acquisition of food; to illness, much of which was similar to that of modern humans but seldom the chronic NCDs of later life; to occasional natural disasters; and to shortage of food.[34-37]

Hominids almost certainly subsisted principally on plant foods supplemented by animal protein of various kinds. *Homo habilis*, for example, was probably an opportunistic omnivore scavenging "animal products such as birds' eggs, larvae, lizards, and small game"[38] rather than hunting bigger prey. A systematic food-sharing economy and possibly some division of labor developed gradually based on cooperative foraging of meat and plant foods.[39-41] Such activities provide for "an important part of the diet of present-day hunter-gatherers."[38] Even a modest intake of meat would have aided survival by provision of energy, a full range of amino acids, trace elements, and vitamin B_{12}.[34] A possible early method of attacking prey for food was stone throwing, as observed in the Hottentots in South West Africa and first nation Australians.[42] Stone throwing may well have begun for self-protection, required because of physical vulnerability in comparison to many other animals.

Most recent opinion seems to favor the idea that after Homo males began to take a serious interest in hunting, women, along with child-bearing and care roles, continued to forage and gather, digging with sticks weighted with perforated round stones.[1,39] As the hunters shared their meat, women shared their finds.[39] It has been estimated that the latter contributed more than half of the required subsistence calories and that diets were, as a consequence, very diverse, which increased the likelihood of balanced nutrition.[43,44] The use of fire, evident from at least 1.2 million years ago, increased survival and health because meats could be made more edible and the toxicity of plants reduced. Dietary modifications led to natural selection pressures regarding particular attributes such as lighter jaws and cutting as opposed to grinding teeth, but also to an increasingly complex and larger brain, smaller colon, and the modulating role of insulin in optimizing dietary glucose.[34]

"Many archaeological sequences … show that knowledge of agriculture and domesticated plants existed long before there was a real shift from hunting and gathering."[45] Indeed, recent debate has suggested that there are no clear-cut distinctions between hunter-gatherers per se and horticulturists who also hunt and gather,[46] and between hunting and herding.[47] Rather a distinction can be made between "immediate return economies," characterized as "hand to mouth" existence, such as that lived by the Hadza, who live in Tanzania,[48] and "delayed return economies" in which a time investment for the future is part of daily life.[49]

Agriculture is an example of a delayed return economy. As it became dominant, and according to the societies and cultures in which they lived, males shifted the focus of their doing from hunting to farming. Recall from Chapter 1 that the range of food, at least initially, was reduced in diversity, leading to an initial increase in mortality and morbidity even though agriculture eventually provided better continuous access to food. The advent of farming heralded a change in role for many females, who increasingly became engaged in household occupations that supported the farmer and extended the nature of the food to be eaten.[50,51] In many instances, agriculture gave a different focus for combined activity too, for both individual and communal good, sometimes incorporating celebration and fun. For example, Ashton reports that as a part of all aspects of farming activities, working parties among the Basuto "are gay, sociable affairs comprising about 10 to 50 participants of both sexes."[52] In Western agricultural societies also, leisure, as well as work, was long associated with seasonal and communal food tasks.

Some hunter-gatherers did not adopt an agrarian lifestyle. This was not because they lacked the intellectual capacity to progress, as evidenced by their complex social organizations and ingenious methods of obtaining foodstuffs.[53] The successful survival of the Inuit of northern Canada in an inhospitable environment is a case in point.[54] Their health and well-being did not deteriorate until recent times when Western industrial values were imposed upon them and impacted on their sources of food. Three possible reasons for the retention of a hunter-gatherer way of life are isolation, climatic conditions not conducive to profitable agriculture, and resistance to change.[53] Coon, the Harvard anthropologist, suggests that societies retaining hunter-gathering economies had an eminently satisfactory way of living together in small groups, free from tedious routine, and all the food they needed.[53] He argues that adopting agriculture would have imposed a "whole new system of human relationships that offer no easily understood advantages, and disturbs an age-old balance between man and nature and among the people who live together."[53]

Some authorities suggest that the demands of living in harsh environments with few tools other than an expanding brain made what the people of traditional societies had to do very arduous and virtually continuous; that for millions of years, the struggle for existence allowed them little time for activities not immediately concerned with survival.[55,56] However, from study of modern hunter-gatherer societies, Coon found most individuals were "jacks of all trades," living and working mostly outdoors, their senses acute and, like their bodies, well exercised.[53] Their schedules and routines would be seldom monotonous and often adventurous.[53] Others agree that this simple, but obviously effective, economy provided a very successful and persistent quality of life, with Marshall Sahlins of the University of Chicago naming it "the original affluent society ... in which all the people's wants are easily satisfied."[57] In the 1840s, Edward John Eyre remarked on the few hours it took for first nation Australians, "without fatigue or labor," to procure sufficient food to last the day.[58] Studies of the !Kung San who live on the northern fringe of the Kalahari Desert provide evidence of such observations.[59] Until recently, when this lifestyle was eroded, adults from 15 to 60 years of age only spent about 2.5 hours daily providing their necessities of life even during a time of drought.[59] Now only a few continue in traditional ways, under pressure from the government to change.

The acquisition of sufficient food and income to supply basic biological needs is now a matter of huge concern for the majority of people, especially those living in developing countries. Many still engage in subsistence occupations similar to those of early economies, but in ever degrading ecosystems changed forever by people's doings. Famine, disease, and death are constant companions that cannot be easily remediated because of the ravages of affluent nations and multicorporate greed. The call for ecologically sustainable lifestyles and a more equitable distribution of resources between the "haves and the have-nots" are responses to this continuing crisis, as is the increasing concern of WHO and public health in nutritional matters across the world.[60] In more affluent societies, advanced social welfare systems provide income for food and other essential commodities without a doing requirement. It could be argued that this, too, may be damaging to physical, mental, or social health in the long term. The number of young people in such societies who do not work to provide for their own needs is increasing and alongside it physical, mental, and social illness is manifest through increasing violence, substance abuse, and suicide.

The 6 ancient rules for health recognized that doing (exercise, action, or motion) and food relate in terms of health outcomes. From time to time this is remembered. Rabinowitch, in 1939 for example, proclaims "occupation, diet and income are intimately related."[61] He outlines "work cannot be performed without expenditure of energy. ... Man obtains his energy from his food. ... When engaged in any occupation ... the primary factor which governs the need for food is the degree of muscular activity. ..."[61] Simply providing food or income without the doing component also adds to the illness outcomes. At one extreme, it contributes to problems of obesity, such as cardiovascular disorders and diabetes, and at the other, it leads to decreasing opportunity and skill to provide the means of continuing to acquire provisions. The WHO publication *The Social Determinants of Health: The Solid Facts* recommends "support for sustainable agriculture and food production methods that conserve natural resources and the environment," and the development of a "strong food culture for health, especially through school education, to foster people's knowledge of food and nutrition, cooking skills, growing food and the social value of preparing food and eating together."[62] This publication reminds us that in the present day it is global markets that control food supplies. This can reduce local job opportunities, food being marketed that does not always meet local health requirements, and perhaps, lead to monopolies and reduction of quality in the long term. Food has become a political issue. In terms of income, and on a personal as well as a population level, the links between food and health are clear. Added to that, though, are other factors such as the links between unemployment, illness, and premature death and the links between health and well-being, job satisfaction, and security.

Shelter

There is little evidence about the earliest forms of shelter, although it is possible to speculate that natural features of landscapes would be used to provide protection from the elements and predators. *Homo habilis* is credited with building the first known stone shelters in Olduvai Gorge and of carrying food to such camp sites for processing and sharing.[63] This has been queried because the site is an area that crocodiles might have inhabited, with Davidson and Noble claiming that there is insufficient evidence of built shelters or regular use of fire prior to 125,000 years ago.[64] They further suggest that this may have been the time when systematic hunting also started.[64]

There is reasonable acceptance that meat eating, clothing, and a capacity to build some form of shelter and to make fire enabled early expansion into colder environs. Evidence in the Central Russian Plains of semipermanent dwellings with vaults, arches, and buttresses, constructed of mammoth bones from about 30,000 years ago, indicates that fixed habitation probably occurred in some regions for thousands of years before the rapid spread of agriculture through most of the world from about 10,000 years ago.[65] As time progressed, a variety of shelters were constructed according to environment in terms of materials available and climatic conditions. These ranged from igloos built of ice, tents made of hide, conical birch bark structures, earth and turf, and wooden or stone structures to simple bark shades demonstrating the practical nature of hunter-gatherer health and well-being practices.

Although it appears common sense that improved shelter enabled better nurture and care of the young, aged, and sick when this was required, the nature of the shelter and surrounding circumstances can herald wider changes that create difficulty in terms of adjustment. For example, the !Kung San's transition from a hunter-gatherer lifestyle to agriculture has led to the dispersion of shelters from villages clustered around a central and publicly shared space to more isolated shelters "owning" the land around them. This has changed the complex support mechanism of the older type of communities. There has been a tendency for individuals to accumulate material goods, as well as a marked rise in birth rate. It has also resulted in an apparent decrease in both social and sexual egalitarianism, a more rigid defining of male and female roles, and changed play behaviors of the children.[59] Such change can provide a starting point for social illness to occur. Similar changes and difficulties can be recognized in other cultures that have changed more slowly through agrarian, urban, and industrial evolution. Changes in size, density, and type of shelter continue with little input from research about whether such shelter meets the occupational needs and natures of people and the health consequences of not doing so.

It is recognized in *The Universal Declaration of Human Rights* that housing is a fundamental aspect of an acceptable standard of living. The WHO housing and health program seeks to "assess and quantify the health impact of housing conditions," "identify health priorities in housing," "develop methodologies for a cost-benefit analysis for housing rehabilitation for health gain," and "focus on specific priority technical topics."[62] Recognized as a social determinant of health, housing is acknowledged as a major environment affecting physical, mental, and social well-being in either a supportive or limiting way even though the relationship between environmental quality, health, and well-being is not yet fully understood.[62]

Education

What is best for the safety and development of offspring is of vital importance to the species. Human young have a lot to learn and, compared with other animals, a long childhood. Learning by observing, imitating, and playing creatively provides education about doing with regard to self-care, safety, and survival. It also provides the experience of fun and the development of skills and self-worth, which are potential motivators for continued doing. Learning that occurs in the first formative years of life has significant lifelong effects; it provides children with models for their own future survival, as well as the protection and guidance of adults before being burdened with their responsibilities. As the species became more complex, the years of childhood, play, and education extended and changed. For example, until recent times, play and education were an integral part of the day-to-day occupations of adults and children, taking place in an environment relevant to the families' work and leisure activities. Today, in postindustrial societies, children and, often, young infants, are separated from their families for much of their waking day, and education is provided according to socially and politically devised criteria. The effects of this change have not been assessed in terms of adult engagement in, or value given to, doing. There are some who challenge the present segregation of education from parents and think that it may be connected with the numbers of dropouts from education systems that no longer appear to satisfy the "doing needs" of young people.

The need to promote education is fundamental according to *The Universal Declaration of Human Rights*. In line with that, United Nations Educational, Scientific and Cultural Organization's (UNESCO's) *Strategic Objectives for Education for 2002–2007* seeks to improve the quality of education through diversifying contents and methods and "the promotion of universally shared values"; to promote "experimentation, innovation and the diffusion and sharing of information"; and to promote "best practices as well as policy dialogue in education" particularly with regard to children affected by crisis.[66] This UN organization claims that "education has sometimes contributed to the outbreak of violent conflict," and is seeking "ways in which education can prevent such conflict or its recurrence" and to "inculcate universal values of peace and tolerance" through diverse programs.[66]

Peace

Leakey suggests that "man is not programmed to kill and make war, nor even to hunt: his ability to do so is learned from his elders and his peers when society demands it."[59] His argument is based on no evidence of inflicted death and warfare being found before the advent of temple towns, making "this ... too recent an event to have had any influence on the evolution of human nature."[59] Hunter-gatherers, like most modern humans, lived in social groups. Various reasons have been given, including affiliation, coercion,[67] dependency, dominance,[68] nepotism,[69-71] reciprocity, self-esteem,[72] and sex,[1] as well as the need to meet biological needs through group activity. Social groups offer some protection against predators, and Bruner observes "there is no known human culture that is not marked by reciprocal help in times of danger and trouble, by food sharing, by communal nurturance for the young or disabled, and by the sharing of knowledge and implements for expressing skill."[73]

Within modern hunter-gatherer societies, such as those of first nation Australians, Kalahari Bushmen, and the Birhhor of Northern India, survival needs and peaceful coexistence are major determinants of group size, usually between 20 and 70 people.[74] "A group of about 25 has a good chance of surviving for perhaps 500 years" and appears to be compatible with minimal conflict.[41] To avoid inbreeding, these groups usually form part of larger tribes of about 500 to 800 people.[41] Humans group together for the purposes of achieving large-scale occupations and for the enjoyment that can be experienced from being with and doing things with others. People with similar interests find pleasure and challenge in discussing and sharing their enthusiasm.

Lorenz asserts that not all would have been peaceful, describing "war between the generations" as part of a "species-preserving function to eliminate obsolete elements hindering new developments."[75] In puberty, young people go through a stage of "physiological neophilia" in which everything new is attractive. When somewhat older, they experience a revival of love of tradition or "late obedience." Lorenz's explanation has some merit in that physiological neophilia at an age when physical and mental capacities are acute will facilitate experimentation and exploration across a wide spectrum of activities, which may well provide survival and health advantages. Additionally, later development, growth, and adaptation may be based on successful experiences and individual interest, enhancing personal capacities, health, and well-being.

With greater population density came an apparent need for territorial defense and the ever-recurring occupation of war.[76] In contrast to Leakey, Lorenz argues that, in common with other animals, humans are innately aggressive in order to maintain sufficient space for existence, to ensure the strongest males father offspring, and to establish a pecking order.[75] Others propose that an inevitable consequence of tribal bonding is hostility to other tribes.[77] It is true that people have expended vast amounts of mental and physical effort, as well as resources, on the development and accumulation of weapons. These may be seen as an expression of a human need to feel safe, of innate aggression, or a need to develop tool technology without being able to foresee the possible consequences of the technology produced. The weapons of war are an aspect of tool technology developing beyond and to the detriment of human well-being. This may be a reflection of the planlessness of evolution: that adaptation to one set of environmental conditions millions of years ago may prove to be a handicap in another type of environment.[78] The expression of capacities through doing that includes ongoing experimentation and technological development is a strong force, especially when valued highly by society. The brain's ability to override biological needs with a highly developed cognitive capacity responsive to sociocultural influences has disadvantages as well as advantages.

In the present day, conflict is a major health problem; in southeast Asia alone, some 20,000 people lose their lives because of it each year. It is therefore apparent that "health workers in conflict areas need to learn how to function effectively without getting caught up in the disputes or be exploited by the warring parties" and to "bring parties together to solve serious health problems in conflict situations."[79] In a message to a health professionals training workshop on "Health As a Bridge for Peace" in Colombo, the Director-General of the WHO claimed, "health workers in conflict zones may defuse tension and build bridges for peace" because health can be "the perfect olive branch which is acceptable to almost all peoples."[80] Many have already reported that "health" has brought about cooperation and, sometimes, even reconciliation. The workshop was the first of its kind to be organized by WHO, and obviously met a recognized need being called for by health professionals in the field in Africa, Eastern Europe, and South America.

A Stable Ecosystem and Sustainable Resources

There is a closeness of fit between hunter-gatherer people and their environments. They:

Have had the energy, hardihood, and ingenuity to live and live well in every climatic region of the world not covered by icecaps. They have done so with stone tools and no firearms. In every well-documented instance, cases of hardship may be traced to the intervention of modern intruders.[53]

It is generally accepted that the advent of permanent settlements and the agrarian revolution were closely associated with environmental and climatic conditions that prevailed in different locations. Those that provided adequate food and shelter year-round probably supported resident populations, reducing to a great extent nomadic ways of life. Theories suggest that when the Pleistocene ice age ended, a major climate change occurred that produced environments conducive to agriculture, and that increasing social complexity resulted in a need for more formalized food production because the food-procuring system of small nomadic communities became inadequate. It is also possible that the developing occupational capacity of humans was instrumental in the change. That is, as humans experimented with material resources, their skills expanded; they began to challenge the environment and adapt it to meet their own needs and comfort. This possibility is supported by the fact that as agriculture developed, so did the diversity of human doings.[81]

A disadvantage of the human capacity for occupational experimentation is that agriculture changed the earth as a result of deforestation, land clearing, ploughing, and irrigation schemes such as blocking or moving river beds.[82] As part of the agricultural process, domestication of animals "involved an accelerating process of elimination of the great diversity of wild animals and plants to replace them with a few species that could be easily managed and manipulated."[83] It has also resulted in the proliferation of some to bad effect.[83] "Erosion and the alteration of the balance of species became inevitable."[82]

In the first chapter, it was noted that agrarian development and the permanent built environment that grew alongside it prevented the re-establishment of natural ecosystems, providing conditions that were conducive to hyperinfestations of disease organisms. For thousands of years throughout the world, infectious diseases caused ongoing morbidity, with periodic plagues resulting in catastrophic numbers of people dying. Perhaps that is indicative of the major problems still to come unless it is recognized that people's doing, ecological functioning, and health are inextricably related.

In a recent press release,[84] the WHO claims that damage to ecosystems poses a growing threat to human health, and a 2005 report from the Millennium Ecosystem Assessment (MA) showed that "some 60 percent of the benefits that the global ecosystem provides to support life on Earth (such as fresh water, clean air and a relatively stable climate) are being degraded or used unsustainably."[84] While ecosystems are acknowledged as the earth's life-support system, it is recognized that the relationship between people's health and environmental change is complex. Indirect, "displaced in space and time," and "dependent on a number of modifying forces" the links are however "fundamental to human health and indispensable to the well-being of all people everywhere in the world."[84] It is hypothesized that erosion of ecosystems could lead to an increase in existing infectious diseases and increased risk of the emergence of new diseases.[84]

Social Justice and Equity

Who and how what individuals did or did not do was determined in the early days of human evolution has long been a point of debate. Whether any such division was equitable or just is a more modern debate. Rowley-Conway believes that although early hominids probably lived in small groups with a structure similar to that of chimpanzees, their form of scavenging required "no division of labor and does not imply sharing or any other social behavior approaching our own."[85] A division of what needed to be done according to gender, though, may have been the case because of the differences in terms of reproductive biology, fat-to-muscle ratio, and greater variation in size than is common today, that together are known as sexual dimorphism. In sexually dimorphic primate societies, monogamy is rare.

The extent of sexual dimorphism and the maturation rates of early humans set some parameters to the debate about social justice and equity,[86] and others reflect concerns of the modern societies from which the ideas emanate, such as power relations, monogamy, and the nuclear family.[87] The question of why men, generally, do one thing and women do another remains one of the often-addressed issues in terms of social justice and equity today, with scientists questioning the contribution of biological versus sociocultural factors. They often turn to the study of evolution in their search for answers. Lampl argues "all human societies have defined roles for men and women that are both overt or active roles and passive roles that are learned by imitation and instruction as children."[87] Although by about 100,000 years ago dimorphism was similar to that found in modern humans,[87] evidence from primate ethology and ethnology of foragers demonstrates that male specialization in hunting and defense gives a "selective advantage to larger males" with resultant sexual dimorphism.[88] Additionally, there may be differences in the capacity to do various tasks between genders because of hormonal differences, which are under the control of genetic influences. Not only do levels of testosterone, estrogen, and progesterone account for differences in male and female activity, behavioral, anatomical, and neurological studies reveal there are significant gender differences in cerebral organization. These include cerebral maturation rates, cerebral laterality, language, and spatial capacities.[89] The necessity for women to assume responsibility for tasks in a sequential order of those nearest to home to those farthest afield was due to the need for women to work close to camp because of child-rearing restraints.[90] There may well have been a selective advantage for women who demonstrated child-rearing, food-gathering and preparing, and fine manipulative skills. Boserup found sexual division of labor in all the traditional societies she studied but no common pattern; what was considered a natural occupation for women was seemingly determined by the fact that they had "undergone little or no change for generations."[91]

In terms of inequality between social groups of quantity, quality, choice, or obligation in terms of what they did or did not do, it has been observed that in early hunter-gatherer lifestyles there would be few exemptions from some kind of labor except for the very young. Some believe that everyone would be primarily a hunter or gatherer and tool/household-implement-maker, even those with extracurricular activities, such as shamans, chiefs, or warriors.[92] Even if that was the case, many of the complex features of our own way of life that may provide a basis for inequities to occur, such as social inequality, occupational specialization, long-distance exchange, and technological innovation, appear to have originated with hunter-gatherers.[76] These claims are supported by finds that raise the possibility of "status by heredity rather than achievement,"[41] long distance trading long before the establishment of agriculture or towns, and the early establishment of economic systems with "ritual exchange obligations."[76] With the formation of cities, it is possible to trace developments in architecture, art, writing, commerce, religion, increased technological innovation, and social administration that helped communities cope with socioenvironmental stress, uncertainty, and unpredictability.[76] The stressors seem to have arisen from within communities living in much larger, specialized populations than they had been used to and also in response to possible dangers from both inside and outside the community. Neff observes that during this period what people did began to acquire distinctions and qualifications and an increasingly complicated infrastructure of evaluative meanings, including a differentiation between labor and leisure.[56]

Such complications have accelerated and increased in complexity as the years have passed, technological expertise has increased, and populations have grown out of proportion to the rest of the natural world. Social injustices and inequities have thrived and grown in those conditions, and illness and death are daily results. In terms of occupational injustice, people are prevented from gaining access to or participating in education, training, and citizen activities because of racism, discrimination, stigmatization, hostility, and unemployment. This is noted in the section Social Exclusion in WHO's *The Social Determinants of Health: The Solid Facts.* Its theme reads as follows: "Life is short where quality is poor. By causing hardship and resentment, poverty, social exclusion and discrimination cost lives. The chances of living in poverty are loaded against some social groups."[62]

SUMMARY

Within communities throughout time, food, income, shelter, education, peace, the ecosystem, and social justice and equity can be recognized as closely related to health and illness. It is probable that community leaders addressed issues relating to health on a daily basis, although they probably thought of it in other terms. That remains the case today when political decisions are made with the well-being of a nation in mind. Erroneously, most appear to only accept decisions as "health" related if medical experts make them. Lack of confidence or understanding about the impact of wide-ranging policies on health outcomes has grown. In part, this may result from the prescriptive nature of "medicine." In the past, health experts of many persuasions, rulers, their advisors, philosophers, shamans, priests, "mouthpieces for the gods," monks, wise-women, physicians, nurses, and anyone who cared to assume the mantel of expert, all prescribed in some way to what people needed to do to be healthy or to overcome illness.

Throughout their existence, it is what people have done that has provided the prerequisites for health and for survival. Although less obvious in postindustrial societies, the evidence that this remains the case is all around us. Because what people did was altered by changes within natural, sociocultural, and political environments, the experience of health was also changed. This, too, is ongoing. Both those factors require more adequate understanding. Additionally, it could be advisable to include greater emphasis in education of health professionals and others on natural mechanisms and ways of meeting prerequisites for health.

Rules for Health

AN ANCIENT "DOING" APPROACH

An important question to consider at this point is whether or not the place of doing has ever been recognized for its contribution to health or whether its economic importance has always been dominant. Consideration of classical Greek medicine from this point of view is a good place to start because its role has been of immense importance throughout millennia to the present day, even though much of its teachings are overlooked or considered outdated.

Authorities in ancient Greece held a holistic view about health that included the everyday doings of its peoples, and because it made great distinction between labor associated with the requirements of living and other forms of doing, it is interesting to consider in relation to the view taken here. The Greek city-states were established by conquest during the third and second millennia BC when the Greek citizen "managed to divest himself of all need to labor," leaving this to slaves, free peasants, artisans, and craftsmen who were usually the indigenous people of conquered domains.[56] Labor and work were regarded as "brutalizing the mind, making man unfit for thinking of truth or for practicing virtue; it was a necessary evil which the visionary elite should avoid."[81] In contrast, the domain of the citizen was doing intellectual, political, social, and war-like pursuits deemed worthy of free men while maintaining "a conscious abstention from all activities connected with merely being alive."[81] Aristotle, concurring with these cultural norms, argued that without labor it is not possible to provide all the necessities of life, but that to master slaves is the human way to master necessity and thus, is not against nature. This opinion was in line with his view of occupation as an aspect of health. In terms of doing, being, and becoming, he believed that labor, manual work, and the banausic arts were deleterious to the body; that because of the monetary component, minds became preoccupied and degraded and that personal development was hindered. However, he approved unconditionally of money earned through medicine, architecture, teaching, and land ownership.[93,94] Hannah Arendt (1906–1975), an authority on the Greco-Roman world, recognized the lack of modern day theory about animal laborans (ie, the labor of the body) and homo faber (ie, the work of our hands) that she found surprising because of the present-day attitude about work as "the source of all values."[95]

Because of the imposed boundaries to what citizens could do, the state (perhaps unconsciously) found it necessary for the health of its population to supplement the restricted occupational regimen by the establishment of gymnasia. Unlike the present day, when gymnasia have once more become popular (labor-saving devices now take the place of slaves), the Greek centers for the development of athleticism included schools for the arts and intellect as well. In these, citizens strived to attain mental as well as physical excellence, health, and beauty through what they did, along with superior war-making skills.

Literature, philosophy, and stories of the gods were methods of promulgating acceptable and desirable things to do as aids to health in ancient Greece.[96] Some examples include Homer's stated belief in music, sunshine, and fresh air and his valuing of crafts, gymnastics, games, and exercises; stories of Apollo, son of Zeus, the original god of healing, who used music and poetry to relieve pain and depression[96]; and the fables of Hygeia and Asclepius with subsequent oscillation between the ascendances of healing or health practices told in the first chapter.[97,98] In medicine, Hippocrates in *On Regimen: Book 1* provides propositions about food, drink, environment, and labor. This also includes a major digression into occupational health issues about a wide range of trades. His *On Regimen: Book 2* addresses similar topics, including labor and rest, sleep and waking, inactivity and repose, fatigue from unaccustomed or excessive exercise, and natural exercise and that which is ill timed.[96] These obviously relate to the ancient rules of health according to the non-naturals.

The medieval version of the non-naturals that provided health rules for Europeans from the 11th to the 19th century was attributed to Claudius Galen, who was particularly interesting in terms of an occupational perspective of health. While the majority of physicians throughout the decades appear to have concentrated on the category that is concerned with food and drink, Galen paid great attention to motion and rest.[99] Indeed, in the classic 17th century *Anatomy of Melancholy*, Burton claims that "Galen prefers Exercise before all Physick, Rectification of diet, or any Regiment in what kinde soever; 'tis Natures Physician."[100] Galen based many of his prescriptions on graded physical occupations of a sporting nature and manual labor for both physical and mental disorders; for the strengthening of cognition, intellect, and body; for the maintenance of health; and for alternative ways of making a living if deemed necessary.[101]

The Classical ideal that doing what was required to stay alive was inferior to a conscious abstention from it was challenged in medieval Christian societies. This was, in part, due to monastic rule, which saw labor as one honorable way of serving God and attaining spiritual health. For example, rule XLVIII of the Benedictine order ordained that "idleness is the enemy of the soul and therefore, at fixed times, the brothers ought to be occupied in manual labor, and again at fixed times, in sacred reading."[102] Such views were based, in part, on the Hebrew notion of God as one who works and the commandment of 6 days of labor followed by a day of rest on the Sabbath.[103] Because early mortality was the norm and an ever-present possibility following what would now be considered minor illnesses, faith in the afterlife tended to give an understandable primacy to spiritual rather than physical health. Additionally, more credence was given at that time to doing the right thing because disease was often attributed to sin.[96] Earlier than the formal publication of the *Regimen Sanitatis Salernitanun*, the influence of Classical medicine was still evident within the health services provided by monasteries. Benedict had founded his monastery at Monte Cassino, close by Salerno where the *Regimen* came into being, and it was there that he wrote his "Rule" organized around alternate periods of prayer, labor, and rest that are compatible with knowledge of the 6 non-naturals.

Health care in much of Europe remained centered around monasteries for centuries. In contrast, dissolution of monasteries in Britain led to the disappearance of health services for many with physical, mental, or social disorders and chronic and degenerative conditions for close to 100 years. The number of homeless and workless swelled the number of beggars so that the environment became a health hazard for beggar and citizen alike. This led to unprecedented action by concerned citizens, perhaps as a result of exposure to the ideas of the *Regimen Sanitatis*. Apparently recognizing the health benefits of productive doing, they approached King Edward VI (Figure 3-1), the son of Henry VIII, for the gift of Bridewell Palace as a hospital of occupations. They successfully petitioned "...have compassion on us, that we may lie no longer in the street for lack of harbour, and that our old sore of idleness may no longer vex us, nor grieve the commonweal."[104] Two governors oversaw the hospital occupant's work in "sciences profitable to the commonweal"[104] making gloves, coats, silk lace, shoes, nails, knives, brushes, and so forth after they had been admitted and "so be preserved from perishing."[105]

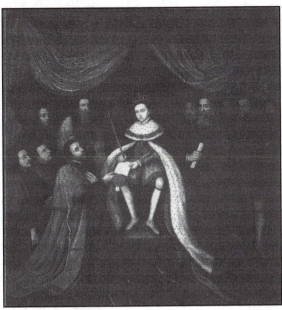

Figure 3-1. Edward VI signing petition for Bridewell Hospital of Occupations. (Reprinted with permission of Bridewell Royal Hospital.)

Apart from this unique establishment, which spawned replicas in some provincial British towns and throughout Europe,[105] in England it was not until the Elizabethan Poor Law Act of 1601 that it was fully recognized that the care of all the poor, infirm, and homeless rested with the government. Work was central within it for reasons of economy, self-respect, and health—action and rest being deemed central to health's preservation as the non-naturals prescribed. When work was not otherwise available, local parish authorities were required to provide it and to supply raw materials for that purpose. The original concept of local initiatives being most useful in community care was revisited in the 20th century and in the oft use phrase "think globally, act locally."[96]

While that initiative provides an example of how social health issues related to doing were tackled according to the ancient rules of health, other initiatives aimed at physical health demonstrate adherence to the same rules. Ambroise Pare (1510–1590), regarded by the French as the Father of modern surgery,[106] described the health-giving nature of doing in terms of the non-natural "motion and rest." The benefits of moderate and well-timed doing were explained in terms of strengthening respiration and body-limb function, increased tolerance, improved digestion and nourishment, expulsion of wastes, and internal cleansing.[107] He prescribed moderate doing that involved all body parts, before food, that ceased when the doer was red, perspiring, weary, or breathing heavily, that were accompanied by cooling down activity and followed by night-time rest. Pare explains "… we see the members of a mans body by a friendly consent are always busied, and stand ready to perform those functions for which they are appointed by nature, for the preservation of the whole, of which they are parts. …"[108] At about the same time, Hieronymous Mercurialis (1530–1606) was advocating occupation as exercise for health (Figure 3-2).[109]

Bernadino Ramazzini (1633–1717), born in Italy a century later, provided empirical evidence of the relationship between what people do and their health. In a monumental literary work, he compiled the earliest substantial research on matters of occupational health and safety. His work preempts the modern day preoccupation with direct cause and effect of illness that is rare but not unknown in the case of specific occupations. Figure 3-3 endeavors to capture the essence of his approach.

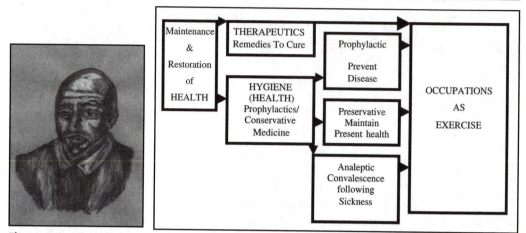

Figure 3-2. Hieronymous Mercurialis. Flow chart of occupation as exercise for health according to Mercurialis. (Reprinted with permission from Wilcock AA. *Occupation for Health. Volume 1. A Journey From Self-Health to Prescription.* London: British College of Occupational Therapists; 2001:184. Reproduced by kind permission of the British Association and College of Occupational Therapists.)

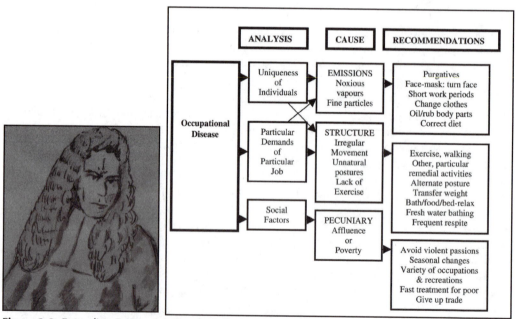

Figure 3-3. Bernadino Ramazzini. Ramazzini's occupational health approach. (Reprinted with permission from Wilcock AA. *Occupation for Health. Volume 1. A Journey From Self-Health to Prescription.* London: British College of Occupational Therapists; 2001:197. Reproduced by kind permission of the British Association and College of Occupational Therapists.)

In England, Cheyne, basing his 18th century medical texts on the rules of the 6 non-naturals, also recognized the value of doing as both a reward and a cost of living in terms of population health and of wear and tear on body and mind. With something of the concern of a present-day occupational scientist or, perhaps, epidemiologist, Cheyne obviously studied the nature of occupation and its effects on productivity and health. In common with many modern thinkers, he claims that many people are able to engage better in intellectual occupations after a night's sleep. He addressed doing as part of mental health[110] and prescribes specific occupations for health in general.[111]

> To restore this decay and wasting of animal bodies, nature has wisely made alternate periods of labor and rest, sleeping and watching, necessary to our being; the one for the active employments of life, to provide for and take in the materials of our nourishment; the other to apply those materials to the proper wasted parts, and to supply the expenses of living.
>
> All the nations and ages have agreed that the morning season is the proper time for speculative studies, and those employments that require the faculties of the mind.
>
> We proceed in the next place, to the consideration of exercise and quiet, the due regulation of which is almost as necessary to health and long life, as food itself.
>
> Of all the exercises that are or may be used for health (such as walking, riding a horseback or in a coach, fencing, dancing, playing at billiards, bowls or tennis, digging, working at a pump, ringing a dumb bell) walking is the most natural, as it would not spend too much of the spirits of the weakly.
>
> *George Cheyne, 18th Century*

Robert Burton also addressed occupation for mental health in his famous and all encompassing work *The Anatomy of Melancholy*. Throughout his text, and backed up by endless references, he advocates the health-giving effects of doing. For example, he claims, "Nothing better than Exercise (if opportunely used) for the preservation of the Body: Nothing so bad, if it be unseasonable, violent or overmuch."[100] Maintaining that idleness—lack of occupation—is a "sole cause of this (depression) and many other maladies,"[100] Burton concludes his great work by stating, "Be not solitary, be not idle," thus drawing attention to another important dual health consideration—occupation and relationships.[112]

Some might argue that such ideas can be considered precursors of what is usually called the "Protestant work ethic," a concept originating with Max Weber, who sought to understand the religious and idealistic roots of modern capitalism.[113,114] Just as it was work that was recognized as a way to spiritual health in medieval times, so it was the work ethic rather than freely chosen doing that was in ascendance as agriculture gave way to industrialization. From the turn of the 18th century in the Occident, the health advantages of people's occupational nature was subjected to perhaps their greatest challenge. With remarkable speed, doing became focused on paid employment, increasingly within capitalist forms of industry. Indeed, in England, which led the change to industry, there was a "steady assimilation of small professional and business families, diverse in point of both wealth and activity" on whom "primarily, depended the viability and growth of the national economy ... social flexibility and stability ..."[115,116] This new middle class, "frequently self-made and always dependent on aggressive use of their talents, ... were genuine 'capitalists' in terms of the investment of their labor and their profits in entrepreneurial activity, whether commercial or professional," dominated what people were required to do or were not able to do.[115] Occupation as integral to accepted rules for health became largely disregarded, replaced with the entrepreneurial fascination with pragmatics and applied technology that lingers today. So, too, does modern economics, which also developed at this time. Indeed, it is one of the most influential forces on doing in the modern day as it is on health.

Adam Smith (1723–1790), whose *An Inquiry Into the Nature and Causes of the Wealth of Nations* is considered the foundation of classical economics, proposed that the key to increasing a nation's wealth was by the accumulation of capital and the division of labor, both of which would increase with the freeing of trade.[117] He held that the division of labor would enhance workers' specialist skills because "the difference of natural talents... is not ... so much the cause, as the effect of labor. The difference ... seems to arise not so much from nature, as from habit, custom, and education."[117] However, he also recognized that the division of labor could decrease the quality of work.[118] In the broad sense, division of labor has led to modern exchange economy (ie, specialization followed by exchange between specialists, a fundamental aspect of all modern economies).[119] While it appears that the vast majority of the population has accepted that material wealth provided by occupational specialization is logical and acceptable, one could raise the basic question of whether division of labor and specialization is conducive to health and well-being, notwithstanding material wealth. This is not a straightforward question because there are many dimensions to specialization, resulting from the development of personal and professional skills to specialization that is imposed by a system. In the former, strengths and capacities can be developed but in the latter, there may be a minimizing of individual development except for minute and meaningless actions, as in some industrial processes, and for the majority of workers little opportunity to explore a wide range of occupations and discover their individual potential.

With the advent of modern medicine in the 20th century, coming hard on the heels of the sanitarians and the hygienists of the previous century, and the ushering in of epidemiological gold standard research, earlier rules based on what had worked for millennia were, more or less, relegated to the scrap-heap. The relationship between what people did or did not do, what they ate or did not eat in relation to their activity, where they did what they did, and what they felt about it was the concern of a minority of hardy souls. Unfortunately, in a time of reductionist, test-tube experimentation, older empirical knowhow based on observation became less valued. Slowly, however, the tide is turning and once again we see the emergence of guidelines about living healthily. The greatest source of these on a holistic front is the WHO.

MODERN: WORLD HEALTH ORGANIZATION DIRECTIVES FOR DOING WELL PHYSICALLY, MENTALLY, AND SOCIALLY

In the first chapter, the 5 major directions of the OCHP were identified as the modern action "rules for health." Public health practitioners and population health occupational therapists require skills in advocacy, mediation, and enablement to empower people toward understanding, acceptance of, and action toward these directives that are focused on everything that people do in their daily lives without being selective. Table 3-2 outlines the "doing" directives within the strategies.

Table 3-2

World Health Organization Directives for "Doing" Health

Building Healthy Public Policy	Creating Supportive Communities	Strengthening Community Action	Developing Personal Skills	Reorientation of Health Services
Direct policy makers to be aware of the health consequences of decisions made	Recognize the inextricable links within societies that are complex and interrelated	Empower communities to own and control their endeavors and destinies	Support personal development through the provision of information and education for health	Share the responsibility for health promotion with those within and outside health services
Direct policy makers to place health promotion on all agendas	Encourage reciprocal maintenance through a socio-ecological approach	Empower communities to set priorities, make decisions, and plan strategies to improve health	Enhance life skills to increase available options for people to control their health and environs	Work with individuals, communities, and governments toward health promotion
Foster equity through coordinated health, income, and social policies	Take care of each other, our communities, and our natural environment	Promote concrete and effective community action	Enable life-long learning and preparation for life stages and coping with possible illness	Move increasingly beyond clinical and curative services toward health promotion
Foster joint action for safer and healthier goods and public services	Foster global responsibility toward conservation of natural resources	Draw on existing community resources for self-help and social support	Facilitate skill development in school, home, community, and work settings	Embrace an expanded mandate sensitive to and respectful of cultural difference
Foster joint action for cleaner, more enjoyable environments	Advance the organization of work and leisure to help create a healthy society	Develop flexible systems to strengthen public participation on health matters	Promote action in educational, professional, commercial, and voluntary bodies	Open channels between health and social, political, economic, and environs sectors

(continued)

Table 3-2

World Health Organization Directives for "Doing" Health (continued)

Building Healthy Public Policy	Creating Supportive Communities	Strengthening Community Action	Developing Personal Skills	Reorientation of Health Services
Identify and inform of obstacles to adoption of healthy public policies and ways to overcome them	Generate safe, stimulating, satisfying, and enjoyable living and working conditions	Seek access to information, learning opportunities, and funding support		Engage in health research and make changes in professional education and training
	Systematically assess action health impact of changing environs work, technology, energy production, and urbanization			Refocus on the total needs of the individual as a whole person

Building healthy public policy is recognized as the fundamental key to improving population health across the globe. Specifically, from the perspective taken here, the general political lack of appreciation of the relationship between what people do and their health, as evidenced in recent years, requires urgent attention. To appreciate that fact, readers are asked to consider again the prerequisites of health—peace, shelter, education, food, income, a stable ecosystem, sustainable resources, social justice, and equity—and reflect on the doing/health aspects of policies that have been enacted recently about those factors. There have been policies, for sure, but each has been separate and little attention has been paid to people's occupational natures and needs and the health impacts of such lack of consideration.

What people do on a daily basis is dependent on public policy, legislation, systems of justice, fiscal measures, taxation, organizational structures, and sociocultural values that are well informed and appropriately constructed with population health and well-being in mind. The economy, in monetary terms, is important in today's world, but it can be argued that, despite what politicians espouse, it is less important than individual, community, population, and environmental health and that depends to a large extent on what people do. It is not only the provision of sound medical care that is essential to reducing illness, it is also the provision of sound and vigilant population health and, most importantly, lifestyles that satisfy basic needs. That requires power brokers and policy architects to formulate and enact health and well-being policies that consider what people do, as well as balancing the "state's power to act for the community's common good and the individual rights to liberty, autonomy and privacy."[120] Drawing the attention of the policy makers to the doing components of the prerequisites of health is a job worthy of serious attention and rigorous action. When it occurs, praise should be unstinting but that should not preclude attention to the outcomes of the policy or critical analysis of the effects.

Jones suggests "healthy public policy includes a good measure of health protection and prevention and builds on public health traditions. The main distinction is on getting the health sector to work with other sectors and agencies."[121] Economic matters often appear beyond the realm of concern of many health professionals who become totally involved in their daily practice and tend to cope (and complain to each other) when policies of a national or local nature appear to prevent the best outcomes. It needs to be remembered that it is people who enact economic policies, so there will be mistakes as well as successes. Indeed, there has been a persistent stream of questioning of the ill effects that accompany the goods proclaimed by classical economics. For example, Lionel Robbins, a mid 20th century economist of the English neoclassical school, suggested that economists "have nothing to say on the true ends of life and that their propositions concerning what is or what can be involve in themselves no propositions concerning what ought to be."[122] Post-Ricardian economics have also been criticized for defending and rationalizing the interests of capitalism at the cost of impartiality, with Marxist writers describing as "vulgar economics" that which concentrates on "surface phenomena," such as "demand and supply to the neglect of structural value relationships."[123]

More than a few socio-cultural-political institutions and policy enactments fail in enabling people to experience or develop through what they do in ways that meet different biological needs or natures as a matter of health. Rather, the majority concentrate on doing as an economic issue. It can therefore be queried whether socio-cultural-political systems have recognized sufficiently occupational difference as a means to promote health and as an important aspect of social justice.[124] Occupational justice, which can be considered a subset of social justice, is concerned with what forms of enabling, mediating, or advocating are needed to create a "doing environment" that is both just and health-promoting for all, recognizing the need to empower people regardless of difference.[125]

Townsend and Wilcock suggest that occupational justice would be served only if all people have appropriate support to engage in doing in a way that provides meaning for them and is health enhancing. To attain occupational justice everywhere will require different policies and resources for different groups.[124]

Some of the strength of population/community health has dissipated in the Western world because of philosophical acceptance of individualism[126] that emerged with the growth of capitalism. Even when no obvious social illnesses appear to exist, the type of economy, regulations, injustices, cultural or spiritual values, habits, and routines may restrict or be disadvantageous to some people's doing potential in the practical, everyday world.[127] This is true, even if collectively individuals are viewed as active agents who hold the power to ensure that resources are allocated toward visionary or ideal goals.[128] Change imposed on older economies more in tune with ecosystems may be counterproductive if not considered carefully with adequate and thorough consultation. If driven by more affluent nations or multicorporate organizations, such change could create more population health problems than bonuses. Structural or attitudinal change will automatically alter a population's activities and lifestyles without necessarily providing health or lifestyle benefit. Recognition of social illness and occupational injustices requires a different mindset to recognition of individual physical or mental disorder that can be medically diagnosed.

The ancient "rules of health" recognized the importance of environmental factors but did so without the present day understanding of either physiological or ecological determinants. The modern directive of the OCHP not only recognizes the inextricable links between people and their environment, it builds upon them and recommends a socioecological approach to health as the overall guiding principle for "the world, nations, regions and communities alike."[33] The protection and conservation of natural resources is as central to health promotion as healthy public policy is. Assisting all people to understand how what they do or do not do impacts the environment is important in terms of future health. Healthy environments are more than protection of unpolluted utilities, the development of which was so important in the early days of public health. They encompass the natural, the communal, the personal, and the built environments; space, comfort, beauty, and facilities that encourage healthful doing have to be considered, as well as clean air and water. Such ideals advocated by the new public health inspired the healthy cities movement instigated by the WHO Regional Office for Europe in 1987. The healthy cities approach is defined as:

> One that is continually creating and improving those physical and social environments and strengthening those community resources which enable people to continually support each other in performing all the functions of life and achieving their maximum potential.[129]

In recommending "systematic assessment of the health impact of a rapidly changing environment, particularly in areas of technology, work, energy production and urbanization,"[33] the OCHP directives encourage occupation-focused initiatives tied to the everyday world of what people do. How education, media, commercial factors, gender issues, attitudinal factors, and the changing patterns of work and leisure impact on health need to be addressed in a holistic interactive way as well as separate issues. All people, by action or by default, have an influence on the design, development, and effectiveness of the communities in which they live. Suitably empowered, population groups in communities can influence societal values and thereby instigate opportunities for people to engage in doing what is health giving rather than illness producing and that meets a community's perceived needs rather than those of bureaucracy. Wass suggests that the development of more flexible systems will assist in strengthening public participation and direction in health matters.[130] These should provide support to community members and the concept of "localism" and assist communities with the provision of resources and the planning of action. "Finding the balance between working with communities through community development and working for communities is an ongoing challenge for health professional workers. Finding the appropriate balance between these requires critical reflection."[130]

An interesting example is provided by a study that analyzed the beliefs about best practice in supported hostel accommodation. In-depth interviews were conducted with people from a range of disciplines, acknowledged by their peers as experts in the field of dementia care. These revealed that best practice meets the needs of staff and management as occupational beings as well as residents despite the latter's progressive decline of cognitive and functional capacities. An enabling approach driven by residents' needs emerged as both a feature and a strategy of best practice.[131] To be health promoting, the needs of the entire community required attention. While it is tempting to restrict population health intervention to those who are deemed ill according to medical science criteria, the latter example supports the WHO premise that all people need to be the ongoing recipients of public and private health-promoting ways of life. This includes opportunity for doing well.

The early development of personal skills is largely in the hands of families and educational institutions but, as has been observed earlier, the separation of children from families at an early age has been the norm in developed countries since the industrial revolution. This means that skill development is largely undertaken in group situations when individual approaches are more difficult. There are political imperatives on what children should learn, at least within schools that receive public funding. That suggests there may be restrictions on availability of some forms of occupational learning. Indeed, that factor is causing problems at present in postindustrial economies where there is a shortage of skilled tradespeople and an overabundance of young people who dropped out of school early because it failed to interest them or who left past the age of wanting to take up a trade apprenticeship. Is it coincidental that some years ago technical education was downsized in schools? The greatest impact of such a move could have been on those with little interest in more intellectual activities. If that was the case, such broad-based policies failed to take into account the occupational needs of a large part of populations in an attempt to ensure other goals, perhaps related to social equity, were met. Another more cynical possibility is that it may have appeared to provide as a political expedience a decrease in unemployment statistics. Some of the most interesting and successful recent "social" programs that have been instigated in Australia have been those that address problems of youthful antisocial behavior by offerings that teach them trades or skills. An occupational justice of difference is important to bear in mind in impoverished, third world communities as well as affluent ones. Community recognition and utilization of the strengths and capacities of individual members can be advantageous to everyone's well-being.

The importance of enabling "people to learn throughout life, to prepare themselves for all of its stages and to cope with chronic illness and injuries"[33] calls for culturally appropriate education that does not reinforce power differentials. A number of commentators fear that approaches within a health promotional framework have the potential to be characterized by professional dominance.[121,132,133] Gorin and Arnold advise that population health practitioners require belief in:

> ... the strengths and capabilities of the client, who defines and determines health care decisions. The provider remains a resource and facilitator of this process. The client is the expert, and the provider offers useful and meaningful information and skills.[120]

To achieve a state in which all individuals, community groups, and governments, as well as health professionals, recognize the importance of ongoing health-promoting ways of life and doing is a daunting task. It demands not only research, but also sensitivity, mutual respect, and a refocus on the total needs of people and environment.

SUMMARY

Together the ancient and modern rules of health provided the development and substance of health determinants and foundations for future action. The former relate more specifically to personal requirements (often based on individual "doing") such as food, water, exercise, and rest according to biological needs and in relationship to each other. The latter concentrates more on the global, ecological, national, political, and public health issues in broad terms. Both are useful so that population health can be tackled and enhanced from a minute and particular perspective to a holistic one.

Determinants of Doing as a Factor in Well-Being or Illness

The theme of the chapter introduced the prerequisites of health as peace, shelter, education, food, income, a stable eco-system, sustainable resources, social justice, and equity. The exploration of those in terms of the things that people do and have done in their everyday lives throughout human time has indicated not only the doings but the health and illness consequences of such doing. These are summarized in Table 3-3.

To draw this chapter to a close, some form of summation is required because the issues discussed are complex in the extreme. To do that, Table 3-3 links the underlying determinants of what people are obliged, want, or need to do and the possible health or illness outcomes. The ideas about doing and health that have been explored in the chapter sustain the view that there are not only indicators to the positive or negative effects that result from what people do, but also underlying factors that can positively or negatively influence the doing.

It is therefore necessary to outline in a linear way the main points emerging from this and earlier chapters, starting with human characteristics and biological needs. These fundamental attributes were instrumental, over millennia, in developing national, political, institutional, and cultural organizations that underlie the experience of what people do. They also changed the environment. Progressing through the consequences of such development in terms of the WHO prerequisites for health, we come to the possible illness or well-being consequences. Figure 3-4 provides a simplified depiction of the complex relationship between doing and illness or physical, mental, and social well-being.

Human characteristics and biological needs are the foundation stones of health and the driving forces behind cultural evolution. These have led to the establishment of different economies; political systems; and national values, policies, and priorities. Four distinct types of underlying determinants of health through doing are categorized:

1. The ecosystem and weather patterns.
2. The type of economy, such as nomadic, agrarian, industrial, postindustrial, capitalist, or socialist.
3. National policies and priorities, such as toward war or peace, economic growth, sustainable ecology, wealth and power of multinational organizations, or self-generated community development.

Table 3-3

The Prerequisites: Health and Illness Consequences of Doing

Prerequisites	Examples of Doings	Examples of Health	Examples of Doings	Examples of Illness
Peace	Creating supportive environs, reciprocal practical help to others, peaceful negotiation	Community development, social well-being	War, terrorism, rioting, anti-social behavior	Death, poverty, head injury, muscle-skeletal trauma, mental illness, social/environmental disruption
Shelter	Building/maintaining/providing adequate safe shelter for all people to suit environs, home-making	Community development; physical, mental, and social well-being; and child security	Destruction of homes for sociopolitical gain, not providing affordable, safe public housing	Death, stress, depressive illness, respiratory disorders, social unrest, and disease
Education	Family activities, participation in community life, attending places of learning	Community development; physical, mental, and social well-being; and child and others' personal development	Not providing appropriate, engaging, or any education, dropping out of education	Poverty, mental, social, and occupational deprivation and depression
Food and income	Work to provide for needs of self and others, home-making, food production, eating healthy	Physical, mental, social, and occupational well-being	Not working (nonavailable or bludging), over or under eating, substance abuse, sitting, watching electronic screens	Poverty and malnutrition; social and occupational deprivation, alienation, and imbalance; NCDs; infectious diseases; obesity; depression

(continued)

Table 3-3

The Prerequisites: Health and Illness Consequences of Doing (continued)

Prerequisites	Examples of Doings	Examples of Health	Examples of Doings	Examples of Illness
A stable ecosystem, sustainable resources	Conserve water; grow food, native plants, and trees; reuse/recycle rather than throw away; support and develop local resource-friendly economies; walk; use public transport	Community development; physical, mental, social, environmental, and occupational well-being	Throw away, chop down, pollute natural environs, self-drive, support multi-national firms that exploit overseas environments and cultures	Poverty from occupational exploitation and deprivation, death of eco-systems, gradual and increasing loss of earth's ability to provide for future health needs of all people
Social justice and equity	Provide opportunities according to occupational interest and skill, reward people (no discrimination) for exceptional contributions in any field, intellectual or practical	Community development; physical, mental, social, and occupational well-being	Segregate, ignore, deprive, or abuse others; reward only those with a particular type of skill; legislate to prevent some people being unable to provide for their needs	Poverty and malnutrition; death; social and occupational deprivation, alienation, imbalance, and apartheid; mental illness

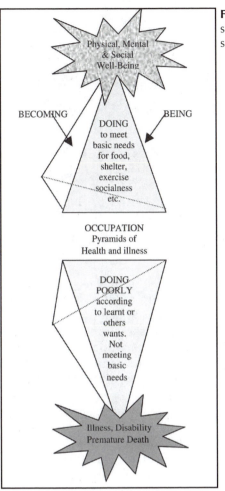

Figure 3-4. Simplified depiction of the complex relationship between doing and illness or physical, mental, and social well-being.

4. Dominant cultural and spiritual values about what things must be done and not done, and how things must be done; about such ideas as social justice and equity as they relate to occupation, how different aspects of doing are perceived, the work ethic, individualistic or communal conventions, and dominant health or healing ideologies (Figure 3-5).

These underlying factors lead to management of the environment and the ecology that may be detrimental or sustaining. They also give rise to the particular state and public institutions, commercial enterprises, and utilities of any given society. For example, the type of economy has direct influence on the availability and use of technology in daily life; how labor is divided between classes, genders, and age groups; the type and extent of health services; and employment opportunities. National priorities have direct influence on legislative and fiscal institutions that provide rules by which people live; on whether people live in fear or hope. Government agencies and policies provide the background to whether commercial enterprises flourish or have no chance; on attitudes and materialism; and on relationships and doings between communities and individuals within their boundaries, and with other nations. Cultural and spiritual values will impact upon such institutions and activities as the media, local regulations, social services, job creation schemes, education, worship, and health care systems.

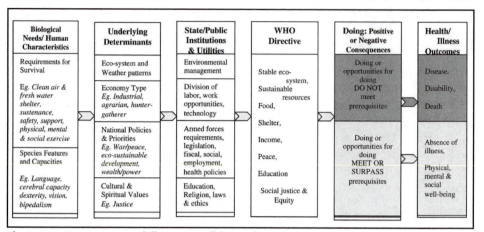

Figure 3-5. Determinants of illness or well-being through doing.

State and public institutions, and the utilities provided by them, can also provide positive or negative influence upon national, community, family, or individual health by providing or restricting equitable opportunity to engage in doing that provides for the prerequisites of health and at the same time exercises and nourishes the mind, body, and spirit. Being able to contribute to population health in a way that is socially valued yet maintains natural resources and recognizes the rights of all living organisms is important yet easily neglected. Underlying determinants may act as deterrents, often in the name of economic advancement. The effects of the underlying factors may not be the same for all communities or for all individuals.

The positive or negative consequences of doing or the opportunity to do to meet the prerequisites for health are many. Positively, they can result in increased energy and alertness; increased flexibility, interest, contentment, or commitment; the ability to relax and sleep; improved relationships; openness to new challenges; and a willingness to learn and grow from completing necessary tasks. More conventional health status indicators, such as appropriate height:weight ratios and normal blood pressure, cholesterol, and lung function, can result from a range of doing as can increased life expectancy.[11] At the other end of the continuum and because of ecological degradation, the type of economy, national priorities and policies, and spiritual and cultural values create a flow-on effect that can also lead to unhealthy outcomes. As well as lack of food, shelter, or income, examples might include health risk factors such as loneliness, overcrowding, or lack of opportunity to exercise regularly through doing whatever is required to meet the prerequisites. There may be imbalance between diet and activity, ongoing unresolved stress, or the development of health risk behaviors such as substance abuse. Such risk factors can lead to early, preclinical health disorders such as stress; boredom; burnout; depression; decreased fitness, brain, or liver function; increased blood pressure; and changes in sleep patterns, body weight, and emotional state. All can ultimately result in disease, disability, or death.

SUMMARY

Health and well-being result from being in tune with our "occupational" species' nature. Being responsive to biologically driven needs and doing to provide the requirements of living have, in the past, been central to maintaining homeostasis, preventing illness, and promoting health. It is relatively easy to see that there is a correlation between obvious survival occupations and health because what people do has direct bearing on their type of shelter and their access to food, clean air, and water, which are recognized by WHO as prerequisites of health. The correlation between ill-health or the natural health benefits of people's engagement in other types of occupations is obscure and complex, and research is limited despite the benefits being recognized in the OCHP.

Doing entails more than simply acquiring requirements for survival. Because physiological and innate biological mechanisms are informed, stimulated, influenced, and adapted by conscious social processes, these too become very influential determinants of human health. For positive health, people need what they do to offer meaning, choice, satisfaction, a sense of belonging, purpose, and achievement. These enable individuals, families, communities, and populations to flourish and provide the species with a survival advantage. This is discussed in the next chapter about "being" as part of occupation.

References

1. Leakey R, Lewin R. *People of the Lake: Man: His Origins, Nature, and Future.* New York: Penguin Books; 1978:38,39,120.
2. Lobkowicz N. *Theory and Practice: History of Concept from Aristotle to Marx.* London: University of Notre Dame Press; 1967:9.
3. Petrovic G. Praxis. In: Bottomore T, ed. *A Dictionary of Marxist Thought.* 2nd ed. Oxford, UK: Blackwell Publishers; 1991:435.
4. Marx K. Economic and philosophical manuscripts, 1844. In: Livingstone R, Benton G, trans. *Karl Marx: Early Writings.* New York: Penguin Classics; 1992.
5. *The Oxford English Dictionary.* 2nd ed. Vol XII. Oxford, UK: Clarendon Press; 1989:130,633.
6. Compact Oxford English Dictionary. 2005. Available at: http://www.askoxford.com/concise_oed. Accessed June 22, 2005.
7. Comstock D. A method of critical research. In: Bredo E, Feinberg W, eds. *Knowledge and Values in Social and Educational Research.* Philadelphia: Temple University Press; 1982:370-390.
8. Lather P. Research as praxis. *Harvard Educational Review.* 1986;56(3):257-277.
9. Kotarbinski T. The goal of an act and the task of the agent. In: Gasparski W, Pszczolowski T, eds. *Praxiological Studies: Polish Contributions to the Science of Efficient Action.* Dordrecht, Holland: D. Reidel Publishing Co; 1983:22.
10. World Health Organization. Global Strategy on Diet, Physical Activity and Health. Chronic Disease Information Sheets. World Health Organization Documents and Publications: Accessed December 2005.
11. Glass TA, et al, Population based study of social and productive activities as predictors of survival among elderly Americans. *BMJ.* 1999;319:478-483.
12. World Health Organization. *International Classification of Functioning, Disability and Health.* Geneva: Author; 2001.
13. Christiansen CH. Occupation and identity: becoming who we are through what we do. In: Christiansen CH, Townsend EA, eds. *Introduction to Occupation: The Art and Science of Living.* Upper Saddle River, NJ: Prentice Hall; 2004.
14. Maslow AH. *Motivation and Personality.* New York: Harper and Row; 1970.
15. Harvey AS, Pentland W. What do people do? In: Christiansen CH, Townsend EA, eds. *Introduction to Occupation: The Art and Science of Living.* Upper Saddle River, NJ: Prentice Hall; 2004:87.
16. Christiansen CH, Townsend EA, eds. *Introduction to Occupation: The Art and Science of Living.* Upper Saddle River, NJ: Prentice Hall; 2004:15.
17. Arnoff MS. *Sleep and Its Secrets: The River of Crystal Light.* Los Angeles, Calif: Insight Books; 1991.
18. Lieberman P. Evolution of the speech apparatus. In: Jones S, Martin R, Pilbeam D, eds. *The Cambridge Encyclopedia of Human Evolution.* New York: Cambridge University Press; 1992:136-137.
19. Sassin JF, Parker DC, Mace JW, Gotlin RW, Johnson LC, Rossman LG. Human growth hormone release: relation to slow wave sleep and sleep waking cycles. *Science.* 1969;165:513-515.
20. Shapiro CM, Bortz R, Mitchell D, Bartel P, Jooste P. Slow wave sleep: a recovery period after exercise. *Science.* 1981;214:1253-1254.
21. Foret J. To what extent can sleep be influenced by diurnal activity? *Experientia.* 1984;40:422-424.
22. Moore JC. *The Lifespan in Relation to the Nervous System.* Melbourne, Australia: Australian Association of Occupational Therapists; 1994:188.

23. Pearlman CA. R.E.M. sleep and information processing: evidence from animal studies. *Neuroscience and Neurobehavioural Reviews.* 1979;3:57-68.
24. Smith C. Sleep states and learning: a review of the animal literature. *Neuroscience and Neurobehavioural Reviews.* 1985;9:157-168.
25. Gay J, Farnworth L, Alcorn K. *The Use of Time and Its Meaning for Forensic Psychiatric Patients.* International Forensic Health Conference. Melbourne, Australia: 1999.
26. Molineux M, ed. *Occupation for Occupational Therapists.* Oxford, UK: Blackwell Publishing; 2004:59.
27. Fowler MJ, Sullivan MJ, Ekstrand BR. Sleep and memory. *Science.* 1973;179:302-304.
28. Fox R. *The Search for Society.* New Brunswick, NJ: Rutgers University Press; 1989:179.
29. Winson J. *Brain and Psyche: The Biology of the Unconscious.* Garden City, NY: Anchor Press/Doubleday; 1985.
30. Campbell SS. Duration and placement of sleep in a "disentrained environment." *Psychophysiology.* 1984;21(1):106-113.
31. Foley R, ed. *Hominid Evolution and Community Ecology.* London: Academic Press; 1984.
32. Klein RG. *The Human Career: Human Biological and Cultural Origins.* Chicago, Ill: University of Chicago Press; 1989.
33. World Health Organization, Health and Welfare Canada, Canadian Public Health Association. *Ottawa Charter for Health Promotion.* Ottawa: Author; 1986.
34. McMichael T. *Human Frontiers, Environments and Disease: Past Patterns, Uncertain Futures.* Cambridge, UK: Cambridge University Press; 2001:31,47.
35. McNeill WH. *Plagues and People.* London: Penguin Books; 1979:13,25.
36. Douglas M. Population control in primitive peoples. *Br J Sociol.* 1966;17:263-273.
37. Birdsell JB. On population structure in generalized hunting and collecting populations. *Evolution.* 1958;12:189-205.
38. Buranhult G, ed. *The First Humans: Human Origins and History to 10,000 BC.* St. Lucia, Australia: University of Queensland Press; 1993:59.
39. van der Merwe NJ. Reconstructing prehistoric diet. In: Jones S, Martin R, Pilbeam D, eds. *The Cambridge Encyclopedia of Human Evolution.* New York: Cambridge University Press; 1992:369-372.
40. Wing ES, Brown AG. *Paleonutrition: Method and Theory in Prehistoric Foodways.* New York: Academic Press; 1978.
41. Isaac GLI. The food sharing behaviour of protohuman hominids. *Sci Am.* 1978;238(April):90-106.
42. Isaac B. Throwing. In: Jones S, Martin R, Pilbeam D, eds. *The Cambridge Encyclopedia of Human Evolution.* New York: Cambridge University Press; 1992:358.
43. Lee RB, DeVore I. *Man the Hunter.* Chicago, Ill: Aldine Publishing Co; 1968.
44. Dalberg F, ed. *Woman the Gatherer.* New Haven, Conn: Yale University Press; 1981.
45. Binford LR. Subsistence—a key to the past. In: Jones S, Martin R, Pilbeam D, eds. *The Cambridge Encyclopedia of Human Evolution.* New York: Cambridge University Press; 1992:365-368.
46. Ellen RF. *Environment, Subsistence and System.* New York: Cambridge University Press; 1982.
47. Ingold T. *Hunters, Pasturalists and Ranchers.* New York: Cambridge University Press; 1980.
48. Foley R. Studying human evolution by analogy. In: Jones S, Martin R, Pilbeam D, eds. *The Cambridge Encyclopedia of Human Evolution.* New York: Cambridge University Press; 1992:336.
49. Woodburn J. Hunters and gatherers today and reconstruction of the past. In: Gellner E, ed. *Soviet and Western Anthropology.* London: Duckworth; 1980.
50. Ember CR. The relative decline in women's contribution to agriculture with intensification. *American Anthropologist.* 1983;85(2):285-304.
51. Burton ML, White DR. Sexual division of work in agriculture. *American Anthropologist.* 1984;86(3):568-583.
52. Ashton H. The Basuto. In: Parker S, ed. *Leisure and Work.* London: George Allen and Unwin; 1983:131.
53. Coon CS. *The Hunting Peoples.* London: Jonathan Cape Ltd; 1972.
54. Thibeault, R. Fostering healing through occupation: the case of the Canadian Inuit. *Journal of Occupational Science.* 2002;9:153-158.
55. Waechter J. *Man Before History.* Oxford, UK: Elsevier-Phaidon; 1976.
56. Neff WS. *Work and Human Behaviour.* 3rd ed. New York: Aldine Publishing Co; 1985.
57. Lewin R. *In the Age of Mankind: A Smithsonian Book of Human Evolution.* Washington, DC: Smithsonian Books; 1988:190.
58. Eyre JE. *Journals of Expeditions of Discovery Into Central Australia and Overland.* London: T and W Boone; 1845.
59. Leakey R. *The Making of Mankind.* London: Michael Joseph Ltd; 1981:226-229,242.

60. World Health Organization. The Declaration of Alma Ata. International Conference on Primary Health Care, Alma Ata, USSR; 1998.
61. Rabinowitch IM. Calories and occupation. In: Canadian Medical Association, ed. *Nutrition in Everyday Practice*. Toronto: Canadian Medical Association; 1939:1,4.
62. Wilkinson R, Marmot M, eds. *Social Determinants of Health: The Solid Facts*. Copenhagen, Denmark: World Health Organization Regional Office for Europe; 2003:28.
63. Jelinek J. *Primitive Hunters*. London: Hamlyn; 1989:24.
64. Davidson I, Noble W. When did language begin? In: Buranhult G, ed. *The First Humans: Human Origins and History to 10,000 BC*. St. Lucia, Australia: University of Queensland Press; 1993:46.
65. Jelinek J. *Primitive Hunters*. London: Hamlyn; 1989:66.
66. UNESCO. The Promotion of Education in Situations of Emergency, Crisis and Reconstruction. Available at: http://portal.unesco.org/education. Accessed May 2, 2006.
67. van den Berghe PL. Sociobiology. In: Kuper A, Kuper J, eds. *The Social Science Encyclopedia*. London: Routledge; 1985.
68. Argyle M. *The Psychology of Interpersonal Behaviour*. Harmondsworth: Penguin Books; 1967.
69. Alexander RD. *Darwinism and Human Affairs*. Seattle, Wash: University of Washington Press; 1979.
70. Chagnon N, Irons W, eds. *Evolutionary Biology and Human Social Behaviour*. North Scituate, Mass: Duxbury Press; 1979.
71. Symons D. *The Evolution of Human Sexuality*. New York: Oxford University Press; 1979.
72. Trivers RL. The evolution of reciprocal altruism. *Q Rev Biol.* 1971;46(1):35-57.
73. Bruner JS. Nature and uses of immaturity. *Am Psychol.* 1972;August:687-708.
74. Liljegren R. Animals of ice age Europe. In: Buranhult G, ed. *The First Humans: Human Origins and History to 10,000 BC*. Australia: University of Queensland Press; 1993.
75. Lorenz K. *On Aggression*. London: Methuen; 1966:52.
76. Lewin R. *In the Age of Mankind: A Smithsonian Book of Human Evolution*. Washington, DC: Smithsonian Books; 1988.
77. Morris D, Marsh P. *Tribes*. London: Pyramid Books; 1988:9.
78. Lorenz K. *The Waning of Humaneness*. London: Unwin Paperbacks; 1983.
79. Uton Muchtar Rafei, Regional Director, SEAR. World Health Organization Regional Office for South East Asia; Health As a Bridge for Peace. Press Release. 1999.
80. World Health Organization Regional Office for South East Asia; Health As a Bridge for Peace. Press Release. 1999. (WHO home page: <http://www.who.int/>).
81. Parker S. *Leisure and Work*. London: George Allen and Unwin; 1983.
82. Hole F. Origins of agriculture. In: Jones S, Martin R, Pilbeam D, eds. *The Cambridge Encyclopedia of Human Evolution*. New York: Cambridge University Press; 1992:373-379.
83. Clutton-Brock J. Domestication of animals. In: Jones S, Martin R, Pilbeam D, eds. *The Cambridge Encyclopedia of Human Evolution*. New York: Cambridge University Press; 1992:380-385.
84. World Health Organization. Global Environmental Change. Press release. WHO/15, 29th March 2005. (WHO home page: <http://www.who.int/>).
85. Rowley-Conway P. Mighty hunter or marginal scavenger? In: Buranhult G, ed. *The First Humans: Human Origins and History to 10,000 BC*. Australia: University of Queensland Press; 1993:61-62.
86. Potts R. The hominid way of life. In: Jones S, Martin R, Pilbeam D, eds. *The Cambridge Encyclopedia of Human Evolution*. New York: Cambridge University Press; 1992.
87. Lampl M. Sex roles in prehistory. In: Buranhult G, ed. *The First Humans: Human Origins and History to 10,000BC*. Australia: University of Queensland Press; 1993:30-31.
88. Burton ML, White DR. Division of labor by sex. In: Kuper A, Kuper J, eds. *The Social Science Encyclopedia*. London: Routledge; 1985:206.
89. Kolb B, Whishaw IQ. *Fundamentals of Human Neuropsychology*. 3rd ed. San Franscico, Calif: WH Freeman and Co; 1990:4,123.
90. Brown JK. A note on the division of labor by sex. *American Anthropologist.* 1970;72(5):1073-1078.
91. Boserup E. *Women's Role in Economic Development*. New York: St. Martin's Press; 1970:15.
92. Herskovits MJ. *Economic Anthropology*. New York: Knopf; 1952.
93. Aristotle. Politics. In: Barnes J, ed. *The Complete Works of Aristotle*. Rev Oxford trans. Princeton, NJ: Princeton University Press; 1984.
94. Aristotle. Politics VIII,2,1337b7-14
95. Arendt H. *The Human Condition*. Chicago, Ill: University of Chicago Press; 1958:83-85.
96. Wilcock AA. *Occupation for Health. Volume 1. A Journey from Self Health to Prescription*. London: BCOT; 2001.
97. Hygeia. *Grolier Multimedia Encyclopedia*. Grolier Electronic Publishing Inc; 1995.

98. Dubos R. *The Mirage of Health: Utopias, Progress and Biological Change*. New York: Harper and Row Publishers; 1959.

99. Georgii A, ed. *Ling's Educational and Curative Exercises*. London: Renshaw; 1876:11.

100. Burton R. *The Anatomy of Melancholy*. Oxford: Henry Cripps; 1651:84,86,216.

101. Macdonald EM. *World-Wide Conquest of Disabilities: The History, Development and Present Functions of the Remedial Services*. London: Bailliere Tindall; 1981:43-44.

102. Bettenson HS, ed. *Documents of the Christian Church*. New York: Springer; 1963.

103. Exodus 20: 9-11. *The Holy Bible*. Authorized King James version. London: Oxford University Press; 1972.

104. *A Short History of Bridewell and Bethlem Hospitals*. London: The Bethlem Art and History Collections Trust; 1899:3-7.

105. Slack P. *From Reformation to Improvement: Public Welfare in Early Modern England. The Ford Lectures Delivered in the University of Oxford 1994-1995*. Oxford: Clarenden Press; 1999:20-25.

106. Isaacs A, ed. Pare, Ambroise. In: *Macmillan Encyclopedia*. London: Macmillan; 1990:926.

107. Johnson T. *The Workes of that Famous Chirurgion Ambroise Parey*. Translated out of Latin and compared with the French. Printed by Th Cotes and R Young; 1634:34-35.

108. Pare A. The Authors dedication to Henry the third, the Most Christian King of France and Poland. 1579. In: Johnson T. *The Workes of that Famous Chirurgion Ambroise Parey*. Translated out of Latin and compared with the French. Printed by Th Cotes and R Young; 1634.

109. Blundell JWF. The Muscles and their Story from the Earliest Times (an Adaptation of the 'Ars Gymnastica') including the Whole Text of Mercurialis, and the Opinions of other Writers Ancient and Modern on Mental and Bodily Development. London, UK: Chapman & Hall; 1864.

110. Cheyne G. *The English Malady*. London: Strahan and Leake; 1733.

111. Cheyne G. *Essay of Health and Long Life*. London: George Strahan; 1724.

112. Burton R. *The Anatomy of Melancholy*. 12th ed. London: Thomas Davison, Whitefriars; 1821;2:601.

113. Weber M. *The Protestant Ethic and the Spirit of Capitalism*. Parsons T, trans. London: George Allen and Unwin Ltd; 1930.

114. Kalberg S. Max Weber. In: Kuper A, Kuper J, eds. *The Social Science Encyclopedia*. London: Routledge; 1985:892-896.

115. Langford P, Harvie C. The eighteenth century and the age of industry. In: Morgan KO, ed. *The Oxford History of Britain*. Vol IV. Oxford, UK: Oxford University Press; 1992:42,44-45.

116. Morgan KO, ed. *The Oxford History of Britain*. Vol V. Oxford, UK: Oxford University Press; 1992.

117. Smith A. (1776). In: Campbell RH, Skinner AS, Todd WB, eds. *An Inquiry Into the Nature and Causes of the Wealth of Nations*. Chicago, Ill: University of Chicago Press; 1976.

118. Raphael DD. *Adam Smith*. Vol 1. Oxford, UK: Oxford University Press; 1985:17.

119. Bannock G, Baxter RE, Rees R. *The Penguin Dictionary of Economics*. 2nd ed. New York: Penguin Books; 1978.

120. Gorin S. Contexts for health promotion. In: S. Gorin S, Arnold J, eds. *Health Promotion Handbook*. St. Louis, Mo: Mosby; 1998:40,74.

121. Jones L. The rise of health promotion. In: Katz J, Pederby A, eds. *Promoting Health: Knowledge and Practice*. Hampshire, UK: MacMillan; 1997:72.

122. Robbins L. *Politics and Economics, Papers in Political Economy*. London: Macmillan; 1963:7.

123. Desai M. Vulgar economics. In: Bottomore T, ed. *A Dictionary of Marxist Thought*. 2nd ed. Oxford, UK: Blackwell Ltd; 1991:574.

124. Townsend EA, Wilcock AA. Occupational Justice. In: Christiansen CH, Townsend EA, eds. *Introduction to Occupation: The Art and Science of Living*. Upper Saddle River, NJ: Prentice Hall; 2004.

125. Daniels N, Kennedy BP, et al. Why justice is good for our health: the social determinants of health inequalities. *Daedalus*. 1999;128(4):215-251.

126. Lukes S. *Individualism*. Oxford, UK: Basil Blackwell; 1973.

127. Wilcock AA, Whiteford GE. Occupation, health promotion, and the environment. In: Letts L, Rigby P, Stewart D, eds. *Using Environments to Enable Occupational Performance*. Thorofare, NJ: SLACK Incorporated; 2003.

128. McGary H. Distrust, social justice, and health care. *Mt. Sinai J Med*. 1999; 66(4):236-240.

129. Frumkin H, Frank L, Jackson R. *Urban Sprawl and Public health: Designing, Planning, and Building for Healthy Communities*. Washington, DC: Island Press; 2004:203.

130. Wass A. *Promoting Health: The Primary Care Approach*. Marrackville, New South Wales: Harcourt; 2000:174.

131. Pols V. Experts Views of what is Best Practice in Dementia Care for Hostel Residents. Unpublished masters thesis, University of South Australia, Adelaide, South Australia.

132. Carey P. Community health promotion and empowerment. In: Kerr J, ed. *Community Health Promotion: Challenges for Practice.* London: Harcourt; 2000.
133. Peterson A, Lupton D. *The New Public Health: Health and the Self in the Age of Risk.* London: Sage; 1996.

Suggested Reading

A Short History of Bridewell and Bethlem Hospitals. London: The Bethlem Art and History Collections Trust; 1899.

Burton R. *The Anatomy of Melancholy.* Oxford: Henry Cripps; 1651.

Cheyne G. *Essay of Health and Long Life.* London: 1724.

Glass TA, Mendes de Leon CF, Marotolli RA, Berkman LF. Population based study of social and productive activities as predictors of survival among elderly Americans. *BMJ.* 1999;319:478-483.

Jones S, Martin R, Pilbeam D, eds. *The Cambridge Encyclopedia of Human Evolution.* New York: Cambridge University Press; 1992

Wilcock AA. *Occupation for Health. Volume 1. A Journey from Self Health to Prescription.* London: BCOT; 2001.

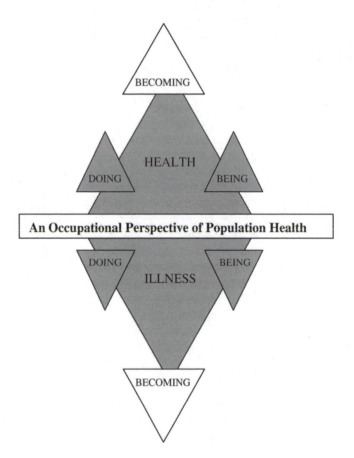

Occupation: Being Through Doing

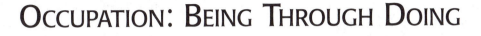

Theme 4:
Health depends on validation of "the uniqueness of each person and the need to respond to each individual's spiritual quest for meaning, purpose and belonging"
WHO, *Health for All in the Twenty-First Century,* 1998

The chapter addresses:
* Being as a determinant of population health
    * Defining the concept
    * Its place in public health
* Being through doing: biological needs, natural health, and finding meaning
    * Biologically based capacities
        * Consciousness
        * Creativity
    * Survival pressures
    * Recognition of people's occupational natures
        * From Marx, Ruskin, and Morris to occupational therapy and beyond
* Being through doing: ancient and modern rules for health
    * How changing values about meaning affected views of health in earlier times
        * Mental health
    * How modern values affect "being through doing" as an agent of health
        * Paid Employment
* Determinants of "being through doing" as factors in well-being or illness

In this chapter, how people feel about what they do is explored. This is an extremely important aspect of occupation that is intimately related to health. I explain it as the "being" component. From observation and from analysis of reports throughout history and in the current press, people who do too little and have too much time for contemplation or too much to do and have too little time for rest or personal and spiritual expression both experience lack of well-being that can be of a physical, mental, or social nature. A balance between doing and being appears to be important. Also intimately related to becoming, being is, perhaps, the most difficult for people to come to terms with in the fairly "concrete" world of health care. In conceptual terms, assisting people to do things is fairly straightforward, and helping them to grow into what they would like to become is, at least, understandable. Being, on the other hand, although a frequently used word, is a concept that has taxed the minds of great philosophers and is seldom addressed in post-modern health care with its emphasis on the minute and the measurable, except perhaps minimally, by professions such as occupational therapy or behavioral psychology. In order to shed light on some of the mystique that surrounds the word and to begin to appreciate its place in occupation-focused public health, the concept requires some clarification.

Apart from introducing it as a determinant of population health, in common with earlier chapters, "being through doing" will be considered in terms of how it can meet biological and natural health needs. To achieve this, the higher-order capacities of consciousness and creativity are considered because these appear important for people to find meaning in what they do. These capacities are, of course, relevant to issues already discussed in the last chapter. They are also fundamental to the next chapter, which considers self-actualization through what people do. Then, the survival pressures that empower or retard people's approaches to seek meaning, purpose, and satisfaction in line with their particular capacities are addressed; and following on from that, it is natural to search for evidence about population recognition of occupational natures and needs. Discussion about one strand of such recognition is provided by considering the connection between social activists (Marx, Ruskin, and Morris), the advent of feminism, and the genesis of occupational therapy and beyond. The section on ancient and modern rules for health considers how changing values about meaning affected views of health in earlier times, and as an example, looks particularly at the development of occupation's use in mental health. The chapter concludes by expanding the determinants of well-being or illness introduced in the last chapter to include the idea of "being through doing."

Being as a Determinant of Population Health

DEFINING THE CONCEPT

In the context it is used here, the meaning of "being" is described in dictionaries as the essential nature of someone; their essence or substance, soul, spirit, psyche, or core; their inner person or persona; such as in "his whole being is musical."[1,2] That is, it refers to the quality, state of existence, or the qualities that constitute living.[3] Aristotle was one of the first philosophers known to inquire into the nature of "being," and his view encompassed the idea that the "true essence of an object is independent of matter, so its 'being' is independent of the material world."[4] More recently from the 19th century, existentialist philosophers such as Hegel, Heidegger, and Sartre have also considered the concept of being. Hegel wrote extensively about it describing, for example, a state in which people can allow themselves to be absorbed and can find repose. He called that "being-within-self."[4] However, he determined that it was difficult to find the true meaning because once it is stripped of all predicates (an object's existence is defined by its relation to other objects and the actions it undertakes), it is simply nothing. Heidegger continued the search to find the meaning of being and distinguished different modes for objects and people with the latter being described as Da-sein (there-being), while Sartre distinguished between being-in-itself and being-for-itself to ground his concept of freedom ontologically.[4]

Like existential philosophers, psychologists have found the concept intriguing. Maslow, a trailblazer in the field, suggests that existential notions of being address the concept and experience of identity in the science of human nature. He prefers the term *identity* to *essence, existence,* or *ontology* because it is easier to understand. He speaks of the value of existentialism resting on experiential knowledge rather than "systems of concepts or abstract categories or a prioris."[5] Maslow came to describe being as the "contemplation and enjoyment of the inner life," explaining that "being in a state of being needs no future because it is already there."[5]

As the last chapter highlighted the functional aspects of doing involved in acquiring the prerequisites of survival and health, it dealt with the rational as opposed to Romantic concepts. Rationalism grew from Enlightenment ideas at the time modern science and research gained a foothold in popular thought. Enlightenment thinkers saw "the world as a wondrous machine and valued rational intelligence and man's power to understand and exploit nature."[6] Economic rationalism of the present day incorporates similar ideology. The dominance of rationalist views explains to some extent why the notion of being is difficult to appreciate in health terms. Being is, essentially, a concept compatible with the Romantic school of thought that emerged in the 18th century. Romantics held an organic view of nature in which people were perceived as "playful, creative, inspired and unpredictable beings."[6] These capacities were upheld as worthy of celebration and enhancement in contrast to rationalists who sought to control them.[6] Both rational doing and Romantic being are aspects of human identity, health, and well-being because of the interconnectedness of the human brain and the dependence on the external environment. Both demand expression and fulfilment in order for people to experience physical, mental, and social well-being and to be able to resist disease as far as it is possible.

In the introduction to this section of the book, I included a figure depicting how students of occupational science and therapy had identified the need for satisfaction, meaning, fulfilment, and purpose as part of a doing-to-being continuum.[7] Other concepts can be added. These include states of being associated with having choice and energy and being challenged, finding balance and opportunity and being free, being creative and finding enjoyment, being committed and being able to cope. The word *being* is frequently used alongside occupational roles to express the essential nature or interests that drive individuals. We talk about people, for example, "being" parents, "being" students, "being" a breadwinner, or "being" a football player, and we talk about well-being.

Its Place in Public Health

Existential philosophy and psychology advance the notion that meaning, choice, and purpose are necessary to well-being. This suggests that lack of meaning, choice, or purpose will result in the opposite (ie, "being" ill). Roger Crisp comments that while philosophers' use of "well-being" is usually applied to how good a person's life is for him or her, the "popular use of the term usually relates to health,"[8] and so it is not surprising that well-being is the starting point of the WHO definition of health. The theme of this chapter highlights the WHO directive that health is dependent on more than the acquisition of the prerequisites discussed in the last chapter. It also encompasses the view that people need to find meaning and purpose in their lives and to experience a sense of belonging. More than this, it accepts that each person is unique and will have differing needs.[9]

These views address the "being" attributes of engagement in occupation and are closely related to what many researchers in the area describe as quality of life. Literature pertaining to the latter addresses a range of attributes that can be related to the "doing" aspects discussed in the last chapter, such as basic needs, freedom, safety, and security. Other attributes to be discussed in the next chapter are items such as enhancement, expectations, possibilities, hopes, and fulfilment. In terms of being, as well as the basic aspect of a person's unique identity, "quality of life" literature has mentioned such attributes as ability, adaptation, belonging, control, diversity, enjoyment, flexibility, happiness, knowledge, opportunities, pleasure, satisfaction, self-esteem, socialness, and spirituality. In a negative sense, it has pointed to distress, isolation, mismatches, and stress.[10] In terms of occupation, it can be claimed that people experience well-being at times of absorbing interest, even when physical, social, and mental capacities are stretched to meet a challenge. At such times, people are said to be able to resist disease and seem impervious to many problems and difficulties that beset them.

Many of the attributes mentioned above can be directly related to mental health. As the WHO sets forth, "Mental health is not just the absence of mental disorder."[11] It is also a state of well-being dependent on people realizing their abilities, coping with the normal stresses of life, working productively and fruitfully, and making a contribution to their community. This type of well-being is dependent on environments that enhance psychosocial, emotional, cognitive, and physical development of children and adolescents and that create opportunities for everyone, including people as they work, those who are unemployed, or the aged.[11] Less obvious perhaps is the relationship between physical or social illness and realizing abilities, coping with stress, working productively, and contributing to communities. It is, in fact, attributable to the interconnectedness of brain mechanisms. This results in whatever affects one aspect of health having a flow-on effect to the others. Unhappiness, for example, can lead to physical disorders or social problems, perhaps as often as it manifests in a depressive illness.

Public health practitioners of whatever discipline have to be cognizant of, and attentive to, the possible causes of disorder due to the interactive physiology and nature of people. While research into the minute and particular aspects of cause and effect is important, of no less importance is research into the holistic interaction between systems, people, and the social and natural environment.[5] Occupation and being, as well as doing, are important parts of this whole and must not be overlooked.

Being Through Doing: Biological Needs, Natural Health, and Finding Meaning

Frankl, in *Man's Search for Meaning*, pronounced that central to both quality of life and the human condition is the quest for meaning.[12] If that is so, finding meaning is central to being and will be tied to both biological needs and natural health. Meaning appears to rely on people making use of their inherent capacities and abilities as well as meeting their spiritual needs. Some basic biological features or capacities that set humans apart from other species have already been discussed, and that discussion requires expansion to take the relationship between being and health into account. This discussion will first describe what is meant by "capacities" and go on to consider the natures of consciousness and creativity that are particularly relevant to being human.

BIOLOGICALLY BASED CAPACITIES

Meaningful and purposeful use of time is part of our biological heritage, evident from very early in evolution. As Selye observes, "our brain slips into chaos and confusion unless we constantly use it for work that seems worthwhile to us," however much "the average person thinks he works for economic security or social status."[13] Capacities critical to complex, self-initiated being through doing that appear to go beyond meeting the prerequisites of health require consideration. Apart from food to maintain the body and neuronal systems, there appears to be a need for food to nourish minds, spirits, and physical attributes that arise from differences attributable to unique DNA. The substance of such food is provided by what people want to do but are not obliged to do to meet their particular needs as human beings. This ties the quest for meaning with being human.

Texts and articles reviewed in the exploration of "capacity" imply it is central to each of the trilogy of doing, being, and becoming. Words such as *genetic potential, characteristic, trait, talents,* and *ability* are used interchangeably. Dictionaries and thesauruses use words such as *faculty, capability,* and *trait.* These extend our understanding, with capability defined as "power of undeveloped faculty" and faculty as "aptitude for any special kind of action; power inherent in the body or an organ; [and] mental power."[14] Trait has synonyms, such as "characteristic quality, distinguishing mark, attribute, feature, peculiarity, speciality, and idiosyncrasy,"[2,15] but in most instances implies an observable rather than a potential aptitude. Capacity, then, in this context, is used to mean the innate and perhaps undeveloped potential, aptitude, ability, talent, trait, or power with which each individual is endowed. Capacities are the building blocks of occupational beings, each of whom have unique natures and personalities expressed through what they do.

To corroborate the idea of individual variation in capacities, it is useful to consider ideas and evidence from studies relating to human difference. In terms of genetic endowment, the range of human capacities is, on the whole, common to the species, although individual variation is the rule. As geneticists and biologists have come closer to understanding the structure and function of genes by using biochemical technology, ranging from electrophoresis of proteins to very sophisticated analysis of DNA structures, "they have uncovered inherited variation, or polymorphism, at almost every level of organization" to the extent that "it is certain that every human being who has lived or ever will live is genetically unique."[16] The biological processes that have increased genetic variability throughout evolution are "mutation, sexual recombination, genetic drift, gene flow, and increase in population size."[17]

Not least because of the evolutionary pressures of natural selection, capacities differ between genders. Difference is due to hormonal factors under the control of genetic influences and levels of testosterone, estrogen, and progesterone; cerebral maturation rates; cerebral laterality; language; and spatial skills.[18] Differences in cerebral maturation rates appear to result in different capacities regardless of gender. Waber has demonstrated that adolescents who mature early perform better in verbal tasks, and those who mature later perform better on spatial tasks.[19] It is generally understood that men ordinarily mature physically and mentally more slowly than women and that maturation rate is a critical determinant of cerebral asymmetry. Waber's material supports the idea that just as capacities can differ between individuals and genders, so are there differences because of age. Discrete neurophysiological mechanisms start functioning at specific times during ontogenesis. This can be observed when infants become responsive, often quite suddenly, to specific external stimuli.[20] In fact, because "connections among the cells are ... not precisely prespecified in the genes," epigenetic processes start in embryo when "key events occur only if certain previous events have taken place."[21] After birth, apart from obvious physical capacities, such as crawling, walking,[22] and talking, whose appearances are well documented, "at a certain point in ontogenesis, each individual begins to realize his or her own powers to direct attention, to think, to feel, to will, and to remember. At that point a new agency develops within awareness. This is the self."[23]

With knowledge of the self comes an increased need to conform to others of the species and to demonstrate particular skills and capacities that are socioculturally valued.

Capacities:

Change in various ways as an individual grows up, since every competence need [has] not appeared fully formed at birth. Some competencies improve with learning and practice during childhood and youth, and all do not improve at the same rate, or necessarily are perfected during a lifetime.[22]

Expansion of the brain has provided humans with "behavioral possibilities undreamed of in other even closely related species."[17] People have the potential not only for making and using tools but also for talking, planning, dreaming of the future, and creating entirely new environments because[17]:

Inside the cortex lie separate centers with specific functions, which we like to call talents. Mathematical ability is a separate talent from the ability to move gracefully; verbal agility is distinct from the previous two. There is a range of different functions, for smelling, for thinking, for moving, for calculating that the brain possesses.[24]

However, as talents (or capacities) "are not given equally to all of us; people are not as consistent as might have been imagined," Ornstein and Sobel contend that it is necessary to study the collage of "specialized neural systems each of which possesses a rich concentration of certain abilities."[24] This will assist understanding of the brain's generic organization and its concern with health and with talents of a specific nature or tendency.[24] One such study led Gagne to group aptitudes and talents into aptitude domains, such as intellectual, creative, socioaffective, and sensorimotor, and fields of talents, such as academic, technical, artistic, interpersonal, and athletic.[25] He also groups primary capacities, such as seeing, standing, perceiving color, or touching, which are complex physiological processes in their own right; there are other more complex capacities, such as problem-solving, exploration, consciousness, creativity, and so on. These more complex capacities are examples of the integrative workings of many independent and interdependent systems.

Capacities are responsive to inner needs and external variables, as well as being capable of rapid reaction to emergency. They seldom work in isolation, but combine with others according to the environment and experience. They are multifunctional, with the combination of specific capacities increasing the potential variability of what people demonstrate through what they do. Each capacity is "relatively independent of the others," but they may "work in concert."[20] A single mental capacity may represent a "family of competencies" that Harvard psychologist Howard Gardner describes as "frames of mind."[26]

In the last chapter, the evolution of language was discussed mainly in terms of communication. The capacity to communicate is not the only benefit of language. As Percy Bysshe Shelley observed in *Prometheus Unbound*, "He gave man speech, and speech created thought, which is a measure of the universe."[27] Although Piaget argues that "language is not enough to explain thought, because the structures that characterize thought have their roots in action and in sensorimotor mechanisms that are deeper than linguistics,"[28] language allows individuals to explore ideas, to think in abstract as well as concrete terms, and to bring to their occupational pursuits concepts based on their unique life experience and ways of thinking. Lewin suggests "mankind's exaggerated intellectual power focuses on the need to build a better mental construct of reality ... It may have required a complex propositional language, not so much that we could converse with others, but so we could think better."[29]

Thinking about and searching for truths about life and its meaning must have developed along with language. It is probable that intellectual activities of the type now called philosophy first emerged as wonder at the natural world and that early belief systems were based on animals and environmental forces important in survival terms. This speculation is founded on the types of images humans left behind in cave drawings and in ornamentation and the fact that the earliest monumental buildings, such as those in Ur in

Mesopotamia, had religious significance frequently associated with natural phenomena. Early Greek philosophy reflects this dual interest in matters natural and spiritual with Thales (c. 600 BC) reported as saying that "all things are full of gods."[30] It was not until the Sophists came into prominence, shortly before Socrates, that philosophy became interested in mankind apart from nature and in reasoning per se. This interest led to a recurring theme in philosophy and psychology—the debate about the nature of consciousness. Here, it is considered from the perspective of its role in the occupational nature of humans rather than in philosophical history.

Consciousness

Consciousness is example of a "super-capacity" being a combination of, and integral to, many others. It is defined variously in dictionaries: in one as "a quality of the mind generally regarded to comprise qualities such as subjectivity, self-awareness, sentience, sapience, and the ability to perceive the relationship between oneself and one's environment"[31]; in another as "the state of being conscious; inward sensibility of something; knowledge of one's own existence, sensations, cognitions, etc.; and the thoughts and feelings, collectively, of an individual or of an aggregate of people."[32] This latter, particularly, suggests a closeness of fit to definitions of being. It has been described as "the tool of the social animal,"[29] and by Watson as "the capacity to see ourselves and to put ourselves in someone else's place. We are not only self-aware, but conscious of being so."[33] It is "the key ... [and] the power which motivates and drives all human affairs."[33] Consciousness enables us to know what we know and to experience our own feelings and the outcomes of what we do. It "is a kind of continuous apprehension of an inner reality, the reality of one's mental states and activities,"[34] providing us with a model of the world "based on sense and body information, expectations, fantasy and crazy hopes, and other cognitive processes."[35] Philosophers divide it according to experience itself or the processing of the things in experience. The first of these is known as phenomenal consciousness and the second as access consciousness.[36]

Edelman has proposed a biological model of the evolution of consciousness according to his theory of neuronal group selection. The processes of natural selection gave rise to form and tissue patterns, which are the basis of behavior. From this developed a "primary repertoire of variant neuronal groups in the brain"[21] that is involved in selection. Selection "assumes that, during behavior, anatomical synaptic connections are selectively strengthened or weakened by specific biochemical processes,"[21] carving out a variety of functioning circuits. "Correlation and coordination of ... selection events are achieved by 're-entrant' signalling and by strengthening of interconnections between the maps" in the brain.[21] During evolution, this selection process linked the brainstem and limbic system, which take care of bodily functions, internal states, and values, with the thalamo-cortical system, which perceives and categorizes world events. Together, through "value-category" memory, they enable perceptual categorization and the subsequent development of primary consciousness. This, in conjunction with changes to the structure of the brain, such as Broca and Wernicke areas, in quite a short timespan evolved higher order consciousness.[21] Edelman concludes that consciousness depends upon perceptual and conceptual categorization, semantics, syntax, and phonology, all of which allow learning to occur.

In considering the purpose of consciousness, it would seem that awareness of the possible consequences of action is necessary for an organism with free will as a guard to ensure survival, although individuals are generally unaware of the process. Ornstein hypothesizes that consciousness vetoes or permits every action that is initiated at an unconscious level.[35] It does so despite the "many different kinds of minds" within brain organization.[35] Consciousness and occupation are part of a 2-way process. Complex occupational behavior would be impossible without consciousness, and the types of occupations in which individuals choose to engage can affect states of consciousness. For example, Csikszentmihalyi has found that "when challenges are high and personal skills are used to the utmost, we experience a rare state of consciousness," which he calls "flow."[37] Flow is enjoyable, narrows attention to a clearly defined goal, provides a sense of control over actions although awareness of time disappears, and people are absorbed and involved. "The activity can be wildly different, but when people are deeply involved [in] meeting a manageable challenge, the state of mind they report is the same the world over."[37-39]

Consciousness, from Csikszentmihalyi's viewpoint, depends particularly on 3 other capacities. He believes "attention, awareness, and memory ... act as a buffer between genetic and cultural instructions on the one hand, and behavior on the other."[23] His view that "consciousness frees the organism from its dependence on the forces that created it and provides a certain [if precarious] control over our behavior"[23] is similar or complementary to that already described. Consciousness, in fact, negates the need for a multitude of separate genetic programs to link stimuli and responses and "increases the possibilities" between "programmed instructions and adaptive behaviors."[23] The "self-system" has a main goal to "ensure its own survival."[23] To this effect, "attention, awareness, and memory are directed to replicate those states of consciousness that are congenial to self and to eliminate those that threaten its existence."[23] On the down side, consciousness has given humans enormous independence and power, with the potential to destroy the environment from which they evolved and on which they depend, and "it is by no means certain that [this] choice and control ... will serve us better than the blind instructions of our genes."[23] Consciousness has the unenviable role of prompting humans to consider the consequences of what they do. It is central in the balancing act between occupational achievement, health, and illness in both the short- and long-term.[40-42] Its watchdog role is made complex by its susceptibility, just as other capacities, to enculturation.

Raising the consciousness of people about lifestyle issues relating to ill health is an integral part of other agendas, such as those aimed at health education, cultural awareness, feminism, social justice, or sustainable ecology. This book is aimed at raising consciousness about the critical relationship between occupation (doing, being, and becoming) and health that is poorly understood. This broader consciousness raising is important as part of a holistic view of health and well-being.[43-45] Advocates of transpersonal psychology, for example, believe that an "optimal state of consciousness" is central in the achievement of positive health because it enables "deep states of relaxation, increased inner awareness, ... body-mind self-awareness" and makes effective choices more accessible.[46,47] They link psychological and physiological states, incorporating notions from many Asian religions. Similar to the pragmatic view that the brain minds the body, the "psychophysiological principle" claims that every conscious or unconscious change in either physiologic or mental-emotional state is accompanied by an appropriate change in the other and that health can be facilitated by awareness and self-regulation of normally unconscious processes.[47]

Creativity

Creativity, like consciousness, is one of the most complex of human capacities. Like capacity, the ideas about creativity that will be introduced here are relevant to both the last chapter on doing and the next chapter on becoming through doing and being. It is subject to many different interpretations, resulting—as it does—from the amalgam of a rich variety of other capacities. Gordon suggests "to create is one of man's most basic impulses."[48] Jung classified it as 1 of 5 major instinctive forces in humans,[49] and Sinnott argues that it is in "inherent creativeness" of the ordinary affairs of people that the "ultimate source" of creativeness is to be found.[50]

Creativity is a capacity that has excited much interest and discussion, yet sources seldom agree on a definition, with one paper written in 1953 offering no fewer than 25.[51] The word derives from the Greek *krainein*, meaning to fulfill, and the Latin *creare*, meaning to make.[52] Dictionaries describe it as the "ability to bring into existence or being, to originate, to beget, to shape, to bring about, to invest with new character, and to be inventive."[14,53] On the Web, definitions and descriptions encompass creativity as a mental phenomena, skill, tool, vision, or action capable of originating and developing innovation, inspiration, or insight as interpretation, writing, science, problem solving, and lateral thinking.[54] A recent theory offered by Schmid, who advances a concept of creativity integral to an occupational perspective of health based to some extent on the earlier version of this work, proposes, "humans have both the innate capacity to be creative and the biological need to express it. When creativity is adequately expressed through everyday activities, it has a major impact on health and well-being."[55]

William Morris suggested that creativity is an integral part of the human contest with nature:

> But a man, making something which he feels will exist because he is working at it and wills it, is exercising the energies of his mind and soul as well as of his body. Memory and imagination help him as he works. Not only his own thoughts, but the thoughts of the men of past ages guide his hands; and, as a part of the human race, he creates.[56]

The extent of early humans' creativity has been hard to assess. Lewin, who traces examples back perhaps 300,000 years, suggests that the creation of paintings, carvings, and engravings represents a true abstraction of thought and mind[29]; others disagree. Although early humans appeared to possess very little in the form of creative artifacts, this may be a consequence of an "inescapable conflict between mobility and material culture."[57] For example, the !Kung and other first nation peoples carry only about 12 kilograms each when they travel, so most of their culture is carried in their heads. This reminds us that creativity is much more than the manufacture of material artifacts and the making of stories, music, and dance. It includes those intellectual and abstract reasoning skills so dear to philosophers and academics and the evidences of culture that is carried in the minds and recreated regularly throughout history. Sinnott suggests that the biological basis for creativity is the "organizing, pattern forming, questing quality" of life itself, which, when applied to behavior and the complexity of the human brain, results in an almost infinite number of new mental patterns.[50] Whatever form creativity takes, it requires abstract conceptualization that some describe as the ultimate human gift.

Marx's suggestion that labor is the collective creative activity of mankind appears compatible with the idea that it was an integration of creative abstract occupations and tool technology that evolved eventually into high technology through cultural evolution. High technology is the epitome of human creativity, yet the products of the industrial and technological age have had a serious effect on many forms of individual creativity. For example, although not true of all people, many no longer make products that they need, preferring to buy, and many seldom create their own entertainment, preferring to watch and listen to prepackaged material. Similarly, the creative behavior of many children has changed with the advent of television or personal computers as hours are spent in viewing or manipulating images rather than experimenting, playing, or creating their own.

Many psychologists, from different branches, have offered theories about creativity.[5,48,58-61] Psychoanalytic theorists have suggested that Freud and Adler accepted the view of creativity held early this century that limited the concept to the arts.[61,62] The arts were held to be socially acceptable activities that were an outlet for sublimation of libidinal energy and other unconscious conflicts, drives, and needs. Creativity was seen as stemming from neurotic tendencies, offering the resolution of guilt feelings and compensation for feelings of inferiority.[63-65] Despite this, Freud recognized parallels between the creative nature of children's play and the creative artist, and, along with others of the psychoanalytical school, suggested that creative people were subject to both better health and more sickness than the average.[62,66]

Humanist and Gestalt psychologists hold the view that creativity is much more than innate talent or genius exemplified by exceptional individuals in the arts. They have linked creativity evident in all aspects of life with individual potential, and the experience of health.[67] The Institute of Personality Assessment at the University of California has identified particular traits as characterizing creative people. They are described as intuitive, open, spontaneous, expressive, independent, self-accepting, flexible not authoritarian, and autonomous, functioning best when working independently on their interests. They are relatively free from fear and are not interested in detail but in meaning and implications, with the ability to synthesize and integrate material and experiences. They have well-developed intrinsic values and are goal directed.[68] Indeed, the links between creativity (and, by inference, occupation that provides meaning and purpose) and mental health appear strong; for example, high creativity has been found to correlate with a high degree of normal mature positive self-esteem.[69]

Creativity in occupation can be observed when people are solving the problems of daily life or engaged in intellectual, artisan, playful, or sociocultural activity or technological advancement. It is one of the inherent capacities that emerge or peak at different parts of the life cycle.[59,70-73] However, creativity can often be regarded as behavior outside "mainstream conventional mores and habits," and despite the apparent links with health:

> *Creativity rather like motherhood and apple-pie, gets much praised in principle, but much derided in fact. Popular legend sees creativity serve as a refuge for the outsider with imagination—a stable society prefers the majority of its citizens to respect convention and not to "rock the boat." Similarly, a manager of employees may sing the praises of creativity and innovation while showing reluctance to implement radically different and potentially disruptive ways of operation.*[54]

Reynolds reports that recent studies support the notion of creativity affecting mental and physical health and well-being in a positive way, but that limited research experience of investigators and poor agreement on definitions of creativity makes it difficult to be conclusive.[74] Examples she provides include studies of older people engaged in artwork that have reported positive effects on self-esteem, personal growth, and community involvement[75,76] and a study of a choir that found most of the 84 subjects reported social benefits, about three-quarters reported emotional improvements, and just over half experienced improvements in physical health.[77] While more conclusive research is evidently needed, the extensive range of physical characteristics and of higher cortical capacities that are central to consciousness and creativity appear to prompt, motivate, and enable an infinite variety of occupational exploration, experimentation, interest, choice, and skill, as well as imbuing people with the need for purpose and meaning. Indeed, the complexities of what people do, and if they feel their lives are meaningful because of what they do, enables many to adapt to and survive healthily and happily in many different environments.

SURVIVAL PRESSURES

Survival pressures would have provided motivation, opportunity, and meaning for engagement in a variety of individual and community occupations that addressed the obvious health risks of the day. In pursuit of such, early humans could develop capacities and talents as they engaged in a range of physical, mental, and social exercise in tune with nature. Hunter-gatherer societies, however, left a legacy of more than stone tools to demonstrate the range of occupations valued by them. Deep in caves, they drew and colored images, usually depicting creatures and humans who were a part of their world. They carved throwing sticks and other implements, along with creating "new and stylistically more complex tools," and there is archeological evidence of "a rich ceremonial life based on complex concepts and rituals."[78] From that evidence and from study of hunter-gatherer people of recent times, it is possible to suggest that early in human history no formal differentiation or value loading existed between labor, leisure, or self-care in the lives of early humans; that doing was not restricted to acquiring the absolute essentials for survival; and that finding meaning and satisfaction was achieved through many forms of doing, not only those related to continued existence.

The mixed economy of hunting and gathering brought with it time for leisure,[57,79,80] Wax observing, "I do not believe that any Bushman could tell us—or would be interested in telling us—which part of activity was work and which was play."[81] The arbitrary separation of doing leisure from doing work appears to have occurred fairly recently, with more time available for leisure in hunter-gatherer societies than in agrarian or industrial societies.[82] Both hunter-gatherer and early agrarian societies seem to have operated in such a way that a natural balance between activity and rest occurred. Their economic activities had built-in leisure components, such as singing and telling stories while they worked.[83] In some recent hunter-gatherer societies, there is no generic word for work or doing but many for specific occupations such as hunting.[84,85] Such a lack of distinction could be advantageous to health and well-being in that individuals are able to develop their own traits and capacities according to biological need and opportunity without subjugating their choice of what to do to economic efficiencies or regard for sociocultural "rules" that have made occupational choice so complex in present times.

With the gradual extension of agriculture, people continued to engage in doing more than was essential to survive. They sought satisfaction, meaning, and perhaps joy through the use of creative talents that also changed methods of acquiring the necessities of life. Evidence of this early use of doing more than was necessary is provided not only by development of hammers, axes, wheels, and boats; by activities such as spinning, weaving, mining, metal working, and bread and beer making; by the building of houses and towns; but also by the use of "words, symbols and probably numbers."[86] As their skills expanded, humans experimented with material resources, began to challenge the environment and adapt it to meet their own perceived needs and comfort, and they changed their social structures and behaviors to accommodate such change. As agriculture developed, so did the diversity of occupations, along with an expansion of goods and services regarded as necessary.[83]

It is possible to trace occupational developments in "being" as distinct from "essential doing" from the time that architecture, art, writing, commerce, religion, increased technological innovation, and social administration became recognizable in modern terms since the formation of cities, between 10,000 to 6000 years ago. Administrative functions, organization, and control of cities in those early days, often combined with religious activity and monumental architecture, developed to help communities cope with socioenvironmental stress, uncertainty, and unpredictability.[29] The stressors arose from within communities living in much larger, specialized populations than they had been used to, and also in response to possible dangers to the community from outside. Neff observes that during this period, occupation began to acquire distinctions and qualifications and an increasingly complicated infrastructure of evaluative meanings, including a distinction between labor and leisure and, one can surmise, between doing and being.[85]

Other forms of occupation apart from labor serve the built-in need to exercise, maintain, and develop the capacities inherent to each individual. Leisure, in postmodern societies, for example, frequently serves as the mechanism for children and adults to exercise their bodies, to be social, to develop their creativity, to fulfil "wishes at the fantasy level," and to sort out problems, as well as having a crucial role in teaching and maintaining "fluency with roles and conventions."[87] Its difference from work in meeting basic human needs is related directly to how it is valued by societies. The ennobling of one aspect of occupation over others may have done disservice to the need to be true to self. It has the potential to deprive individuals of a balanced use of their innate capacities, of using some and not others to the detriment of overall well-being. The more holistic notion of the preindustrial society of the Baluchi of Western Pakistan has much to recommend it; there, occupation is divided into the sphere of obligatory duty and the sphere of one's own will, with the latter being the valued domain in which individuals choose to spend energy and creativity.[81] In terms of labor, the valued domain in the postmodern world, Neff believes it takes on a "servile" nature when subjugation of one people to another is part of the equation. To dominant groups, it may appear "degrading to perform certain kinds of work"; however, "it is not work itself that is degrading but the power relationships and social structure which surround it."[85]

Until the industrial revolution, as Jones observed, "labor/time-absorbing employment was the norm in human experience."[86] Then, even social and celebratory customs as an integral part of work diminished, and the division between work and leisure became clearer. This division was not absolute or the same for each individual,[88] and in many traditional workshops, ritual patterns of fellowship and celebration continued.[89] However, the change was so evident that it encouraged entrepreneurs to recognize the commercial potential of separated entertainment, which has led to one of the most powerful industries of the present day.[90] The separation of work from leisure is also demonstrated in the way leisure was deplored by Victorian explorers who perceived, in their encounters with hunter-gatherer peoples, that their "nonwork ethic" was a major reason for lack of progress.

RECOGNITION OF PEOPLE'S OCCUPATIONAL NATURES

At the time of the Industrial Revolution, the extreme dichotomy of economic and social conditions and the nature of occupations led intellectuals as various as Karl Marx, John Ruskin, and William Morris to consider the effects of the industrial era on the occupational nature of humankind. Some of their ideas were similar to those expressed by Renaissance Utopians, that what people do can provide their being with a source of joy if it is creative and provides pleasure in the exercise of a range of skills.[91,92] The brief account of the views of Marx, Ruskin, and Morris that follows demonstrates a connection between these eminent authorities and the establishment of occupational therapy as a health profession in both North America and the United Kingdom. This connection explains how occupational therapy practice in health care holds what are often unrecognized concerns about the nature of humankind and issues of occupational justice and public health.

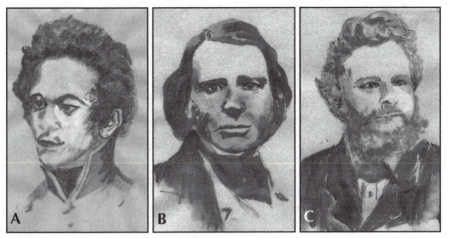

Figure 4-1. (A) Karl Marx. (B) Ruskin. (C) Morris.

From Marx, Ruskin, and Morris to Occupational Therapy and Beyond

Karl Marx (Figure 4-1) in his early works formulated a "materialistic theory of history," arguing that it is social and economic conditions, rather than metaphysical or religious ideas, that drive human history and determine how people live.[93-965] Marx had not intended these papers for publication but following a Soviet translation in 1932, they created enormous interest and provided new insights on his concepts of alienation and the self-creation of humanity. Influenced by Hegel, who described "labor as man's act of self-creation,"[97] Marx founded much of his philosophy on the idea that "free conscious activity constitutes the species character of man."[92] He discussed praxis as the free, universal, creative, and self-creative activity that differentiates humans from other animals and by which they make and change themselves and their world.[92] To do that, such occupation should uphold dignity, enable fulfilment, and contribute to well-being. When work is simply a process to earn a wage for subsistence and is destructive to physical or intellectual potential, workers are alienated by it. It is a contradiction of the nature of humankind, economic conditions having become more powerful than individuals.[92] Fischer comments on this argumen by stating, "the reduction of labor to empty wage earning is now accepted without question."[97] Marx criticized the capitalist industrial society because it prevented individuals from being able to cultivate their unique talents, alienated them from their species' need to be active, productive beings, and, in fact, led to misery, exhaustion, and mental debasement. The concepts of alienation, of people as creative beings, and that compulsion and subservience can act against the health-giving biological function of occupation were major themes of Marx's theories.

Ruskin (1819–1900) and Morris (1834–1896) differed from Marx in that they came to social criticism from the viewpoint of creative artists.

Ruskin (see Figure 4-1) was a well-known art critic who experienced bouts of illness as a young man and found that a simple occupational regimen of walking, reading, writing, and painting was remedial.[98] Later in his life, starting with the publication of *Unto This Last* in 1862, Ruskin turned to writing about and experimenting in the field of political economy.[99] Like Coleridge[100] and Carlyle,[101] he challenged classical political economists as ignoring the human factor. His central theme was that the quality of life that citizens enjoy is the true measure of a nation's prosperity, rather than the accumulation of wealth for its own sake. He attacked the boredom and monotony of the Victorian industrial system and the disconnection between leisure and work, and he advocated that training schools should be established at government expense for all children.[102] These schools should teach the laws of health, habits of gentleness and justice, and the "calling" by which each would live. In conjunction with these, he proposed that the government should establish factories and workshops, producing high standard goods, to run in competition with private business. Any person out of employment should be admitted immediately to a government school, trained, and given work for wages. For those unable to work, he proposed special training schemes or "tending" in the case of sickness. For those who objected to work, he suggested they be compelled to work in less desirable jobs, their wages retained until each learned to respect the laws of employment.

Morris (see Figure 4-1) was the most notable of Ruskin's followers. He was influenced by Marx to the extent that he joined a Marxist socialist group and later formed his own socialist organization. Known, in the main, these days as a poet, architect, painter, printer, and craftsman, Morris was also a notable social reformer.[103] As a craftsman, he deplored the machine age and the fact that commerce had become a "sacred religion," turning work from a solace into a burden, and for the majority a mere drudgery.[104] He accepted that "Nature does not give us our livelihood gratis; we must win it by toil of some sort or degree,"[105] but he also believed that the necessary work of society could be accomplished without overstrain or difficulty. Arguing against the "stifling overorganization common to both capitalist and socialist versions of modern industrial society,"[106] Morris suggested that most work could be done with actual pleasure in the doing.[105] His descriptions of a fictional Utopia are based on his ideas of work in which people are free and independent and where poverty, exploitation, competition, and money all disappear.[107] He recognized the importance of all people being fulfilled and satisfied and finding meaning through doing, and that this was a health issue. Morris wrote, "There are two types of work—one good, the other bad; one not far removed from a blessing, a lightening of life; the other a mere curse, a burden to life."[105] Of the first he explained, "... to all living things there is a pleasure in the exercise of their energies, and that even beasts rejoice in being lithe and swift and strong," and that "worthy work carries with it the hope of pleasure in rest, the hope of pleasure in using what it makes, and the hope of pleasure in our daily creative skill."[105] He described the second type as "worthless"; "mere toiling to live, that we may live to toil."[105] Anticipating an ecological view of health-giving being through doing Morris argued:

> Wealth is what Nature gives us and what a reasonable man can make out of the gifts of Nature for his reasonable use. The sunlight, the fresh air, the unspoiled face of the earth, food, raiment, housing necessary and decent; the storing up of knowledge of all kinds, and the power of disseminating it; means of free communication between man and man; works of art, the beauty which man creates when he is most a man, most aspiring and thoughtful—all things which serve the pleasure of people, free, manly and uncorrupted. This is wealth.[105]

It is also health through doing and being in tune with the natural world.

Marx, Ruskin, and Morris believed that meaningful and purposeful occupation is basic to human nature. They saw that the economic, industrial, and commercial use of this innate characteristic was destructive both to individuals and to humankind in the long term. The challenges aimed at changing the values of industry and commerce led by socialist comment achieved some success, but social inequities and conditions of work have remained the major focus of debate and action. The basic ideological arguments about the nature of doing and being and the human need for purposeful creative

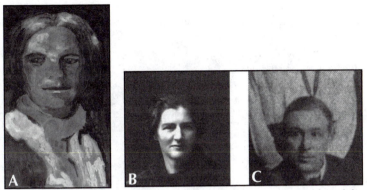

Figure 4-2. (A) Octavia Hill. (B) Elizabeth Casson. (Reproduced by kind permission of the British Association and College of Occupational Therapists.) (C) George Barton.

occupation were and still are, on the whole, overlooked. Mainstream socialism "became enmeshed in the 'quasi-socialist machinery' of party politics" and followed the Fabian vision of a technocratic society with enlightened leadership.[106,108] Workers continued, in better conditions, to be servants of machines and, for many people, there was little opportunity for meaning or creativity or even the chance to be involved in a total process of production.

George Barton (Figure 4-2), a founder of the American Occupational Therapy Association, who had studied with Morris, provides one link in the chain connecting an occupation-focused social activism with the establishment of occupational therapy early in the 20th century. Another important link in the connection is provided by Octavia Hill (see Figure 4-2), granddaughter of physician and public and social health pioneer Thomas Southwood-Smith, mentioned earlier, who was, herself, a 19th century social activist in housing, the settlement movement, a pioneer of the use of occupation for social health, and a close friend of Ruskin. In England, Hill influenced the occupational philosophy of Elizabeth Casson (see Figure 4-2) whom she employed and who went on to establish the first school of occupational therapy in the United Kingdom.[98,109] Another contact was Alice Peck, a Canadian who visited Hill's Social Housing Schemes when at high school in England. There, she saw crafts being used to assist migrant women in skill development and was so impressed that during the World War I she returned to England as a volunteer teacher of craftwork in a hospital. Later, back in Montreal, she established the use of crafts in military hospitals before the formal advent of occupational therapy in Canada.[110] American Jane Addams (Figure 4-3) met Hill when researching settlement houses in England before she went on to found her own settlement house in Chicago, known as Hull House. It was there that the first recognized school of occupational therapy in the United States was established and where Eleanor Clark Slagle, a founder and pioneer of the profession, both trained and taught.

Hull House was developed to meet the social, economic, and health problems of new immigrants and assist them to adjust into the American industrial society of the turn of the century. The settlement movement, which aimed at developing and improving community life as a whole rather than providing particular social services, began when Samuel Barnett and his wife, who was also an employee of Hill, settled at Toynbee Hall in a poor area of London in 1884. The movement quickly spread to America—Neighborhood Guild, New York (now University Settlement) being established in 1886 and Hull House

Figure 4-3. Jane Addams. (Reprinted with permission from Jane Addams Memorial Collection [JAMC neg. 20], Special Collections, The University Library, The University of Illinois at Chicago.)

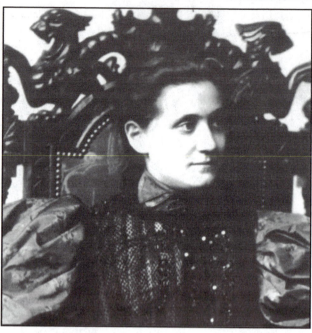

in Chicago in 1889.[111] The movement continued to grow throughout Europe and Asia, and it can be seen as a forerunner to today's community development movement. In settlement houses, a mix of local and imported people engaged in crafts, cultural activities, and worker and homemaker education. Together, the activities and the socialist ideals that were espoused formed a natural link with the Arts and Crafts Movement. Hull House provided the venue for many mutual aid, professional, trade, educational, athletic, theatrical, and musical organizations and groups[112] and was a center in which, from its inception, civic betterment, investigative research, and joint ventures with activist scholars from the University of Chicago toward social reform took place.[113] Addams described the Hull House Settlement as:

> *An experimental effort to aid in the solution of the social and industrial problems which are engendered by the conditions of life in a great city ... It is an attempt to relieve at the same time, the over accumulation at one end of society and the destitute at the other.*[114]

Hull House was founded and developed by women. As such, it was important in the history of women in the helping professions and feminism that has been accepted by the WHO as an aspect of social equity and a prerequisite of health.[115] Feminism grew from the same Enlightenment ideas that sparked humane and moral treatment, with early feminist activists concerning themselves with securing legal rights for women in education, marriage, and employment; with anti-slavery; with evangelical movements; and later with the struggle for votes.[116] Jane Addams, who was educated at one of numerous women's colleges in the American northeast, in an 1892 paper to the Ethical Culture Societies in Plymouth, Mass, applied her own experience to that of other educated young people. Many "have been shut off from the common labor by which they live which is a great source of moral and physical health. They feel a fatal want of harmony in their lives, a lack of coordination between thought and action," which can be provided by "a proper outlet for active faculties."[114] She recognized that lack of being through doing is not restricted to the poor and that "this young life, so sincere in its emotion and good phrases and yet so undirected, seems to me as pitiful as the other great mass of destitute lives."[114] Such beliefs formed by her experience, and a meeting with Morris, led to Addams' involvement in the establishment of the Chicago Arts and Crafts Society in 1897.[106]

Charles Norton, the first professor of fine arts at Harvard and a close friend of John Ruskin, is credited with bringing Ruskin's and Morris' ideology to America. Morris' views about work and a simple life away from materialistic, alienating cities found "particularly fertile ground in late 19th century America," which had long been influenced along similar lines by functionalist religious groups such as Puritans and Shakers.[102] Different groups accepted the ideology in different ways.

> *While Simple-Lifers stressed familiar virtues of discipline and work, aesthetes embodied a new style of high consumption appropriate to the developing consumer economy, and educational reformers offered manual training as a therapeutic mode of adjustment to the corporate world of work.*[106]

However, because the Puritan work ethic was so central to American culture, Ruskin's and Morris' conception of a preindustrial, creatively absorbed craftsperson became reinterpreted so that eventually no distinction was made between modern and pre-industrial work habits.[117] American Arts and Crafts leaders, along with their progressive contemporaries,[118,119] drew back from fundamental social change for social justice, favoring instead "a new kind of reform" aimed at "manipulating psychic well-being" and fitting individuals into emerging hierarchies.[106] This notion of "mental and moral growth" was compatible with 19th century American ideas about individualism, which was central to capitalism, its liberal democracy ideology, and values focusing on human rights.[120-122] Historian John William Draper describes the "wonderful, unceasing" activity and social development of the North following the Civil War as "the result of individualism; operating in an unbounded theatre of action. Everyone was seeking to do all that he could for himself."[123] For Ralph Waldo Emerson, America's favorite poet of the late 19th century, individualism was "the route to perfection—a spontaneous social order of self-determined, self-reliant, and fully developed humans."[124] Not for Draper and Emerson the belief of Marx, Ruskin, and Morris, that socialism was the path to fully developed humans in tune with their creative natures.

Similarly, at Hull House, where Ruskin's and Morris' photographs had pride of place, the Arts and Crafts ideology was reinterpreted from a socialist to an individualistic focus.[102] Addams accepted the inevitability of the industrial system, and instead of fighting for social justice against occupational inequities produced by mass production, she sought to revitalize working class lives by education toward personal fulfillment and best use of the industrial economy. This focus accepted the transformation to the 20th century work culture, which separated work from living, from being, and finding meaning and joy through doing, reinforcing the belief that paid employment is, and indeed should be, tedious and demanding.[106]

In terms of the role of women in American society at the time, the direction taken by the women leaders at Hull House was inevitable. To establish positions in which they could exercise their previously untapped capacities and potential, women needed to demonstrate their ability to work within dominant social values, rather than lead massive social change, even if they had perceived this to be necessary, which is doubtful. Establishing a female workforce in the professions and bringing to these a feminine, caring, moral viewpoint that flowed over from their earlier, often unacknowledged, family or charitable duties was, in itself, sufficiently challenging to the social order. In further relation to the origins of occupational therapy, Jessie Luther, who ran the Labour Museum at Hull House and taught craftwork between 1901–1903, continued to work in programs in which occupation was used for therapeutic purposes. In Newfoundland, Canada, she is said to have combined "Settlement" and "Arts and Crafts" philosophy "to create a viable social community" often in contact with Alice Peck mentioned earlier.[110] The interrelatedness of the social activist, occupation-focused pioneers appears to have been remarkable.

Both "Settlement" and "Arts and Crafts" philosophies were of the Romantic school. Hocking describes how Romantic and rationalist concepts informed the origins of occupational therapy on both sides of the Atlantic, but with the decline of the former as economic rationalism gained momentum, occupational therapists "substantially lost touch with their Romantic heritage":

> A key factor in this history was occupational therapists' ignorance of the philosophies on which their practice was founded. The outcome of this disruption to the profession's dual heritage was an era of practice that has been widely characterized as mechanistic. In short, occupational therapists lost the means to express their trust in their client's capacity to overcome their circumstances and to regain their lives and themselves.[6]

Neither the establishment of occupational therapy, nor the capitalist, individualist growth focus, nor the antimodern socialist revolution focus was successful in creating global awareness of the need to consider people's occupational nature in future social or health planning, although all went some way in that direction. The choice of individual education and reductionist medicine rather than social revolt and growth models of health can be viewed as factors leading to the diminution of the development of a broadly based, lasting "population focused occupational perspective." They also delayed careful consideration of Romantic, humanist, and socialist ideas as opposed to rationalist views until the present postindustrial difficulties once more raised some collective consciousness as to their importance. Despite the enormous energy and commitment of strong leaders, the exploration of humans as occupational beings was lost in the zeal to establish practical programs that were based on concepts of how humans' occupational natures could be best fitted to emerging social environments. As part of this process, the burgeoning occupational therapy that grew from humanist and socialist ideas became bound to individualist, medical, or other models for years to come. The other group of health professionals who might have a particular interest in doing, being, and population health—public health practitioners—were tied at that time to a practice geared to civic sanitary conditions and control of epidemics of infectious diseases.

Being Through Doing:
Ancient and Modern Rules for Health

Building on the foundation of the ancient rules for health and the modern directions of the WHO provided in the OCHP that were offered in earlier chapters here, discussion will center on how meanings can change as sociocultural conditions change. This is despite biological need for meaning remaining intact. For example, earlier it was explained how in Ancient Greece the choice of occupation (and the meaning that arose from it) was determined by citizenship or alternate status. That value changed over time, the Stoics (from the 3rd century BC) accepting there was no difference between Greek and others. Seneca (c55 BC–AD 41) reasoned that both had the same basic human nature and need for air and water, living and dying in the same way. In common with earlier ideas, Stoics explained people as social beings only able to experience fulfilment within the community of others and that "social responsibility" rather than the "individual task" was of vital importance. People had "a natural duty" to serve others, "either by taking part in civic affairs or by leading a contemplative life, or by combining these two ways of life."[125]

Irrespective of that was the "obligation to marry, to raise a family and to work"[126]; justice was the ultimate virtue.[125]

HOW CHANGING VALUES ABOUT MEANING AFFECTED VIEWS OF HEALTH IN EARLIER TIMES

Rather than considering a range of examples, I have chosen instead to highlight changes to how mental illness was perceived in the Western world and how the nature and meaning of doing and being altered as part of that.

Mental Health

The story can be picked up in medieval times when monasteries and nunneries provided the majority of institutional health care. Spiritual salvation was central to what people did either in the giving or receiving of treatment and in expectation of a future after death. All strata of societies were advised to engage in moral occupations, to seek solace in prayer, to make supplication through pilgrimage, and to engage in physical and/or charitable work.[98] Mental illness was the work of the devil and, as such, deplored so punitive means were sought to expel the cause. Some treatments that would be considered abusive in the present day were used to eliminate unwanted humors as well as the demonic possession. This continued to be the case for centuries with laws, such as that of 1714 in the United Kingdom that allowed for the "furiously mad and dangerous" to be locked up in a secure place. However, in this law, whipping was expressly forbidden.[127]

Authors of texts addressing mental illness or wellness began to discuss other causes and ways to prevent or improve it. Sanctorius Sanctorius (1561–1636) was a well-known Italian physician who is an example of those who suggested that doing as it relates to being is implicit in relation to affections of the mind according to the ancient rules for health. For example, "continual satisfaction of the mind" and "free perspiration" were said by him to overcome melancholy.[128] Such glimmers of light as those and the nonacceptance of whipping mentioned earlier began to appear from quite an early date and grew as numerous private "madhouses" (nomenclature of the period) were established throughout the 18th century, often catering for quite small numbers of wealthy clients.[129,130] Remedial approaches in these included the punitive in many but not all cases, with the addition of physic or organic therapies such as bleeding, purging, medication, and water immersion. As well, moral management was introduced. This involved behavioral and environmental interventions and the provision of occupation. So, ideas that seem to leap out of nowhere with the advent of moral treatment, in fact, grew gradually over the preceding centuries. John Locke's *An Essay Concerning Humane Understanding* may have been influential, and this equated madness less with passionate animals and more with children unable to think straight.[131] Burton's *The Anatomy of Melancholy* would have been another influential text. The index to that, as well as entries such as "humors what they are," lists a range of ideas about doing and being causes of melancholy such as "idleness"; "poverty and want"; "exercise, if immoderate"; "loss of liberty, servitude, imprisonment"; and "passions and perturbations … how they work on the body." It also advises treatment that incorporates being through doing, such as "recreations good against melancholy"; "walking, shooting, swimming, & good against melancholy"; "mathematical studies recommended"; "gardens for pleasure"; "minde how it works on the body"; and "labour, business, cure of love melancholy."[132]

Growing from moral management, and a product of the Age of Enlightenment, is moral treatment's humane approach to the insane that revolutionized psychiatric institutions during the late 18th and 19th centuries. The genesis, success, and demise of moral treatment provide a fascinating but cautionary tale about changes in beliefs about the

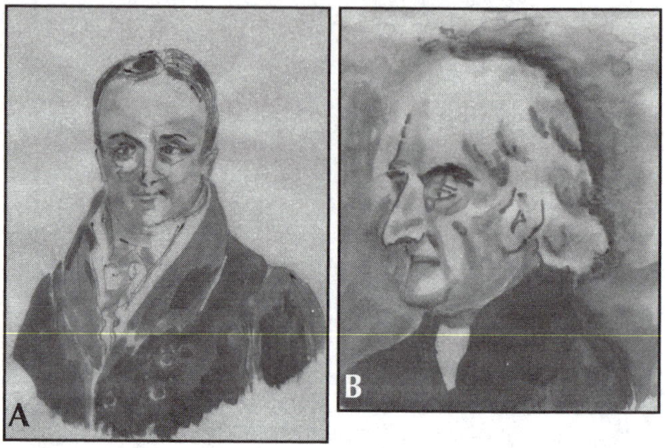

Figure 4-4. (A) Pinel. (B) William Tuke.

causes of illness and the place of occupation in improving people's experience of health: of being through doing.

While in today's terms it certainly appears that much of what moral treatment replaced was immoral, eminent doctors of the mad such as William Cullen argued that "restraining the anger and violence of madmen is always necessary for preventing their hurting themselves or others; but this restraint is also to be considered as a remedy."[133] This treatment, far from being condemned by people of the time, provided entertainment for the curious, when for an example, for a penny, the inmates were exhibited through the open doors of Bethlem Hospital. In fact, even George III, during bouts of mania, was subjected to similar treatment by his physician Francis Willis. "He was sometimes chained to a stake. He was frequently beaten and starved, and at best he was kept in subjection by menacing and violent language."[134] It appears that even whether or not behavior is perceived as humane or inhumane, moral or immoral depends on the context, the world-view, and the values of those perceiving it. Scull argues that "the subjugation of the madman [and] the breaking of his will by means of external discipline and constraint" were consistent with the view that "in losing his reason, the essence of his humanity, the madman had lost his claim to be treated as a human being."[135] In turn, this view was congruent with the theological and supernatural beliefs and values of an agrarian economy in which God and nature dominated and humans, on the whole, did not seek, or think possible, self-transformation. Moral treatment, he suggests, arose as a result of a change in "the cultural meaning of madness," which emerged along with the change from agriculture to industry, from reliance on nature to reliance on human activity, and invention in the transformation of natural resources into marketable products. In fact, as industrialists sought to "make such machines of man that cannot err," they cultivated in workers a new belief in "'rational' self-interest [that was] essential if the market system were to work."[136]

At about the same time as Pinel (Figure 4-4) liberated and removed the prison chains of the insane constrained in the dungeons of Bicêtre in France, William Tuke (see Figure 4-4) established moral treatment in Britain, specifically for members of his faith because of his concerns about what he believed was the inhumane treatment of a fellow Quaker who died in a public asylum.[137] Tuke based the revolutionary approach taken at the Retreat in York on beliefs that self-discipline, hard work, and kindness rather than external control were the keys to rehabilitation of the insane. Reflecting the Quaker work ethic, as well as religious discipline, treatment at the Retreat encouraged individuals to regain self-control through occupation, as "of all the modes by which the patients may be induced to restrain themselves, regular employment is perhaps the most generally efficacious."[138]

Tuke recognized that "in itself, work possesses a constraining power superior to all forms of physical coercion" because of "the regularity of the hours, the requirements of attention, [and] the obligation to produce a result."[137] It is also a requisite of self-esteem, which Tuke valued highly. The program established at the Retreat was the catalyst for the introduction of programs of occupation in the many large public asylums being established throughout the United Kingdom at the start of the 19th century. There were several notable superintendents who, for a period of about 50 years, established occupation as the principle treatment method for the vast majority of patients.[98,109] One of those, W. A. F. Browne, wrote in *What Asylums Were, Are and Ought to Be,* "The whole secret of the new system and of that moral treatment by which the number of cures has been doubled may be summed up in two words, kindness and occupation."[139]

Pinel's "moral" approach differed in several ways from Tuke's, particularly in that his asylum was "a religious domain without religion, a domain of pure morality, of ethical uniformity,"[137] but it, too, recognized the value of occupation:

> It is the most constant and unanimous result of experience that in all public asylums, as in prisons and hospitals, the surest and perhaps the sole guarantee of the maintenance of health and good habits and order is the law of rigorously executed mechanical work.[140]

Ironically he found, "... those whose condition does not place them above the necessity of submission to toil and labour, are almost always cured; while the grandee, who would think himself degraded by any exercise of this description, is generally incurable."[141]

The occupation theme continued in France after Pinel's time; we read, for example, of Leuret, a 19th century French psychiatrist who included manual labor, drama, music, and reading and stressed improvements of habits and the development of a consciousness of society within his treatment programs.[142]

In America at that time, despite a predominantly agricultural economy, a "new liberal philosophy ..." was developing rapidly, so, not surprisingly, it too embraced the concept of moral treatment.[143] In part, this was through the efforts of Tuke's son Samuel,[144] and also through the reforms of Benjamin Rush, who, like Pinel, was inspired by the writings of John Locke. The Worcester State Hospital in Massachusetts, which opened in 1833, served as a proving ground for moral treatment in America, demonstrating "beyond doubt that recovery was the rule."[145] It was introduced in other American asylums for the insane. Thomas S. Kirkebride, for example, implemented moral treatment in the Pennsylvania Hospital for the Insane, a prestigious private institution that he headed for 40 years. He wrote annual reports aimed at prospective customers and their families, among others, in which he detailed more than 50 occupations available to inmates. They included light gymnastics, fancy work, magic lantern displays, and lecture series, and, in order to meet the intellectual and artistic needs of more cultivated clients, "intelligent and educated individuals with courteous manners, and refined feelings" were employed to encourage reading, handiwork, and music in the wards.[146] He assured prospective patrons that cure could be expected in many cases, especially if treatment was prompt, but that even in cases requiring long-term care, moral and humane conditions would apply. In fact, moral treatment was reported as curative by the superintendents of the asylums who ran the programs, with some hospitals, such as the Hartford Retreat, recording success rates of up to 90%.[147] An example of the recovery statistics of patients admitted to the Worcester State Hospital between 1833 and 1852 and used to attract prospective customers is provided in Table 4-1.

The cautionary part of the tale lies in the decline of moral treatment despite its reputed success. Most of the asylums in America in which it was used were small private hospitals. Access was limited to the affluent, but the claims of the curative effects of

Table 4-1

Outcome in Patients Admitted to Worcester State Hospital Who Were Ill Less Than 1 Year

5-Year Period	Patients Admitted	Patients Discharged, Recovered	Patients Discharged, Improved
1833 to 1837	300	211 (70.0%)	39 (8.3%)
1838 to 1842	434	324 (74.6%)	14 (3.2%)
1843 to 1847	742	474 (63.9%)	34 (4.6%
1848 to 1852	791	485 (61.3%	37 (4.7%)

Annual Reports of the Hospital. Reprinted with permission from Bockoven JS. *Moral Treatment in Community Mental Health.* New York: Springer Verlag Publishing Co Inc; 1972:14. Used by permission of Springer Publishing Company, Inc., New York 10036.

moral treatment caused social reformers to push successfully for it to be available to all. Asylums became overcrowded,[143] activity rooms became wards, and because resources were limited, due to a Civil War-taxed economy, the treatment deteriorated into custodial care.[147] Occupational programs also deteriorated. "Reductionist, mechanical" values associated with industrialization replaced those Enlightenment ideas that inspired moral treatment.[148] Medicine was reconsidering the causes of insanity in the light of new physiological knowledge in which ideas about occupation did not seem important. Indeed, it seems almost inevitable that as positivist, medical science developed, doctors would try to make their role in the treatment of the insane fit with their view of their own skills, beliefs, and purpose. The doctor's role in moral treatment in the early days was as a wise authority figure, Pinel and Tuke both asserting "moral action was not necessarily linked to any scientific competence."[137] However, it was from Tuke's and Pinel's programs that "madness" became associated with medicine and from these 18th century ideas that modern notions of rehabilitation have grown. Ironically, understanding of an occupational approach to mental health, as well as physical and social health, has lessened over 2 centuries of use.

Foucault, who describes psychiatric practice as a "certain moral tactic contemporary with the end of the 18th century, preserved in the rites of asylum life, and overlaid by the myths of positivism," points to a gradual "magical" belief in psychiatrists and ultimately to the transfer of the potential to cure from asylum to doctor.[137] It was unavoidable that the natural would be overtaken by the scientific. The reported success of moral treatment was challenged as exaggeration and disappeared from psychiatric practice. Peloquin suggests, "The failure to identify and address the social and institutional changes that had gradually made the practice and success of moral treatment virtually impossible led to the erroneous conclusion that occupation was not an effective intervention."[147]

HOW MODERN VALUES AFFECT "BEING THROUGH DOING" AS AN AGENT OF HEALTH

The historic overview above poses some questions about current views of mental health in terms of an occupation-focused perspective of public health. The WHO, like other authorities noted earlier, measures mental health in terms of quality of life.[11] It seeks to promote it as a primary concern by the development of an assessment tool to be used as an adjunct to the measurement of traditional morbidity and mortality data and to have mental health promotion placed firmly on national agendas. Mental health promotion covers a variety of strategies such as the enhancement of socioeconomic environments and an individual's resources and capacities. The WHO directive recognizes the following[11]:

* Because resources are limited, at present priority is given to acute services for the mentally ill, then to rehabilitation and community services, and last to promoting mental health.

* Multisectoral action is required.

* There is a need to enhance the value and visibility of mental health promotion through policies aimed at all sectors of society. "These would include the social integration of severely marginalized groups, such as refugees, disaster victims, the socially alienated, the mentally disabled, the very old and infirm, abused children and women, and the poor."

* Programs are required at all stages of life to encourage creativity and promote self-esteem and self-confidence.

Such requirements suggest that even in the modern day within advanced health conscious communities, issues about people finding meaning in their lives through what they do are either inadequately recognized or inadequately acted upon.

In terms of health promotion, generally the OCHP and *Jakarta Declaration* called for action that generates living and working conditions that are stimulating, satisfying, and enjoyable as well as being safe and meeting health's basic prerequisites. The call recognizes that leisure, as well as work, is a source of health.[149] There are few public health programs at present in postindustrial societies that address the potential holistic health impact of a range of occupations and the meaning it holds for people. There is ongoing research and there are programs that address illness and safety concerns in paid employment, and there are increasing programs of physical exercise to reduce the incidence of cardiovascular diseases, other NCDs, and more recently, to reverse the obesity epidemic in affluent countries. Even addressing only the limited elements of work and exercise has provided significant pointers to the relationship between what people do, how they feel about it, and their health. Such programs, however, do not entice all people and obesity and other NCDs continue to rise. Programs based on the myriad of factors that constitute doing and being and that have meaning for people could be a sound alternative.

Paid Employment

Because of the preoccupation with work, in this section material relating to the health and illness effects of paid employment is reviewed. This suggests how being through doing (epitomized by meaning) is central to positive or negative health outcomes. Scott, in *The Psychology of Work*, points to the study of tiredness to explain "the overlap between various aspects"[150]; how, for example, manual tasks lead to the build up of lactic acid in muscles that leads, in turn to tenderness, swelling, pain, and physical fatigue. While fatigue in that case is due to excessive work, it can also be a symptom of boredom that emanates from too little to do, lack of variety, or repetition. To complicate the situation, further repetition leads to physical fatigue as well as boredom.[150] Scott and his colleagues set out to examine:

What work really was, why we did it and how it affected us. We saw that man's muscle was the main source of power before the industrial revolution and even now his muscle

*is important though aided by all sorts of means ... Man's work is characterized by ver-
bal communication, at a superficial level even the chatter in the canteen is important.
If silence reigns, then there is something wrong with the work.*[150]

Echoing the thoughts of Marx discussed earlier, Scott claims that although "at first work
appears merely as a source of money—a means of earning a living ... it is the force that
transforms the world and makes it either a better or a worse place in which to live ... and
changes us."[150]

Modern society is "work-oriented in a systematic, non-seasonal way, as it has been
since the industrial revolution."[151] In terms of the present day value accorded to paid
employment, Colish contends it "receives strongly positive valuation as a social virtue"
being "dignified, natural, compatible with virtue ... a means of serving others as well as
a means of exercising one's own ethical integrity."[126] This overt valuing of work, Jenkins
and Sherman argue, has led to leisure not being considered seriously, often being confused with pleasure, and being made to sound "vaguely sinful and hedonistic and frivo-
lous enough to be frowned upon."[151] Despite this, they observe that modern technology
creates a reduction in the availability of paid employment, leaving many people with up
to 100% leisure time. This is made worse because society appears to value technological
progress and the material rewards of employment above all other forms of occupation.
Eventually, Jenkins and Sherman argue, societies are going to have to come to terms
with the idea that the work ethic is fast becoming redundant. A need to blur work and
leisure has been a constant theme of writers concerned with their study for the last 50
years.[83,152-156]

In terms of meaning as opposed to doing for the sake of survival, the value given to
work for work's sake can be seen to be less than health enhancing. To meet the WHO
directives that provide the theme for the chapter, it can be claimed that consideration
should be given to satisfying people's particular talents and capacities in a variety of ways
that contribute to the community. Not to develop new ways forward with such thought in
mind may be a contributing factor in the increasing number of dropouts from education
and the number of young people who do not appear willing to take up paid work, preferring instead to live on social welfare.

Despite affluent societies appearing to have an abundance of occupational choices that
offer opportunity for the exercise and development of physical, mental, and social capacities and talents and to find meaning, the structures, material costs, attitudes held, and
values placed upon different aspects may well affect how successfully people access these
opportunities. Radford, for example, reflects on gender inequalities:

> *In all human societies that we know of, men and women have generally been brought
> up and educated, and have tended to follow different occupations. ... Without much
> doubt, on the whole the range of opportunity available to women has been less than that
> for men, although it has not always been the case that women have necessarily been
> disadvantaged. ...*[157]

There are also inequalities of potential meaning resulting from how the nature of
different work is perceived by society. For example "in all urban cultures and in most
periods manual work has been looked down upon by those with property and power."[158]
Such population feelings can affect willingness to take on such work, thereby preclud-
ing any chance that occupation may provide meaning, albeit unexpected. People may be
restricted in their choice by factors as various as time, lack of resources, lack of awareness,
lack of interest, peer pressure, or place of habitat. "Some people have choice and others
overcome constraints through determination, courage, foresight or with encouragement.
Still others, rather than making a rational choice from a range of alternatives 'find themselves' in jobs that do not fit their interests for a variety of reasons."[157] These might be

associated with what Radford terms *occupational culture*. To describe the latter scenario, he uses another useful term, *occupational fate*.[157] Richard Smith suggests in *Unemployment and Health* that "most employment for most people has, since the industrial revolution, been hard, exhausting, boring, dirty, degrading, and, as Marx said, alienating."[159] Those issues, and many others, are fundamental to health in the long term.

Jahoda found, from study of the unemployed in the 1930s, that employment offered more than financial reward.[160,161] It allowed purpose, a sense of achievement, a daily time structure, social contact outside the family, and social status, and its lack caused boredom, mental despair, apathy, and deterioration.[160] In the late 1980s, she remained convinced about these effects.[161] Similarly, Warr found that employment offers scope for developing new skills and decision making, but that on the down side, the value given to employment causes the unemployed to suffer frequent humiliations and loss of social status.[162] Smith's summary account suggests that unemployment and poor health are strongly associated, that unemployment itself causes some illness, and that health problems are compounded by unemployment; that the poverty, low socioeconomic status, poor education, and housing conditions, associated frequently with both ill health and unemployment, cause difficulties in clarifying the strength of the associations. Unemployment is also associated with high divorce rates, child and spouse abuse, unwanted pregnancies, abortions, reduced birthweight and child growth, perinatal and infant mortality, and increased morbidity in families, though for none of the associations can it be assumed that unemployment itself is the cause.[159]

Smith is supported by many detailed studies. About one-fifth of the unemployed report a deterioration in their mental health since being out of work.[162-164] Studies using standardized questionnaires consistently show that the mental health of the unemployed is poorer than those with work[162,165] and that there is a link between unemployment, suicide, and deliberate self-injury.[166] There is less evidence associating unemployment with psychoses.[167] Fryer and Payne found that 5% of the unemployed they studied reported an improvement in their mental health—some because they escaped from jobs they disliked—while others had found positive aspects to unemployment.[168] The studies linking unemployment with physical illness are limited. However, the British Regional Heart Study has shown higher rates of bronchitis, chronic obstructive lung disease, and ischemic heart disease among the unemployed than among the employed.[169] Beale and Nethercott found a statistically significant 20% increase in medical consultation rates for families of 80 men and 49 women who lost their jobs when a local factory closed compared with controls who did not lose their jobs.[170] A 60% increase in referrals to hospital outpatients was also found. In a 1992 Australian paper, unemployed men were reported as experiencing a 66% higher prevalence of disability, 21% prevalence of recent illnesses, 101% more days of reduced activity because of illness, and of diabetes and respiratory disorders as a cause of death than employed men.[171] Women followed the same trends but not to the same extent.[171] Brenner, a professor at Johns Hopkins University, found a relationship between downward fluctuations in the American economy between 1940 and 1973 and physical and emotional illness.[172,173] He calculated that an unemployment increase of about 1 million people (1% of the population) sustained for 6 years could be linked with increases of 36,887 in total deaths, 4227 in mental hospital admissions, and 3340 in prison admissions. His study indicated that health is vulnerable to subtle economic fluctuations and that it improves and declines with the economy. Scott-Samuel and Moser found unemployment may also be associated with premature death[174-177]; however, Gravelle is unconvinced that this is the case.[178] Work structures that mix labor and leisure lessen drudgery and enable workers to meet their social and psychological needs, although, from a capitalist view combining work and leisure is considered inefficient and uneconomical. Labor is seen as separable from other types of occupation and merely one aspect of the production process.

Despite those factors, engagement in what might be unfulfilling, unsatisfying employment as opposed to unemployment continues to be a strongly held social value. Smith goes so far as to suggest that paid employment has become the central institution mattering more to individuals than "government, education, religion, defense, or health."[159] He believes being unemployed may be worse than "being excommunicated, disenfranchised, illiterate, conquered, and diseased," with many people without paid employment feeling unwanted, as if they no longer belong to society, their impoverished days having neither structure nor purpose.[159]

In postmodern cultures, people have shifted their ideas from expecting to work to provide for their own needs toward an expectation that they have a right to work to provide themselves with material comforts and to meet needs for satisfaction and status. Despite this, paid employment for many people is still not intrinsically satisfying.[179] For example, Winefield and his colleagues, in a prospective longitudinal study of more than 3000 young Australians, found that people dissatisfied with their employment were no better off in terms of self-esteem, levels of depression, or lack of psychological well-being than the unemployed who were, as could be expected, significantly worse off than those satisfied with their employment.[180]

Of people who are unemployed, many experience a reduction in the range of occupational options outside paid work. They may, as a result, experience a doubling of the effects of already limited opportunities to use physical, mental, or social capacities in ways that provide exercise, opportunity, and meaning. This compounds the potential for an ever-decreasing experience of health and well-being. Additionally, lack of significant work may cause mental and social ill health because of the value placed upon it by society. Significant work is conducive to well-being and preventive of illness if it complies with societal values, as well as meeting primary needs and personal meaning.

In terms of mental health, the WHO provides guidelines suggesting "special emphasis should be given to those aspects of work places and the work process itself which promote mental health."[11] As a basis for quality of life within paid employment, WHO identifies 8 areas of action[11]:

1. Increasing an employer's awareness of mental health issues.

2. Identifying common goals and positive aspects of the work process.

3. Creating a balance between job demands and occupational skills.

4. Training in social skills.

5. Developing the psychosocial climate of the workplace.

6. Provision of counseling.

7. Enhancement of working capacity.

8. Early rehabilitation strategies.

In terms of unemployment, and particularly youth unemployment, the WHO calls for strategies to improve work opportunities such as job creation programs, the provision of vocational training, and the development of social and job-seeking skills.[11]

Determinants of "Being Through Doing" as Factors in Well-Being or Illness

Occupationally, well-being through doing embraces the belief that the potential range of people's occupations will allow each of them to be creative, adventurous, and find meaning as they experience all human emotions, explore and adapt appropriately, and without undue disruption meet their life needs through what they do. If well-being is to be attained, doing needs to provide meaning and purpose as well as self-esteem, motivation, and socialization. Other important requirements appear to be sufficient intellectual challenge to stimulate neuronal physiology and encourage efficient or enhanced problem-solving, sensory integration, perception, attention, concentration, reflection, language, and memory.[181,182] Additionally, a balance of occupations between physical activity, intellectual challenges, spiritual experiences, emotional highs and lows, solitary and social in nature, effort, and relaxation is required. This does not imply constant high-powered mental "doing" or "feeling," rather that this should be interwoven with time for simply being at ease with the self.[183] Well-being will be enhanced if people in their chosen or obligatory occupations are able to develop spiritual, cognitive, and emotive capacities; to experience timelessness and "higher-order meaning."[184] Along those lines, John Hersey's admission of "feeling nourished and transformed" as a result of his literary work makes sense.[185] It appears to be important that occupational and social natures and needs are intertwined and taken into consideration as a complementary whole. This requires people's doing and being, enabling the maintenance and development of satisfying and stimulating relationships with family members and associates and within the community in which they live. It also calls for a balance between social situations and time for quiet and reflection. Being through doing will have the most obvious health-promoting effects if socially sanctioned, approved, valued, and endowing social status.

Figure 4-5 provides an overview of the complex relationship between "being through doing" and illness or physical, mental, and social well-being. Human characteristics and biological needs are the foundation stones of the human need to "be" as they are of health and cultural evolution. The need to find meaning, purpose, and a sense of belonging has led to the establishment of unique economies; political systems; and national values, policies, and priorities.

The utilities that emanate from those underlying institutions also provide positive or negative influence upon national, community, family, or individual health by providing or restricting doing that provides meaning and nourishes the mind, body, and spirit. The effects of the underlying factors or facilities that grow from them may not be the same for all communities or for all individuals. The positive or negative consequences of finding meaning, purpose, satisfaction, and belonging from doing are many and various similar to how they were reported at the end of the last chapter. As WHO has claimed, "Health depends on validation of the uniqueness of each person and the need to respond to each individual's spiritual quest for meaning, purpose and belonging."[9]

In this chapter on being true to self through what people do, it has been found that biological characteristics and capacities go beyond provision of the prerequisites of survival. Complex capacities, such as consciousness and creativity, have enabled people to develop unique interests, to seek meaning, to find purpose through what they do, to continually seek out the new and the different, to feel a sense of belonging, and to adapt culturally to many different natural and social environments. A brain capable of meeting a whole range of biological needs and sociocultural adaptations is common to humankind but is

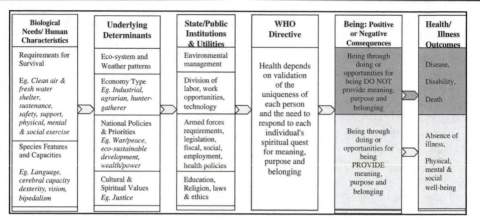

Figure 4-5. Determinants of illness or well-being of being through doing.

also unique in each individual. During the exploration, the place of being through doing in survival, health, and well-being began to emerge, setting the scene for later consideration about approaches to promote health. The next chapter will explore these ideas still further as occupation and health are considered from the perspective of people reaching out toward what they have the potential to become through what they do.

References

1. Landau SI, ed. *Funk & Wagnalls Standard Desk Dictionary*. Vol 1. Harper & Row, Publishers Inc; 1984:58.
2. *Word Finder: Australian Thesaurus*. Sydney, Australia: Reader's Digest; 1983:56.
3. Being. *Merriam-Webster On-line Dictionary*. Merriam-Webster Incorporated; 2005.
4. Being. Wikipedia. (GNU Free Documentation License). Accessed November 2005.
5. Maslow AH. *Toward a Psychology of Being*. 2nd ed. New York: D. Van Nostrand Company; 1968:9
6. Hocking C. *The Relationship Between Objects and Identity in Occupational Therapy: A Dynamic Balance of Rationalism and Romanticism*. Auckland University of Technology: Unpublished PhD Thesis; 2004:137,171,338,339.
7. 1st year students. Occupational Science and Therapy. Deakin University. Geelong, Australia. 2002.
8. Crisp R. University of Oxford/St. Anne's College (Copyright 2001) Accessed April 2005.
9. World Health Organization. *Health for All in the Twenty-First Century*. Geneva: WHO; 1997.
10. Notes on "Quality of Life." Available at: http://www.gdrc.org/uem/qol-define.html. Accessed November 2005.
11. World Health Organization. *Mental Health: Strengthening Mental Health Promotion*. Fact sheet N°220. Revised November 2001; © World Health Organization 2005.
12. Frankl VE. *Man's Search for Meaning*. New York: Pocket Books; 1963.
13. Selye H, Monat A, Lazarus RS. *Stress and Coping: An Anthology*. 2nd ed. New York: Columbia University Press; 1985:28.
14. *The Standard English Desk Dictionary*. 2nd ed. Oxford, UK: Oxford University Press; 1975.
15. Roget PM. *Roget's Thesaurus of Synonyms and Antonyms*. London: The Number Nine Publishing Co; 1972.
16. Jones S. Genetic diversity in humans. In: Jones S, Martin R, Pilbeam D, eds. *The Cambridge Encyclopedia of Human Evolution*. New York: Cambridge University Press; 1992:264-267.
17. Campbell BG. *Humankind Emerging*. 5th ed. New York: Harper Collins Publishers; 1988:86-87,364,365.
18. Kolb B, Whishaw IQ. *Fundamentals of Human Neuropsychology*. 3rd ed. San Franscico, Calif: WH Freeman and Co; 1990:4,123.
19. Waber DP. Sex differences in cognition: a function of maturation rate? *Science*. 1976;192:572-573.
20. Campbell J. *Winston Churchill's Afternoon Nap*. London: Palladin Grafton Books; 1986:166.
21. Edelman G. *Bright Air, Brilliant Fire: On the Matter of the Mind*. London: Penguin Books; 1992:23.
22. Lieberman P. Evolution of the speech apparatus. In: Jones S, Martin R, Pilbeam D, eds. *The Cambridge Encyclopedia of Human Evolution*. New York: Cambridge University Press; 1992:136-137.

23. Csikszentmihalyi M, Csikszentmihalyi IS, eds. *Optimal Experience: Psychological Studies of Flow in Consciousness*. New York: Cambridge University Press; 1988:20-23.
24. Ornstein R, Sobel D. *The Healing Brain: A Radical New Approach to Health Care*. London: Macmillan; 1988:39,57.
25. Gagne F. Toward a differentiated model of giftedness and talent. In: Colabango N, Davis G, eds. *Handbook of Gifted Education*. Gagne, Mass: Allyn and Bacon; 1991.
26. Gardner H. *Frames of Mind. The Theory of Multiple Intelligences*. New York: Basic Books; 1983:290.
27. Shelley PB. *Prometheus Unbound*, II, IV. London: C and J Ollier; 1820.
28. Piaget J. *Six Psychological Studies*. New York: Random House; 1967:98.
29. Lewin R. *In the Age of Mankind: A Smithsonian Book of Human Evolution*. Washington, DC: Smithsonian Books; 1988:174,179-180.
30. Hamlyn DW. *A History of Western Philosophy*. Hamlyn, England: Viking; 1987:15.
31. Consciousness. Wikipedia. (GNU Free Documentation License). Accessed November 2005.
32. *The Macquarie Dictionary*. NSW: Macquarie Library Pty, Ltd; 1981.
33. Watson L. *Neophilia: The Tradition of the New*. Sevenoaks, Kent: Hodder and Stoughton Ltd; 1989:43.
34. Churchland PM. *Matter and Consciousness*. Rev ed. Cambridge, Mass: Bradford Book; 1988:73.
35. Ornstein R. *The Evolution of Consciousness: The Origins of the Way We Think*. New York: Touchstone; 1991:228.
36. Block N. *The Encyclopedia of Cognitive Science*. 2004. Accessed November 2005.
37. Csikszentmihalyi M. Activity and happiness: toward a science of occupation. *Journal of Occupational Science: Australia*. 1993;1(1):38-42.
38. Sato I. Bosozuko: flow in Japanese motorcycle gangs. In: Csikszentmihalyi M, Csikszentmihalyi IS, eds. *Optimal Experience: Psychological Studies of Flow in Consciousness*. New York: Cambridge University Press; 1988.
39. Delle Fave A, Massimini F. Modernization and the changing context of flow in work and leisure. In: Csikszentmihalyi M, Csikszentmihalyi IS, eds. *Optimal Experience: Psychological Studies of Flow in Consciousness*. New York: Cambridge University Press; 1988.
40. Dossey L. Consciousness and health: what's it all about. *Topics in Clinical Nursing*. 1982;3(Jan):1-6.
41. Newman MA. Newman's theory of health as praxis. *Nursing Science Quarterly*. 1990;3(1):37-41.
42. Burch S. Consciousness: how does it relate to health? *Journal of Holistic Nursing*. 1994;12(1):101-116.
43. Grimshaw A. Consciousness raising. In: Bullock A, Stalleybrass O, Trombley S, eds. *The Fontana Dictionary of Modern Thought*. 2nd ed. London: Fontana Press; 1988:166.
44. Koerner JG, Bunkers SS. The healing web: an expansion of consciousness. *Journal of Holistic Nursing*. 1994;12(1):51-63.
45. Smith-Campbell B. Kansans' perceptions of health care reform: a qualitative study on coming to public judgement. *Public Health Nurs*. 1995;12(2):134-139.
46. Dossey BM. The transpersonal self and states of consciousness. In: Dossey BM, Keegan L, Kolkmier LG, Guzzetta CE, eds. *Holistic Health Promotion. A Guide for Practice*. Rockville, Md: Aspen Publications; 1989:32.
47. Green E, Green A. Biofeedback and transformation. In: Kunz D, ed. *Spiritual Aspects of the Healing Arts*. Wheaton, IL: The Theosophical Publishing House; 1985:145-162.
48. Gordon R. The creative process. In: Jennings S, ed. *Creative Therapy*. London: Pitman Publishing; 1975:1.
49. Jung CG. *Collected Works*. Princeton, NJ: Princeton University Press; 1959.
50. Sinnott EW. The creativeness of life. In: Vernon PE, ed. *Creativity*. London: Penguin Books; 1970:115.
51. Morgan DN. Creativity today. *Journal of Aesthetics*. 1953;12:1-24.
52. Young JG. What is creativity? *Journal of Creative Behaviour*. 1985;19(2):77-87.
53. *The Concise Oxford Dictionary of Current English*. Oxford, UK: Clarendon Press; 1911.
54. Wikipedia. Creativity. *GNU Free Documentation License*. Accessed November 2005.
55. Schmid T. *Promoting Health through Creativity: For Professionals in Health, Arts and Education*. Philadelphia: Whurr Publishers; 2005:27.
56. Morris W. 1884. In: Morton AL, ed. *Political Writings of William Morris*. London: Lawrence and Wishart; 1973.
57. Leakey R. *The Making of Mankind*. London: Michael Joseph Ltd; 1981:101-103.
58. Skinner BF. *The Science of Behaviour*. New York: Macmillan; 1953.
59. Amabile TM. *The Social Psychology of Creativity*. New York: Springer-Verlag; 1983.
60. Gardner H. *Creating Minds: An Anatomy of Creativity Seen Through the Lives of Freud, Einstein, Picasso, Stravinsky, Eliot, Graham, and Gandhi*. New York: Basic Books; 1993.
61. Bruce MA, Borg B. *Frames of Reference in Psychosocial Occupational Therapy*. Thorofare, NJ: SLACK Incorporated; 1987.
62. Taylor IA, Getzels JW, eds. *Perspectives in Creativity*. Chicago, Ill: Aldine Publishing Co; 1975.

63. Freud S. *A General Introduction to Psychoanalysis.* Boni and Liveright; 1920:326-327.
64. Freud S. *Creativity and the Unconscious.* New York: Harper and Row; 1958.
65. Freud S. Creative writers and daydreaming. In: Strachey J, ed. *The Standard Edition of the Complete Psychological Works of Sigmund Freud.* Vol 9. London: Hogarth Press; 1959:143-144.
66. Barron F. *Creative Person and Creative Process.* New York: Holt, Rinehart and Winston; 1969.
67. Maslow AH. *Motivation and Personality.* New York: Harper and Row; 1954.
68. Payne WA, Hahn DB. *Understanding Your Health.* 2nd ed. St. Louis, MO: Times Mirror/Mosby College Publishing; 1989.
69. Solomon R. Creativity and normal narcissism. *Journal of Creative Behaviour.* 1985;19(1):47-55.
70. Feldman D. *Beyond Universals in Cognitive Development.* Norwood, NJ: Ablex; 1980.
71. Dennis W. Creative productivity between the ages of 20 and 80 years. *Journal of Gerontology.* 1966;21:106-114.
72. Lehman H. *Age and Achievement.* Princeton, NJ: Princeton University Press; 1953.
73. Simonton DK. Sociocultural context of individual creativity: a transhistorical time-series analysis. *J Pers Soc Psychol* 1975;32:1119-1133.
74. Reynolds F. The effects of creativity on physical and psychological well-being: current and new directions for research. In: Schmid T. *Promoting Health through Creativity: For Professionals in Health, Arts and Education.* Philadelphia: Whurr Publishers; 2005,
75. Fisher B, Specht D. Successful aging and creativity in later life. *Journal of Aging Studie*s. 1999;13:457-472.
76. Forthofer M, Hanz M, Dodge J, Clark N. Gender differences in the associations self esteem, stress and social support with functional health status among older adults with heart disease. *Journal of Women and Aging.* 2001;13:19-36.
77. Clift S, Hancox G. The perceived benefits of singing: Findings from preliminary surveys of a university college choral society. *Journal of the Royal Society for the Promotion of Health.* 2001;121:248-256.
78. Buranhult G, ed. *The First Humans: Human Origins and History to 10,000 BC.* St. Lucia, Australia: University of Queensland Press; 1993:98-99.
79. Leakey R, Lewin R. *People of the Lake: Man: His Origins, Nature, and Future.* New York: Penguin Books; 1978.
80. van der Merve NJ. Reconstructing prehistoric diet. In: Jones S, Martin R, Pilbeam D, eds. *The Cambridge Encyclopedia of Human Evolution.* New York: Cambridge University Press; 1992:369-372.
81. Wax RH. Free time in other cultures. In: Donahue W, et al, eds. *Free Time: Challenge to Later Maturity.* Ann Arbor, Mich: University of Michigan Press; 1958:3-16.
82. Sahlins M. *Stone Age Economics.* Chicago, IL: Aldine-Atherton; 1972.
83. Parker S. *Leisure and Work.* London: George Allen and Unwin; 1983:14,17,19,119.
84. Boas F. *The Mind of Primitive Man.* New York: Macmillan; 1911.
85. Neff WS. *Work and Human Behaviour.* 3rd ed. New York: Aldine Publishing Co; 1985.
86. Jones B. *Sleepers, Wake! Technology and the Future of Work.* Melbourne, Australia: Oxford University Press; 1995:11,80.
87. Bruner JS. Nature and uses of immaturity. *Am Psychol.* 1972;August:687-708
88. Lowerson J, Myerscough J. *Time to Spare in Victorian England.* Hassocks: Harvester Press; 1977.
89. Bailey P. *Leisure and Class in Victorian England.* London: Routledge; 1978.
90. Cunningham H. *Leisure in the Industrial Revolution.* London: Croom Helm; 1980.
91. Campanella T. *City of the Sun.* Donno DJ, trans. Berkeley, Calif: University of California Press; 1981.
92. Marx K. *Early Writing*s. New York: Penguin Classics; 1992.
93. Marx K. Economic and philosophical manuscripts. In: *Early Writings.* New York: Penguin Classics; 1992.
94. Bottomore T. *A Dictionary of Marxist Thought.* 2nd ed. Oxford, UK: Blackwell Ltd; 1991.
95. Marx K, Engels F. *The German Ideology.* London: Lawrence and Wishart; 1964.
96. Marx K. *The Holy Family.* London: Lawrence and Wishart; 1957.
97. Fischer E. *Marx in His Own Words.* London: Allen Lane, The Penguin Press; 1970:31,49.
98. Wilcock AA. *Occupation for Health. Volume 1. A Journey from Self Health to Prescription.* London, UK: COT; 2001.
99. Ruskin J. *Unto This Last.* London: Collins Publishers; 1970.
100. Coleridge ST. *The Friend.* New York: Freeport; 1971.
101. Carlyle T. Sartor Resartus 1833-1834. In: *Sartor Resartus, and On Heroes and Hero Worship.* London: Dent; 1908. Reprinted New York: Dutton; 1973.
102. MacCarthy F. *William Morris: A Life for Our Time.* London: Faber and Faber; 1994:70,71,603,604.
103. Cole GDH. In: Selgman ERA, ed. *Encyclopaedia of Social Science.* New York: Macmillan; 1933.
104. Morris W. Art and socialism. In: Morton AL, ed. *Political Writings of William Morris.* London: Lawrence and Wishart; 1973:110-111.
105. Morris W. Useful work versus useless toil. In: Morton AL, ed. *Political Writings of William Morri*s. London: Lawrence and Wishart; 1973.

106. Jackson Lears TJ. *No Place of Grace: Antimodernism and the Transformation of American Culture 1880-1920.* New York: Pantheon Books; 1981:63,64,67,73,79-81.

107. Morris W. News from nowhere. In: Morton AL, ed. *Three Works by William Morris: News from Nowhere, The Pilgrims of Hope, A Dream of John Ball.* London: Lawrence and Wishart; 1968.

108. Mackenzie N, Mackenzie J. *The Fabians.* New York: Weidenfeld and Nicolson; 1977.

109. Wilcock AA. Occupation for Health. Volume 2. A Journey from Prescription to Self-Health. London: BCOT; 2002.

110. Friedland J. *Why Crafts. Muriel Driver Lecture.* Canadian Association of Occupational Therapists Conference. 2003.

111. Reinders RC. Toynbee Hall and the American settlement movement. *Social Service Review.* 1982;56(1):39-54.

112. Holli MG, Jones P, eds. *Ethnic Chicago.* Grand Rapids, Mich: William B Eerman's Publishing Co; 1984.

113. Fish VK. Hull House: pioneer in urban research during its creative years. *History of Sociology.* 1985;6(1):33-54.

114. Addams J. The Subjective Necessity for Social Settlements. Paper to the Ethical Culture Societies, Plymouth, MA, 1892.

115. World Health Organization. *Jakarta Declaration on Leading Health Promotion into the 21st Century.* 4th International Conference on Health Promotion, Jakarta, Indonesia, 21-25th July, 1997.

116. Grimshaw A. Feminism. In: Bullock A, Stalleybrass O, Trombley S, eds. *The Fontana Dictionary of Modern Thought.* 2nd ed. London: Fontana Press; 1988:312.

117. Pressey EP. New Clairvaux Plantation, Training School, Industries and Settlement. *Country Time and Tide.* 1903;February:121-122.

118. Link AS, McCormick RL. *Progressivism.* Arlington Heights, IL: Harlan Davidson, Inc; 1983.

119. Resek C, ed. *The Progressives.* Indianapolis, Ind: The Bobbs-Merrill Co, Inc; 1967.

120. The course of civilization. United States Magazine and Democratic Review 1839;VI:208ff,211. Cited in: Lukes S. Individualism. Oxford, UK: Basil Blackwell; 1973.

121. Lukes S. *Individualism.* Oxford, UK: Basil Blackwell; 1973.

122. Arieli Y. *Individualism and Nationalism in American Ideology.* Cambridge, Mass: Harvard University Press; 1964:345-346.

123. Draper JW. *History of the American Civil War.* Vol 1. New York: Harper; 1867:207-208.

124. Emerson RW. New England reformers (1844). Summarized in: Lukes S. *Individualism.* Oxford, UK: Basil Blackwell; 1973:29.

125. Stoics. Girling DA, ed. New Age Encyclopaedia. Vol. 27. Sydney, Australia & London, UK: Bay Books; 1983:160-161.

126. Colish ML. *The Stoic Tradition from Antiquity to the Early Middle Ages.* (2 volumes) Leiden: E.J.Brill; 1985;40,41.

127. Porter R. *Mind-Forged Manacles.* London, UK: The Athlone Press; 1987:117.

128. Washington, DC Medicina statica. In: Sinclair J. *Code of Health and Longevity.* Edinburgh: Arch Constable and Co; 1806:184-189.

129. Ferriar J. *Medical Histories and Reflections.* London: Cadell and Davies; 1795:2,111-112.

130. Fox EL. Brislington House, an asylum for lunatics, situated near Bristol. In: Scull A, ed. *Madhouses, Mad-Doctors and Madmen: The Social History of Psychiatry in the Victorian Era.* Philadelphia: University of Pennsylvania Press; 1981.

131. Locke J. An Essay Concerning Humane Understanding. London: Printed for Tho, Basset, and sold by Edw. Mory at the sign of the Three Bibles in St Paul's Church-Yard; MDCXC (1690).

132. Burton R. *The Anatomy of Melancholy.* Oxford: Henry Cripps; 1651:Index.

133. Cullen W. First lines in the practice of physics. In: Hunter RA, MacAlpine I, eds. *Three Hundred Years of Psychiatry.* London: Oxford University Press; 1963:478

134. Bynum W. Rationales for therapy in British psychiatry, 1780-1835. In: Scull A, ed. *Madhouses, Mad-Doctors and Madmen: The Social History of Psychiatry in the Victorian Era.* Philadelphia: University of Pennsylvania Press; 1981.

135. Scull A. Moral treatment reconsidered: some sociological comments on the episode in the history of British psychiatry. In: Scull A, ed. *Madhouses, Mad-Doctors and Madmen: The Social History of Psychiatry in the Victorian Era.* Philadelphia: University of Pennsylvania Press; 1981:108,115.

136. Wedgwood J. Josiah Wedgwood and factory discipline. *Historical Journal.* 1964;1:46.

137. Foucault M. *Madness and Civilization: A History of Insanity in the Age of Reason.* New York: Random House; 1973:247,275-276.

138. Tuke S. *Description of the Retreat.* York: Alexander; 1813:141,156.

139. Browne WAF. What asylums were, are and ought to be. In: Carlson ET, advisory ed. *Classics in Psychiatry: Arno Press Collection.* North Stratford, UK: Ayer Company Publishers Inc; 2001:177.

140. Pinel P. Traite medico-philosophique sur l'alienation mentale. In: Foucault M. *Madness and Civilization: A History of Insanity in the Age of Reason*. New York: Random House; 1973:258.

141. Pinel P. *A Treatise on Insanity*. Birmingham, Ala: Classics of Medicine Library, 1983:195.

142. Leuret F. 1840. On the moral treatment of insanity. In: Licht S. *Occupational Therapy Source Book*. Baltimore, Md: Williams and Wilkins; 1948.

143. Bockoven JS. *Moral Treatment in American Society*. New York: Springer; 1963:172.

144. Corsini RJ, ed. *Encyclopedia of Psychology*. Vol 2. New York: John Wiley and Sons; 1984:162.

145. Bockoven JS. *Moral Treatment in Community Mental Health*. New York: Springer Publishing Co, Inc; 1972:14.

146. Tomes NJ. A generous confidence: Thomas Story Kirkebride's philosophy of asylum construction and management. In: Scull A, ed. *Madhouses, Mad-Doctors and Madmen: The Social History of Psychiatry in the Victorian Era*. Philadelphia: University of Pennsylvania Press; 1981.

147. Peloquin SM. Moral treatment: contexts considered. *Am J Occup Ther*. 1989;43(8):537-544.

148. Serrett KD, ed. *Philosophical and Historical Roots of Occupational Therapy*. New York: The Haworth Press Inc; 1985.

149. World Health Organization, Health and Welfare Canada, Canadian Public Health Association. *Ottawa Charter for Health Promotion*. Ottawa, Canada: Author; 1986.

150. Scott D. *The Psychology of Work*. London: Duckworth; 1970;228-230,233,234.

151. Jenkins C, Sherman B. *The Leisure Shock*. London: Eyre Methuen Ltd; 1981:1.

152. Keniston K. Social change and youth in America. *Daedalus*. 1962;Winter:145-171.

153. Friedlander F. Importance of work versus non-work among socially and occupationally stratified groups. *J Appl Psychol*. 1966;December:437-441.

154. Hollander P. Leisure as an American and Soviet value. *Social Problems*. 1966;3:179-188.

155. Robertson J. *Future Work*. England: Gower Publishing Co; 1985.

156. Pettifer S. Leisure as compensation for unemployment and unfulfilling work. Reality or pipe dream? *Journal of Occupational Science: Australia*. 1993;1(2):20-26.

157. Radford J, ed. *Gender and Choice in Education and Occupation*. London: Routledge; 1998:iv,151.

158. Applebaum H. *The Concept of Work, Ancient, Medieval and Modern*. New York: State University of New York Press; 1992:125.

159. Smith R. *Unemployment and Health: A Disaster and a Challenge*. Oxford, UK: Oxford University Press; 1987.

160. Jahoda M. *Employment and Unemployment*. New York: Cambridge University Press; 1982.

161. Jahoda M. Economic recession and mental health: some conceptual issues. *Journal of Social Issues*. 1988;44(4):13-23.

162. Warr P. Twelve questions about unemployment and health. In: Roberts R, Finnegan R, Gallie D, eds. *New Approaches to Economic Life*. Manchester: Manchester University Press; 1985.

163. Colledge M, Bartholomew R. *A Study of the Long Term Unemployed*. London: Manpower Services Commission; 1980.

164. Jackson PR, Warr PB. Unemployment and psychological ill health: the moderating role of duration and age. *Psychol Med*. 1984;14:605-614.

165. Dowling PJ, De Cieri H, Griffin G, Brown M. Psychological aspects of redundancy: an Australian case study. *Journal of Industrial Relations*. 1987;29(4):519-531.

166. Platt S. Unemployment and suicidal behaviour: a review of the literature. *Soc Sci Med*. 1984;19:93-115.

167. Jaco EG. *The Social Epidemiology of Mental Disorders*. New York: Russell Sage Foundation; 1960.

168. Fryer D, Payne R. Proactive behaviour in unemployment: findings and implications. *Leisure Studies*. 1984;3:273-295.

169. Cook DG, Cummins RO, Bartley MJ, Shaper AG. Health of unemployed middle aged men in Great Britain. *Lancet*. 1982;i:1290-1294.

170. Beale N, Nethercott S. Job loss and family morbidity: a study of factory closure. *Journal of Royal College General Practitioners*. 1985;280:510-514.

171. Enough to Make You Sick: How Income and Environment Affect Health. Australian National Health Strategy Research paper, No 1, Sept 1992.

172. Brenner MH. Health costs and benefits of economic policy. *Int J Health Serv*. 1977;7:581-593.

173. Brenner MH. Mortality and the national economy: a review, and the experience of England and Wales. *Lancet*. 1979;ii:568-573.

174. Scott-Samuel A. Unemployment and health. *Lancet*. 1984;ii:1464-1465.

175. Moser KA, Fox AJ, Jones DR. Unemployment and mortality in the OPCS longitudinal study. *Lancet*. 1984;ii:1324-1329.

176. Moser KA, Goldblatt PO, Fox AJ, Jones DR. Unemployment and mortality: comparison of the 1971 and 1981 longitudinal census sample. *BMJ*. 1987;294:86-90.

177. Kerr C, Taylor R. Grim prospects for the unemployed. *New Doctor.* 1993;Summer:23-24.
178. Gravelle H. *Does Unemployment Kill?* Oxford, UK: Nuffield Provincial Hospitals Trust; 1985.
179. Aungles SB, Parker SR. Work, *Organisations and Change: Themes and Perspectives in Australia.* Sydney, Australia: George Allen and Unwin; 1988.
180. Winefield AH, Tiggerman M, Goldney RD. Psychological concomitants of satisfactory employment and unemployment in young people. *Soc Psychiatry Psychiatr Epidemiol.* 1988;23:149-157.
181. Lilley J, Jackson L. The value of activities: establishing a foundation for cost effectiveness. A review of the literature. *Activities, Adaptation and Aging.* 1990;14(4):12-13.
182. Foster P. Activities: a necessity for total health care of the long term care resident. *Activities, Adaptation and Aging.* 1983;3(3):17-23.
183. do Rozario L. Ritual, meaning and transcendence: the role of occupation in modern life. *Journal of Occupational Science: Australia.* 1994;1(3):46-53.
184. Rappaport R. Ecology, Meaning, and Religion. Richmond, Va: North Atlantic Books; 1979.
185. Hersey J. Time's winged chariot. In: Fadiman C, ed. *Living Philosophies: The Reflections of Some Eminent Men and Women of Our Time.* New York: Doubleday; 1990.

Suggested Reading

Campbell J. *Winston Churchill's Afternoon Nap.* London: Palladin Grafton Books; 1986.
Edelman G. *Bright Air, Brilliant Fire: On the Matter of the Mind.* London: Penguin Books; 1992.
Jackson Lears TJ. *No Place of Grace: Antimodernism and the Transformation of American Culture 1880-1920.* New York: Pantheon Books; 1981.
Jones B. *Sleepers, Wake! Technology and the Future of Work.* Melbourne, Australia: Oxford University Press; 1995.
MacCarthy F. *William Morris: A Life for Our Time.* London: Faber and Faber; 1994.
Maslow AH. *Toward a Psychology of Being.* 2nd ed. New York: D Van Nostrand Co; 1968.
Ornstein R. *The Evolution of Consciousness: The Origins of the Way We Think.* New York: Touchstone; 1991.
Smith R. *Unemployment and Health; A Disaster and a Challenge.* Oxford, UK: Oxford University Press; 1987.
Pinel P. *A Treatise on Insanity.* Birmingham, Ala: Classics of Medicine Library; 1983.
Tuke S. *Description of the Retreat.* York: Alexander; 1813.
Winefield AH, Tiggerman M, Goldney RD. Psychological concomitants of satisfactory employment and unemployment in young people. *Soc Psychiatry Psychiatr Epidemiol.* 1988;23:149-157.
World Health Organization. *Mental Health: Strengthening Mental Health Promotion.* Fact sheet N°220. Geneva: WHO; 2005.

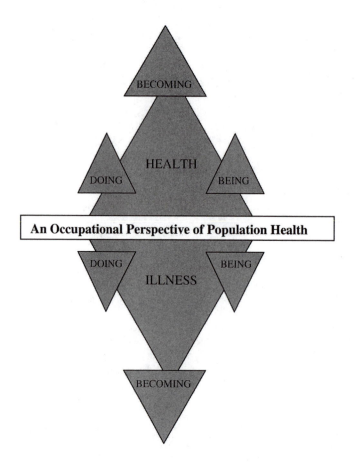

OCCUPATION:
BECOMING THROUGH DOING AND BEING

Theme 5:

To reach a state of complete physical, mental and social well-being, an individual or group must be able to identify and to realize aspirations..."
WHO, *Ottawa Charter for Health Promotion,* 1986

The chapter addresses:
* Becoming as a determinant of population health
  * Defining the concept
  * Its place in public health: holism and health promotion strategies toward all people being able to achieve physical, mental, and social aspirations and potential
* Becoming: biological needs, natural health, and reaching potential
  * Biological bases for need to reach potential
  * Natural health and reaching potential
* Aging and becoming: ancient and modern rules for health
  * An example from the past
  * UN and WHO ideology about active aging
* Lack of becoming as a factor in illness
  * Occupational deprivation
  * Occupational alienation
  * Occupational imbalance

Explored in this chapter is the need for people to aim toward total physical, mental, and social well-being through focusing on becoming what each has the capacity to be. It builds onto and adds a sense of future to the notions of doing and being. Play, fantasy, and dreaming are integral to becoming and can be regarded as adaptive behavior aimed at creating new ways forward despite Freud's linking of them as escapist.[1] At every point in their lives, every day, people can either grow or diminish; their "becoming" can be strengthened, stagnant, or sick. That total well-being is dependent on continual becoming is a serious aspect of occupation that is frequently overlooked or considered outside the medical, and therefore health, field.

From observation and from reports of people who live to a good old age, it appears that most have or had deep interests and continue with what are often considered youthful doings throughout their lives. To them, more than just doing and being appears to be important in the ongoing experience of physical, mental, and social health. The frequent stories of people who have been committed to careers of great interest dying shortly after retirement support that notion. Without ongoing or new interests that provide as much purpose and meaning as their career once did and the potential to continue the self-actualization process, such people are often unable to thrive. The implication of these observations is that health can be enhanced if people hold aspirations and allow these to inspire, guide, and assist the utilization of capacities in ways that keep them exercised and working well. For this reason, the guidelines from the UN and WHO about "Active Aging" that are in accord with these observations are addressed in the section about health "rules."

"Becoming" is a concept, perhaps, almost as difficult as "being" for people to accept as relevant in the fairly "concrete" world of health care. This is despite the "romantic" and possibly understandable notion of helping people with medical problems to have some future aim to pin their hopes on so that there is personal purpose and meaning to exercise body, mind, and spirit. As in the last chapter, to clarify some of the mystique that surrounds the word, and to begin to appreciate its place in occupation-focused public health that is applicable to all people whether or not they have a medical problem, the concept requires some explication.

Becoming as a Determinant of Population Health

Ah, but a man's reach should exceed his grasp,
Or what's a heaven for?[2]

DEFINING THE CONCEPT

In a pragmatic sense, becoming can be defined as to become (somehow different), to grow, for something to come into being. Becoming is an ever-incomplete process. People never become; throughout life they are always becoming different—for better, for worse—even if they cease trying to become. As Anne Wilson Schaef explains, "Life is a process. We are a process. Everything that has happened in our lives … is an integral part of our becoming … awareness of every aspect of ourselves allows us to become who we are."[3] She talks about a "living, moving, evolving energy" and about the way things are done rather than what is done or the results of doing.[4]

The topic of becoming was touched on in Chapter 1 when, during the discussion on mental well-being, the focus of humanist psychologists as influenced by existentialism was outlined.[5-8] The rhetoric of this humanist approach became "equated with productiveness, social adjustment, and contentment—'the good life' itself," and extended consideration to the further reaches of the human psyche.[9] The humanist tradition can be said to stem from the "mental hygiene movement," founded in America in 1909 with which occupational therapy was closely related, and it upholds the Renaissance tradition of human achievement and the ideals of the Age of Enlightenment. The central concept of these approaches is that well-being depends upon the meeting of individual potential.

Maslow was identified as the 20th century front-runner in this sphere of interest. He identified 2 terms—*self-actualization* and *full humanness*—to describe the state that is synonymous with what it being described here as "becoming." In a way, similar to his view, becoming is seen here as an aiming toward the highest level of personal development;

that ultimate well-being is about people recognizing and striving toward their potential by utilizing their personal capacities and strengths as fully as possible.[10] Maslow explains that the characteristics of self-actualizing people are discovered, not invented:

> *These are potentialities, not final actualizations. Therefore they have a life history and must be seen developmentally. They are actualized, shaped or stifled mostly (but not altogether) by extra-psychic determinants (culture, family, environment, learning, etc.).*[11]

Humanist and Gestalt psychologists hold that the potential to self-actualize is given to all human beings at birth.[12] Rogers and Maslow go so far as to propose that self-growth motivates creativity and that creativity and the achievement of individual potential are synonymous with health. Rogers describes "man's tendency to actualize himself, to become his potentialities" as the mainspring of creativity,[13] and Maslow observes "that the concept of creativeness and the concept of the healthy, self-actualizing, fully human person seem to be coming closer and closer together, and may perhaps turn out to be the same thing."[10] Maslow reached this conclusion following a study of self-fulfilled, mentally healthy subjects. The aim of his research was to determine the attributes and components of a basically healthy intrinsic nature and to discover how people are enabled toward growth and self-actualization. He described the healthiest and most effective people as transcenders. Such people are responsive to beauty, holistic in their perceptions of humanity, motivated by the satisfaction of being and service values, able to adjust well to conflict situations, and more likely to accept others with an unconditional positive regard. They are less attracted by the rewards of money and objects and work whole-heartedly toward goals and purposes. They tend to fuse work and play and have more peak or creative experiences. It also appears that, for most people, developing creative potential requires incubation, education, diligence, nurture, and opportunity, despite some evidence of particular individuals having the ability to overcome detrimental circumstances in order to actualize their occupational creativity.[14-17]

There are numerous references to potentialities from many different spheres that have been collected on the World Wide Web.[18] Three of those that relate to the idea of becoming through doing and being, and that come from authors with a range of occupational interests are provided in Table 5-1.

Becoming is intimately related to concepts of self; it is often an expression of autonomy[19]; it is also an expression of the values within societal structure. A way of communicating what people think they are about, it allows them to demonstrate what they can do. Becoming is also about what people believe they can contribute to their own growth through doing and what they can offer the community that is a special gift from them, that by its provision alters their place within societal structure. Aiming toward potentialities provides people with the chance to portray themselves as more than their outward appearance and everyday behavior; it allows the expression of attitudes, beliefs, and values in ways that demonstrate self-definition. Engaging in occupation that people perceive as self-actualizing provides opportunity for self-evaluation and grounds the senses of competency and moral worth. Becoming is both an agent of self-creation and a product of socializing forces providing motivation to experience the self as efficacious, competent, and consequential.[20] The latter claim touches on the notion that becoming is problematic for people who seek personal isolation or who find close relationships difficult, and points to why such people who have a particular talent may feel compelled to use it in order to communicate.

The concept of becoming that constitutes this occupational perspective of health includes the ideas of growing or coming into being; of living, moving, evolving energy; of aiming toward the highest levels of personal development and self-esteem; of potenti-

---

Table 5-1
Ideas About Potentialities From
Three Different but Significant American Sources

John Foster Dulles	1888–1959	Mankind will never win lasting peace so long as men use their full resources only in tasks of war. While we are yet at peace, let us mobilize the potentialities, particularly the moral and spiritual potentialities, which we usually reserve for war.[21]
Katherine Anne Porter	1890–1980	Our being is subject to all the chances of life. There are so many things we are capable of, that we could be or do. The potentialities are so great that we never, any of us, are more than one-fourth fulfilled.[21]
Margaret Mead	1901–1978	If we are to achieve a richer culture, rich in contrasting values, we must recognize the whole gamut of human potentialities, and so weave a less arbitrary social fabric, one in which each diverse human gift will find a fitting place.[21]

---

alities; of full humanness; of self-actualization; and that it is an ever-incomplete process. Such ideas are seen as integral to the view that people's occupational natures evolved over millennia with structural changes to body and brain in response to changes of environment, habitat, and survival pressures and as a result of natural selection. It is interesting to compare this with McMichael's description in Chapter 1 of the inter-related and distinctive features of the history of human ecology and disease. Readers may recall that the first 2 of these addressed the encounters of human societies with new environmental hazards and the recurring tension between biological needs and capacities and changes in living conditions.[22] This suggests, yet again, a close relationship between occupation and health.

Late in the evolutionary chain, as human capacities expanded, the need to keep those of a more diverse "intellectual" nature exercised for when they were required, demanded increased and more flexible activity patterns. These activity patterns were superimposed on and integrated with older activity/rest rhythms. Ornstein and Sobel observe that:

> As the brain evolved, its ability to handle the world became increasingly comprehensive. ... The paradox is that as the human brain matures and develops it both enormously increases its ability to find out new things and, at the same time, develops an enormous capacity for getting bored.[23]

The question of boredom is a complex one and will be addressed later when occupational imbalance is considered as an illness and as a cause of illness. That points to the need to recognize becoming as part of the health-illness complex.

ITS PLACE IN PUBLIC HEALTH: HOLISM AND HEALTH PROMOTION STRATEGIES TOWARD ALL PEOPLE BEING ABLE TO ACHIEVE PHYSICAL, MENTAL, AND SOCIAL ASPIRATIONS AND POTENTIAL

The place of becoming in public health relates to the discipline's acceptance that health promotion should be aimed toward all people being able to achieve physical, mental, and social aspirations as the holistic vision of WHO directs. The theme of this chapter from the OCHP is the source of the vision of health that is inclusive of becoming: "To reach a state of complete physical, mental and social well-being, an individual or group must be able to identify and to realize aspirations, to satisfy needs, and to change or cope with the environment."[24]

The vision is encapsulated in the Australian Aboriginal definition of health provided earlier. It prescribed a striving by health services "to achieve that state where every individual can achieve their full potential as human beings."[25] Public health certainly espouses the need to aim toward similar outcomes, but to enact them in the daily scheme of things is more difficult, especially as resources are scarce and becoming is seldom recognized as a priority.

No vision occurs in a vacuum, and there are many earlier sources relating to the belief that health and personal growth are entwined. For example, Alexis Carrel (1873–1944), a French-American physiologist who was a recipient of the Nobel Prize in 1912, when contemplating the benefits and drawbacks of the "modern society" of his era, concluded:

> It is a primary datum of observation that physiological and mental functions are improved by work. Also, that effort is indispensable to the optimum development of the individual. Like muscles and organs, intelligence and moral sense become atrophied for want of exercise ... the physiological and mental progress of the individual depends on his functional activity and on all his efforts. We become adapted to the lack of use of our organic and mental systems by degenerating. ... In order to reach his optimum state, the human being must actualize all his potentialities.[26]

Maslow's ideas echoed these earlier thoughts when he observed "capacities clamor to be used, and cease their clamor only when they are well used. That is, capacities are also needs. Not only is it fun to use our capacities, but it is also necessary for growth."[11] Some empirical research points to the truth of such assertions. For example, in a large, population-based, longitudinal study, Glass and colleagues found "enhanced social activities may help to increase the quality and length of life" and "social and productive activities are as effective as fitness activities in lowering the risk of death."[27] This study corroborates findings from other earlier research.[28,29] The opposite is also a source of anecdotal lore, with Maslow claiming, "The unused skill or capacity or organ can become a disease center or else atrophy or disappear, thus diminishing the person."[11] Certainly, inactivity has been found to be associated with several risk factors associated with the likelihood of cardiovascular disease[30-33] and with other diseases emanating from obesity.

The notion of becoming poses a particular challenge to health workers engaged in institutional or community care or in economically challenged programs for people living in poverty. Often they feel obliged to overlook people's potential growth and simply help them to cope with the here and now. The people they work with in that way can become unable to see what they have the capacity to be and how they might go about it. As Elizabeth Kubler Ross explained about her workshops with the dying, "... we have learned from the dying patient who has been our teacher ... things that regrettably no one helped them accomplish earlier so that they would have been able to say, 'I have truly lived.'"[3]

The question can be asked whether health practitioners compromise their professional becoming when they concentrate on coping services to the neglect of growing services; when they concentrate on risk elimination instead of encouraging and enabling managed risk taking. It is hypothesized that professional groups, as in any other community, will be less effective, become ill, and die a little if the potential and scope of their doing is restricted to a great extent by an outside force. This conjecture is applicable to both practitioners in affluent countries and to those working with many populations in the developing world. Practitioner and community alike frequently experience governance that curtails expression of inherent capacities. Many in socially disadvantaged, war-torn, or ecologically devastated countries are unable to meet even the prerequisites of health because of human enterprise or natural causes. Public health intervention for such situations, if possible, meets prerequisite needs while bearing in mind and attending to the being and becoming needs of whole communities that may assist in the future. The latter thought points to becoming being more than a matter of individual growth. It is the idea that links personal health with community development and suggests how important partnerships with groups in the wider community are in the world of promoting population health or preventing disasters from being ongoing.

Becoming: Biological Needs,
Natural Health, and Reaching Potential

Once again it is important to draw on biological science and history to inform the present and future. As controversial, Chicago-born philosopher, polemicist, and author Francis P. Yockey (1917–1960) explains:

> *The greatest repository of psychology of all is History. It contains no models for us, since Life is never-recurring, once-happening, but it shows by example how we can fulfill our potentialities by being true to ourselves, by never compromising with that which is utterly alien.*[18]

The first part of this section will consider becoming as a biological need, and the second, natural health and survival pressures.

BIOLOGICAL BASES FOR THE NEED TO REACH POTENTIAL

Readers will recall, in one definition of human biological needs in the first chapter, that they are seen as related to health from the standpoint of how organisms are recognized as flourishing.[34] That is, some biological needs have been described as facilitating fulfilment of potential.[34] Additionally, it was explained that instinctive energy of a primitive nature can be redirected toward ends that are perceived to be of particular value, and that the capacity for redirection allows people to make choices, which enable the "highest achievements of humanity."[35,36] The meeting of needs when they focus on becoming provides people with the essence of well-being.

Maslow saw this process as the "... development of the biologically based nature of man, [empirically] normative of the whole species conforming to biological destiny, rather than to historically arbitrary, culturally local value models as the terms 'health' and 'illness' often do."[11] His "Hierarchy of Human Needs" is usually depicted as a pyramid in which self-actualization forms the apex to represent the highest of the needs. People who reach self-actualization sometimes experience a state of "transcendence," described as an increased awareness of self and species potential. People attempt to meet the "deficiency or D needs" of the layers below the apex because they feel anxiety if they do not. The self-actualization needs at the top of the triangle Maslow called "growth needs," "being values," or "B-needs."[10,37] These include needs for justice, truth, beauty, meaning, simplicity, wholeness, and order, some of which have been touched on already in previous chapters. This is not surprising because the division between doing, being, and becoming made in this text is arbitrary and solely for the purpose of understanding the complexity of an occupational perspective of health.

Many people make the mistake of attributing becoming needs only to people who appear gifted with a particular talent such as of an artistic nature. Becoming, however, is a need of all people and can be recognized in many spheres of life while forming the essence of personality. In that vein, Jung proposed:

> *Personality is the supreme realization of the innate idiosyncrasy of a living being. It is an act of high courage flung in the face of life, the absolute affirmation of all that constitutes the individual, the most successful adaptation to the universal conditions of existence coupled with the greatest possible freedom for self-determination.*[38]

Erikson, another psychiatrist, discusses a further aspect of becoming that touches on health. In the book *Identity*, he writes:

> *A man's character is discernible in the mental and moral attitude, in which, when it came upon him, he felt himself to be most deeply and intensely active and alive. At such moments there is a voice inside which speaks and says: "This is the real me."*[39]

These are but 2 of numerous hypotheses about a basic need for becoming: the "third dimension" of occupation. Another that is worthy of consideration is discussed in *Churchill's Black Dog and Other Phenomena of the Human Mind*. In this text, becoming is explained in relation to the need to create order and unity out of complexity and diversity because "human beings have to order their experience, both spatially and temporally, as part of their biological adaptation to reality, and the forces which impel them to do so are just as 'instinctive' as sex."[1]

Storr describes, in ways that resonate with notions about self-actualization, of the biological endowment to discover and to create "new hypotheses which bring order and pattern to the maze of phenomena."[1] In the everyday world, searching for answers to vexed questions is a regular occurrence that also calls upon this extraordinary dimension of futurity that is a part of becoming. Since early in the last century when Wallas described how inspiration appeared to follow a period of incubation,[40] others have also found this to be the case. A process of conscious preparation is followed by a stage of apparently doing nothing and, often following sleep, the emergence of a new illumination and inspiration. Sometimes this happens overnight, and at other times it can take many years. This unconscious problem-solving, creative solution process is an ongoing one that can be the trigger to becoming activity. Perhaps understandably to those who advocate the remedial nature of occupation, the motivating factor that sets people upon the hazardous, often unrewarding task of trying to bring order and meaning to their lives can originate from alienation or despair as well as joy. Creative endeavor that reconciles disparate elements is essentially integrative and some are driven to it by "a need to prevent their own disintegration."[1]

In Sir Ernst Gombrich's *The Sense of Order*, links are also made with exploratory tendencies and the need for "pattern making."[41] By creating order, the need to pay equal attention to every impinging stimulus is reduced, and people only need to take notice of novel stimuli. This explanation meshes with zoologist Watson's determination that humans, in common with some other species such as tigers, wolves, monkeys, and apes, never stop investigating, exploring, or adapting. This need or tendency—neophilia—is aimed at thriving as well as surviving; at becoming as well as doing and being; not without problems it has been a positive and powerful force in evolution to the present day:

We create unnecessary problems, inventing labour-wasting devices to help fill the time between the cradle and the grave. Our basic needs are taken care of by society, so we make difficulties for ourselves. We allow our jobs to become more complex than necessary. We fill our leisure time with more and more elaborate recreations. We tempt fate by courting danger, taking risks. ... We look in our own lives, for more complex forms of expression, experimenting with arts and sciences that give free rein to our gigantic brains. ...[42]

Neophilia "grows from old and well-established roots"[42] and is a need that is experienced throughout life, not solely during childhood and youth. It is easily squashed by external forces of a personal nature, of political initiative, or of environmental circumstance. When the restrictions that are commonly placed on older people "for their health's sake" are touched upon later in the chapter, it is cautionary to recall how little attention is paid to the notion that becoming is a need throughout life, except, perhaps, with regard to those considered exceptional in some field. Among these, there appears to be opposing schools of thought with regard to their mental health specifically. People recognized with special talents that require nurturing tend either to be seen as exceptionally well-balanced or to be liable to instability.[1] In a study of 47 award-winning British writers and artists, it was found that 38% had undergone treatment for affective illness.[43] At the opposite extreme, experimental psychology lends some support to the hypothesis that "creative powers are to some extent protective against mental illness" despite creative people exhibiting "more neurotic traits than the average person."[1] The apparent incompatibility between mental illness and creativity is supported by a decline in the quality and quantity of the work of many creative people if they do become insane.[1] Some creative people such as Balzac, for example, "... keep the devil at bay by manic overwork. Success and public recognition can, in some degree, compensate for inner emptiness by providing recurrent injections of self-esteem from external sources."[1] Additionally, while engaged in creative or other demanding occupations, including paid employment, people can live through and seek out what Maslow defines as a peak experience and Csikszentmihalyi describes as flow.[44]

The biological needs associated with becoming are part of humans' inheritance along with their capacities, talents, personalities, and biological characteristics. The needs are weak in terms of how easy it is for them to be overcome by societal, cultural, and environmental expectations, and much of people's inner nature is repressed or unconscious, though it rarely disappears. Indeed, the pressure to self-actualize, to grow, and to experience well-becoming is a dynamic force that enables improvement. Maslow predicted that if this inner nature is "frustrated, denied or suppressed, sickness results" in some form or other, sooner or later.[11] More recently along those lines, Doyal and Gough affirm "people consist of more than the deterministic relationships between their bodily components."[19] They identify 3 major variables in their exploration of autonomy as a key human need alongside health:

1. The level of self-understanding and cultural expectations
2. The capacity to formulate options
3. The opportunities enabling action

In essence, these relate to people's doing, being, and becoming through the "ability to formulate consistent aims and strategies which they believe to be in their interests and their attempts to put them into practice in the activities in which they engage."[19]

NATURAL HEALTH AND REACHING POTENTIAL

All humans have a common origin and can exist in countless different environments because of their complex and biological characteristics and capacities. For millennia, the characteristics and capacities that form the basis of the need to strive toward becoming what each has the potential to become were the foundation of creative ways to survive in disparate ecosystems. Selection favored the adaptive and creative. As the great Dubos explains:

> *Adaptive patterns of behavior become, of course, increasingly important as one ascends the scale of living things. In higher animals, and more so in man, adaptation expresses itself in instincts, tastes, and habits which help the group and the individual in making use of available resources and in avoiding sources of danger.*[45]

Humans have used their "becoming capacities" for adaptive behavior so effectively that population growth, constant change, and innovation are evident throughout the globe. That means ways of doing that are innovative are still a primary mechanism for survival; doing, being, and becoming are all important to continuity of health and well-being. The interaction between becoming through doing and being, changing occupational structures, and the experience of well-being or morbidity and mortality opens a window into a variety of recurring themes. One that emerges as important is the effect on health of urbanization and technological advancement.

Urbanization started with the acquisition and possession of land following the adoption of agriculture. However, only a small proportion of people have lived in urban centers for the thousands of years since then, and even as late as 1800 only 3% of the world's population were city residents. The Greeks "mistrusted aggregations of more than 10,000 people since they considered anything larger hard to govern and keep healthy."[46] Their cities were complex, innovative, and beautiful, a testament to people's search for more than meeting the needs of shelter, safety, comfort, and social life. Medieval and Renaissance cities were also small, yet are said to have been "architecturally, economically, and intellectually satisfactory and satisfying social entities even though their hygiene was poor and their infant mortality high."[46]

This picture changed as urbanization escalated dramatically and paid employment became segregated from family life and home base. From roughly 1730 until the turn of the 20th century, urban conditions were appalling.[47] Possibly the innovators in the industrial classes reached their potential, but workers were too crowded, tired, and sick to have any chance of meeting those needs.

Lorenz described how he saw overcrowding as deleterious to health; people subjected to the overpopulation of city life experience "exhaustion of interhuman relationships."[36] His argument is that this causes them to lose sight of the species' innate friendliness and social nature that is apparent "when their capacity for social contact is not continually overstrained."[36] A "superabundance of social contacts forces every one of us to shut himself off in an essentially 'inhuman' way and, because of the crowding of many individuals into a small space, elicits aggression."[36] His point of view does more than suggest that aspects of sociality also fit into this becoming sphere. People can exist alone if they can obtain the basic needs for water, food, and shelter; they can do whatever is required of a single person to obtain such prerequisites of health according to the environment; they can find meaning and purpose through those and other solitary activities. Becoming, though, as well as often being an expression of personal strengths and capacities, is usually dependent upon stimulation or feedback from others or is aimed at solving social problems of some kind.

In terms of stimulation, Dubos, in the foreword to *Population, Environment and People*, comments: "I love crowds and cities ... All over the world the largest and most polluted cities are also the ones with the greatest appeal even though their inhabitants uniformly complain of congestion and pollution."[48] There may be truth in the claim that city living "provokes to activity those attributes of the brain which are essentially human, namely the capacity to devote major resources of human endeavor to pursuits and goals that are not material."[46] It is common for people to express strong feelings about their attachment to city living or, alternatively, their desire to "get away from it all." Yet whether or how changes in the size of population groupings affect health has not been the topic of intensive inquiry and may be a major, largely unrecognized factor in occupational imbalance, deprivation, or alienation through restrictions to physical, mental, or social becoming.

As paid employment has assumed high status, many other forms of occupation have become devalued. Additionally, leisure activities have become subject to high technological development and over-regulation. Advances in technology have largely overtaken the value once given solely to human achievements so that a change in the nature of capacities that are applauded is apparent. Effectively, this values material goods at the expense of people and process, and devalues capacities and skills, as well as the goods people can produce by their own efforts. Ironically, although not always linked with capitalist gain, technological experimentation and development have been strong characteristics of the becoming nature of humans throughout history. Our "genetic constitution" is organized in such a way that all people experience the need to engage in exploratory, adaptive, and productive occupational behavior seemingly for the purpose of reducing time spent on necessary occupations in favor of time for self-chosen ones. The effort to save time in order to use it in some other way demonstrates how individuals unconsciously seek to use the range of their capacities. For some people, the range of obligatory activities concerned with their work may meet their biological needs for physical, mental, and social stimulation, exercise, and self-actualization; for others, this may be far from the truth.

Industrial processes and capitalist structures narrowed the range of activity of many individuals to those that were economically efficient and viable, reducing many of the peripheral occupations, often of a social or problem-solving nature, that in earlier economies had provided opportunity to use a wide range of capacities. Industrialization certainly signalled an enormous change from the long period of human occupation based mainly on natural processes through either hunting and gathering or agriculture, to occupations that in some cases appear to be many steps removed from nature and natural needs or processes. Carrel, in his call for the scientific study of mankind, suggested that "it is difficult ... to know exactly how the substitution of an artificial mode of existence for the natural one and a complete modification of their environment have acted upon civilized human beings."[26] People joyfully welcome "modern civilization," adopting new modes of life and "ways of acting and thinking" and laying aside "old habits" because these "demand a greater effort."[26] Most accept that technological change is necessarily an improvement and that the development of machines to reduce occupational effort is inevitable and desirable. In this way, new technology leads to new cultural adaptations, which, in turn, lead to further technological change, and so on. This can be constructive or destructive and, depending on the viewpoint taken, can be either or both.

In technically advanced societies, the industrial era has evolved rapidly into a new electronic era. Arthur Penty, a follower of Morris, is credited with coining the phrase "postindustrial society" at the turn of the 20th century,[49] but social commentators as diverse as Daniel Bell, Alain Touraine, and Barry Jones give us contemporary descriptions.[50-52] To them, postindustrial society is characterized by a change from production to service industries, from manual to professional and technical workers, and to decision-making based on information technology. Those economic changes are part of "a crisis that is simultaneously tearing up our energy base, our value systems, our sense of space and time, our epistemology as well as our economy" and will result in a "wholly new and drastically different social order."[53] The tension between traditional social forms that are still largely in place and modern postindustrial arrangements has been responsible for a period of unprecedented uncertainty and loss of direction for many people. Jones suggests that, despite "universal literacy, an omnipresent media, and a vast information industry," postindustrial society is threatened by its "preoccupation with materialism, a conviction that national and international salvation is to be found in economic growth alone, and emphasis on externalized (consumption-based) value systems."[52] He predicts that if a new labor-absorbing industry comes into being, as has been the case after earlier economic revolutions, it will turn away from technology. Reintroduced will be labor/ time-absorbing work such as education, home-based industries, craftwork, leisure, tourism, and welfare services that will act as a guard against unemployment and the concentration of wealth into fewer and fewer hands.

The value given to technology has caused a devaluation of older members of society. Many are confused by the rapid social and technical changes occurring around them; whereas in agricultural societies they were often viewed as wise counselors and spiritual leaders, in postindustrial societies they have been effectively displaced because their early life experiences are no longer seen as relevant and they are viewed as being part of a "stagnant, marginal social category."[54] The same attitude is evident in dealings with nonmodern technology-based societies. In large part, the lack of understanding and recognition of the human need for occupation and its relationship with health has contributed to humans allowing technological development to drive them rather than the other way around. The driving force at present is based on economic theory rather than on human nature and needs. Countering this could be possible if all people had a better understanding of the purpose and meaning of occupation in a generic sense. Such understanding demands "... a sociological imagination that reminds us of the real range of social behavior ... necessary so that we can collectively decide which kinds of work and which kinds of leisure are appropriate to a good life and create the opportunities for these to be realized."[55]

In fact, from the industrial era forward, occupation for its own sake seems to have lost its efficacy and value, perhaps because it is no longer an integral part of a self-sustaining ecological way of life. This has obscured some biological needs that are germane to the species' survival. The need to use human capacities in a creative, problem-solving, inventive, or adaptive way has led to the domination of occupational technology over the ecology, queries about the survival of the species in the long-term, and ironically to the detriment of present and future use of personal capacities to meet biological potential.

Some commentators argue that when humans become sufficiently focused on these culturally created problems, the same drive that created them will be able to counteract the ill effects. This could already be in process. Indeed, Toynbee suggested in the 1960s that even though "in making ... tools progressively more effective" and the "misuse of them progressively more dangerous," the "World's most powerful nations and governments have shown an uncustomary self-restraint on some critical occasions" demonstrating an "advance in social justice" and an increase in humanitarianism.[56] In present times, there is widespread questioning of the wisdom of continuing with economic policies that place technological development and the expansion of trade before human well-being and diminishing natural resources. Robertson, in *Future Work*, calls for people to reject a future of technological determinism in which technology rather than value systems dictate choice[57]; and Jones suggests that "the most appropriate analogies for economic processes are to be found in biology—with growth, maturation, nourishment, excretion, and decline—rather than physics."[52]

Aging and Becoming:
Ancient and Modern Rules for Health

An Example From the Past

Earlier, 3 factors were identified by Doyal and Gough in relation to people's need for autonomy.[19] These factors are apparent in the brief story that will be told here to illustrate an ancient and aging view of becoming. This tale is told because it provides:

* An example of a personal experience in line with the ancient *Regimen.*

* A link to the modern rules: to UN and WHO ideology about active aging.

Lewis Cornaro, a noble Venetian from an illustrious family, tells his story. Written in Padua in 1558, he reflects on his experiences of good health and relates them to the way he lived his life in his later years. In his younger days, he had been intemperate in his habits and prone to anger in part because family misconduct led to disgrace, a loss of honor, and a subsequent loss of public roles in the service of Venice. When he was about 40, he perceived the ill consequence of his actions and curbed his inordinate appetites and passions. A man of sound understanding, courage, and resolution, he recovered his health and vigor. At a very advanced stage of life, he wrote the story of the irregularities of his youth, his reformation, and his hopes for a long life. He died when over 100 years old seated in a chair and without any pain. Cornaro wrote the first of 3 discourses at the age of 83, the second at 86, and the third at 91. They were published separately and contain lively descriptions of the health, vigor, and perfect use of all his faculties that he enjoyed at an advanced age.[58]

> ... I will therefore give an account of my recreations, and the relish which I find at this stage of life, in order to convince the public (which may likewise be done by all those who know me) that the state I have now attained to is by no means death, but real life; such a life as by many is deemed happy, since it abounds with all the felicity that can be enjoyed in this world.
>
> ... And this testimony they will give, in the first place, because they see, and not without the greatest amazement, the good state of health and spirits I enjoy; how I mount my horse without any assistance, or advantage of situation and how I not only ascend a single flight of stairs, but climb up a hill from bottom, to top, afoot, and with the greatest ease and unconcern; then how gay, pleasant, and good-humoured, I am; how free from every perturbation of mind, and every disagreeable thought; in lieu of which, joy and peace have so firmly fixed their residence in my bosom as never to be part from it. Moreover, they know in what manner I pass my time, so as not to find life a burden; seeing I can contrive to spend every hour of it with the greatest delight and pleasure, having frequent opportunities of conversation with many honourable gentlemen, men valuable for their good sense and manners, their acquaintance with letters, and every other good quality. Then, when I cannot enjoy their conversation, I betake myself to the reading of some good book. When I have read as much as I like, I write; endeavoring in this, as in every thing else, to be of service to others, to the utmost of my power. And all these things I do with the greatest ease to myself, at their proper seasons, and in my own house ...   *(continued)*

... I have my several gardens supplied with running waters, and in which I always find something to do that amuses me. I have another way of diverting myself, which is, going every April and May, and likewise every September and October, for some days, to enjoy ... a convenient and handsome lodge, in which place I likewise now and then make one in some hunting party suitable to my taste and age. ... But what delights me most is, in my journeys backwards and forwards, to contemplate the situation and other beauties of the places I pass through; some in the plain, others on hills, adjoining to rivers or fountains; with a great many fine houses and gardens.

... And if it be lawful to compare little matters, and such as are esteemed trifling, to affairs of importance, I will further venture to say, that such are the effects of this sober life, that, at my present age of eighty-three, I have been able to write a very entertaining comedy, abounding with innocent mirth and pleasant jests.

... And, indeed, if I may be allowed to be an impartial judge in my own cause, I cannot help thinking that I am now of sounder memory and understanding, and heartier, than he was (Sophocles) when ten years younger...

... I find there, before me, not one or two, but eleven, grandchildren, the oldest of them eighteen, and the youngest two; all the offspring of one father and one mother; all blessed with the best health; and, by what as yet appears, fond of learning, and of good parts and morals. Some of the youngest I always play with, and, indeed, children from three to five are only fit for play. Those above that age I make companions of; and, as nature has bestowed very fine voices upon them, I amuse myself, besides, with seeing and hearing them sing, and play on various instruments. Nay, I sing myself, as I have a better voice now, and a clearer and louder pipe, than at any other period of life. Such are the recreations of my old age.

Cornaro L. *A Treatise on a Sober Life.* 1558.

United Nations and World Health Organization Ideology About Active Aging

In line with recognition of the ongoing nature of becoming needs, it is important for population health approaches to encourage older people to do what they can and want to do, rather than tell them what they can't or shouldn't do.

The WHO, in its fact sheet discussing mental health promotion, stated that:

Aging of the population is a highly desirable and natural aim of any society. By 2025 there will be 1.2 billion older people in the world, close to three-quarters of them in the developing world. But if aging is to be a positive experience it must be accompanied by improvements in the quality of life of those who have reached—or are reaching—old age.[59]

It is clear from preceding chapters that it is not just any occupation that is health promoting. People's doing, being, or becoming can lead to either or both negative or positive health outcomes. To ensure that aging is a positive experience, it is imperative to consider whether occupations provide people with sufficient meaningful physical, mental, and social exercise and opportunity to meet their unique becoming needs. Fortunately, the modern rules of health supplied by the WHO and in accord with the UN are more than supportive of this proposition.

At the UN's first World Assembly on Aging in 1982, recognition was accorded to the accumulated wealth of knowledge and experience that makes the aged an asset rather than a liability to society. At that time, the Assembly reaffirmed that the Universal Declaration of Human Rights:

> ... apply fully and undiminished to the aging and recognized that the quality of life was no less important than the longevity, and that the aging should therefore, as far as possible, be enabled to enjoy in their own families and communities a life of fulfillment, health, security and contentment, appreciated as an integral part of society.[60]

The UN's support of older people needing and being enabled to continue to fulfil their occupational becoming in ways that enhance potential and growth was developed further in 1989 and again in 1999 when the International Year of Older People was celebrated. It petitioned nations to establish or strengthen policies aimed at meeting the developmental potential of the aged as well as their humanitarian needs.[61,62] In 2001, governments were again urged to promote healthy, active aging through the development of programs that ensure quality of life.[61]

Picking up on the theme of active aging, the WHO developed a Policy Framework for the second UN World Assembly on Aging held in Madrid in 2002. Based on recognition of the UN principles of "independence, participation, dignity, care and self-fulfillment,"[63] this recommended that policies and programs for older people need to both enable those who are able to continue to contribute to society in important ways and also prevent discriminatory action that can be counterproductive to well-being.[63] The concept is described as allowing "people to realize their potential for physical, mental and social well-being throughout the life course and to participate in society according to their needs, desires and capacities."[63] Active aging, therefore, centers older people firmly within the postmodern vision of fair, ethical, and moral societies. The civic principles of such encourage both freedom of expression and liberty for all people, whatever their age.[64,65] As a matter of social justice, it is claimed that people should be able to enact aspirations and use their talents as well as engage in daily life tasks regardless of difference in age or, indeed, of class, income, race, gender, disability, health status, or similar grouping factors.

Enactment of legislation in countries with codes of social justice in accord with WHO directives appears impressive, but recognizing the principles in terms of everyday life emerges as more difficult. Examples of the call for active and inclusive societies in which rights carry responsibilities and individuals experience opportunities to realize potential can be found in legislation throughout the Western world. In the main, though, discussion in such legislation focuses on people of working age despite the growing numbers of older citizens. Comments in 1990s policies termed "enabling states," such as in Clinton's "blueprint for a new America," omit strategies relating to enabling older people to play an active role as the prime agents of their own development.[66] Rather, their place in the brave new scheme of things was, and is, as passive clients of welfare systems, and comments are often limited to economic concerns, such as provision of pensions and services.[67-70]

A question arising from these modern rules for physical, mental, and social health is why there appears to be so little emphasis in legislation or in health and social welfare literature on active aging. To adopt this humanitarian approach might not only enable older people to improve the quality of their lives in ways that enable them to keep on growing, it might also reduce the numbers it is generally feared will clog the beds available in institutional care. Perhaps it is a reflection on the youth culture of postindustrial societies when everything old is disregarded and thrown away and people spend fortunes on looking young. It is even being said that the sale of antiques is dropping so generalized is the trend. This tendency is widespread despite the growing numbers of older people. Whatever the cause is found to be commonly and patronizingly, active aging as it pertains to the doing, being, and becoming wants and needs of people beyond "paid employment" years is marginalized. This is often in the name of risk management, particularly for those who come into contact with medical, health, and social welfare services. Risk management strategies fail in many respects to recognize that externally imposed strategies can disempower recipients and lead to illness of a kind less obvious in cause than hazards like slipping on mats or rugs. Widespread too is discouragement by family members and caregivers of older people engaging in pursuits of their own choice that are deemed too active. Although apparently altruistic and due to fear of detrimental effects on health that may lead to increasing dependence or of their relative's death, such discouragement can be viewed as discriminatory whether institutionally or privately constituted.[71] Older people have the same rights as others to lead their own lives in the way that ensures their continuing to actualize their potential.

As the UN claims, the aging of populations is a "pervasive, unprecedented and enduring process with profound social and economic implications."[62] To create societies in which all older people can continue to contribute according to their capacities is not without difficulty in capitalist economies. Despite rhetoric to the contrary, such economies embrace action that sustains inequalities because they are largely driven by monetary considerations rather than the enabling or enhancement of human capacities.[71]

Despite this, some older people display a level of well-being that clearly equates to their level of activity, to their meeting personal goals, and to reaching toward their potential. Alex Comfort, in a remarkable book that pre-empts the "active aging" initiatives, explains, "Aging has no effect upon you as a person. When you are 'old' you will feel no different and be no different from what you are now or were when you were young, except that more experiences will have happened."[72]

He supplies an extremely useful definition of agism and some prime examples of older people continuing to become what they had the potential to become.

Ageism is the notion that people cease to be people, cease to be the same people or become people of a distinct and inferior kind, by virtue of having lived a specified number of years. ... Like racism, which it resembles, it is based on fear, folklore and the hang-ups of a few unlovable people who propagate these. Like racism, it needs to be met by information, contradiction and, when necessary, confrontation. And the people being victimized have to stand up for themselves in order to put it down.

At 64 Maggie Kuhn organized an American network of highly vocal older people, dedicated to fighting agism. They were known as the Gray Panthers. A firm believer in experimenting with new life styles she claimed: "the old are isolated by government policy."

Italy's great nineteenth-century composer, Giuseppe Verdi, was 73 when he completed Otello, approaching 80 when he composed Falstaff, a scintillating comedy, very different from his previous works. He retired after completing Stabat Mater, an inspired choral work at 84.

(continued)

Golda Meir resigned as Israel's Prime Minister at the age of 75. She had held the post for five years through two Middle East wars. The following year she was asked to head a committee to rejuvenate the Labour Party.

In Helena Rubinstein's memoirs, *My Life for Beauty,* written when she was in her nineties, she told of creating a beauty business over seven decades that crossed six continents. Claiming work had been her beauty treatment she explained her belief that hard work keeps the wrinkles out of the mind and the spirit, helping to keep a woman young and alive.

Duncan MacLean was 90 when he won a silver medal at the 1975 World Veterans' Olympics by running 200 metres in 44 seconds. A sprinting champion of South Africa from 1905 to 1907 he continued sprinting after his retirement at 80. Prior to that he had toured the world with a comedy song-and-dance act and, in his sixties, took up house painting. His future goal was to run a hundred metres on his hundredth birthday.

Charlie Smith who was officially recognized as the oldest person in the United States in 1972 had been made to retire from his work on a citrus farm when he was 113 because he was considered too old to be climbing trees. For twenty years after that he ran a small store in Florida, until he was 133, living alone at the back of his store, when, on medical advice, he moved into a retirement home.

Comfort A. *A Good Life.* Melbourne, Australia: Macmillan Company of Australia; 1977:35,82,105,109,147,174,182.

Comfort's examples are clear indicators of health and occupational well-being through doing, being, and becoming. They also point to self-chosen risk taking as integral to continued becoming and health enhancement. These indicators are facilitated or inhibited by the same underlying factors identified in the previous 2 chapters. The underlying factors determine in large part for how many years, and in what circumstances, people carry out chosen occupations for growth and self-actualization. In support of the idea that becoming is intimately related to positive health outcomes, Csikszentmihalyi found that an optimal state relating to health and well-being occurs when individuals are challenged by their occupations and have the personal capacities to meet the challenge.[73] The antithesis is that if this does not occur, ill health may be a consequence.

Figure 5-1 provides a paradigm of the complex relationship between becoming through doing and being and illness or physical, mental, and social well-being.

Human characteristics and biological needs are the foundation stones of "becoming," as they are of health and cultural evolution. These have furthered the establishment of different and creative economies; political systems; and national values, policies, and priorities and erect, often by default, division between classes, genders, and age groups in opportunities for engagement in occupation and on attitudes, relationships, and doings within communities. State and public institutions and the utilities should not restrict equitable opportunity for people to engage in doing that nourishes and challenges the mind, body, and spirit. If no restriction occurs, communities are likely to demonstrate increased energy, interest, contentment, and commitment and an increased life expectancy.[27] If it does occur, preclinical social and mental illness such as early institutionaliza-

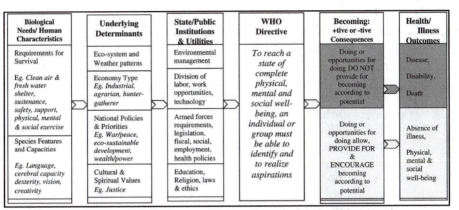

Figure 5-1. Determinants of illness or well-being through doing and being to become.

tion, antisocial behavior, substance abuse, stress, boredom, and depression or preclinical physiological signs such as decreased fitness, increased blood pressure, changes in sleep patterns, and emotional state can occur. All can ultimately result in disease, disability, or premature death.

Lack of Becoming as a Factor in Illness

Since the 1940s, medicine and public health have had an impact on conditions of human life worldwide. In many places, some types of infection have become rare and some extinct and epidemic diseases have declined in importance where they were formally common and serious. It is hard to exaggerate the impact of those changes on human health and outlook.[74] Those medical science advances ensure that more people are provided with a stable base from which to experience becoming, positive health, and well-being. On the whole, though, in many parts of the world, health and well-being seem to sit uneasily amid the rush and stresses of present-day occupational structures that humans have constructed over the years. It is here that public health intervention is required, not least in addressing more thoroughly what and how people do, be, and become.

Morbidity and mortality can result from lack of individual, community, or social awareness about the relationship between what people do, how they feel about it, and whether or not they can actualize their potentialities. This is, in large measure, because of a lack of research based on a sufficiently broad or holistic perspective of occupation and a resultant dearth of intervention strategies from public health, social, political, or national policies. That suggests that understanding the nature of stress as an outcome of unsatisfactory doing, being, and becoming would be useful.

Stress is a basic phylogenic mechanism that under normal circumstances works to maintain physiological equilibrium in times of physical and emotional pressure. If prolonged at an unacceptable level, susceptibility to illness is increased. Adolph Meyer is credited with recognizing, early in the last century, that disease appeared to occur when this regulatory system became subjected to overload,[75] and Hans Selye, in 1936, described the "general adaptation syndrome"[76] in which he hypothesized that the adaptive response can break down due to "innate defects, understress, overstress, or psychological mismanagement."[76] Common stress diseases include "high blood pressure, heart accidents, and nervous diseases."[77] Currently, it is probable that nutritional disorder might join that list. Selye argued that the type of illness experienced as a result of stress expresses an individual's weakest points.[78] This suggests that genetic or familial predisposition, such as mental breakdown, arthritis, or cardiac failure, can be activated by prolonged stress.[79] Work based on Selye's hypothesis has largely sustained it. A well-publicized study by French and Caplan links stress with coronary heart disease,[80] and others have suggested that stress is associated with depressive illness and disorders of the musculoskeletal, digestive, and immune systems.[81]

Roskies and Lazarus propose that the ability to cope with everyday stress has more effect on physical, mental, and social health than stress episodes themselves,[82] and similarly, Moore argued that:

> Long-term chronic stress and especially chronic unpredictable stress can result in an earlier demise or long-term disability (mental and/or physical), unless therapeutic intervention can reverse the individual's way of coping and/or reverse the situations which are causing the stress.[83]

She listed some effects of chronic unpredictable stress as increased heart rate, respiration, muscle tension, and blood-glucose levels; decreased peristalsis, lymphocytes, T and B cells, immune response, destabilization of lysosomes, and hyper-alert states as well as blood pressure. Temoshok argues that there is little empirical evidence either "to support or refute potential biological pathways linking stress factors and disease initiation or progression for any disorder."[84] He suggests that this reflects the complexity of the connections, which probably include person and situation variables, interaction effects including physiological and psychological predispositions, as well as social, cultural, economic, and political contexts.[84] That argument, while challenging the possible direct links between stress and disease, supports the theory proposed here that it is the complex relationship between the outside world and all parts of the brain involved in health and in occupation that can lead to stress-related illness or wellness.

Stress-related illnesses as a result of doing too much or too little (occupational imbalance), finding little meaning or purpose in doing (occupational alienation), and not having opportunities to aim toward becoming (occupational deprivation) have undoubtedly increased during evolution.[85-89] That is despite the obvious benefits of living in today's postindustrial world rather than that of hunter-gatherers and despite longer life expectancy, lower infant mortality, and miraculous advances in technological and pharmaceutical medicine for those living in postindustrial societies. That being so, to conclude this chapter on becoming, the risks of occupational deprivation, alienation, and imbalance will be discussed.

OCCUPATIONAL DEPRIVATION

Deprivation implies dispossession, divestment, confiscation, or taking from, and the influence of an external agency or circumstance that keeps a person from "acquiring, using, or enjoying something."[90] The external agency or circumstance that causes occupational deprivation may be technology, the division of labor, lack of employment opportunities, poverty or affluence, cultural values, local regulations, and limitations imposed by social services and education systems, as well as the social consequences of illness and disability. Particularly relating to becoming aspects of occupation, familiar examples spring to mind, such as prisoners of the state as punishment for criminal activity or as a result of taking refuge in another country, the reluctant retiree, the institutionalized, numerous individuals engaged in caregiver duties, the school leaver or middle-aged process worker unable to find paid employment, or the lonely, battered child with little access to toys or stimulus. It might also be the social impact (or external circumstance) of being confined to a bed or wheelchair because of illness or physical handicap. Illness or disability itself is an example favored by occupational therapists perhaps because of familiarity. However, Whiteford, who is becoming a leader in this new field of exploration,[91-93] claims that on the whole deprivation relates to "external, socially constructed phenomenon based on cultural values that creates exclusion" rather than illness or disability itself.[94]

All types of biological and social deprivation have been associated with failure to make use of occupational opportunities for any age group.[95-97] Infants deprived of the opportunity for learning through doing because of lack of sensory stimulation within their environments fail to develop normally or to thrive.[98-102] In extreme examples where children have been left alone in almost empty rooms and provided with only food and a place to sleep, they have failed to develop even basic skills of walking and self-care. The classic example of child deprivation is the "wild boy of Aveyron" who appeared from the woods of Caune, France in the late 18th century after, probably, at least 7 of his 12 years living alone. Despite 5 years of experimental education by Jean Itard, he never attained normal language or robust health, although he did develop in many ways.[103] The prolonged deprivation experienced by children in Romanian orphanages is a more recent example. Every child in these institutions for over 6 months showed significant developmental delays.[104] Infants were initially found to be functioning at a level between the "at risk" and "deficiency" categories of the total Test of Sensory Functions.[105] Following a 6-month program within an enriched environment, children improved in all but "adaptive motor functions."[106]

For prisoners, the importance of finding meaning through occupation is one factor in their survival odds. In a study of the coping behavior of Nazi concentration camp survivors, purpose was identified as essential to those who survived; one found this by focusing on "where I could find a blanket, something to chew, to eat, to repair, a torn shoe, an additional glove."[107] Frankl, an existential psychiatrist, observed about his own concentration camp experiences that mortality rates were highest among those unable to find purpose.[108] Imagine the deprivation effects of imprisonment on children. As late as 15 years ago in Brazil, minors who roamed the streets between 1979 and 1990 could be taken from their families and placed in dreary places known as "Funamen" (National Foundation for the Well-being of Minors) until they were 18. Here they were without any benefits that education provides.[109] In jails, states of occupational deprivation have been linked with both community and individual disorders, such as prison riots[110] and suicide while in custody.[111] The opposite was the case as, over a period of 7 years, prisoners being studied became increasingly involved in a variety of occupations. That led to decreases of dysphoric emotional states, stress-related medical problems, and disciplinary incidents.[112]

As was reported in the last chapter, many people experience reduced options to do, be, and become because they are deprived of paid employment for a variety of reasons and may, as a result, suffer a decrease in health. The value placed upon paid employment by society increases the potency of the deprivation and is not restricted to the types of employment considered normative in the Western world. An example is provided by the "self-destructive activities such as drinking [and] violence"[113] and poor health experienced by First Nation Australians that occurred alongside loss of traditional occupations. Aboriginal elders, particularly from remote areas, disturbed by the phenomenon "asked that 'sit-down' money be replaced by money for work done by those who were unemployed" (sit-down money is welfare or dole money).[113] The Community Development Employment Project Scheme came into being, providing "an increase in the health of communities, ... more people involved in physically active tasks, a decrease in alcohol consumption, an increase in cleanliness, and better nutrition."[114] This is a rare example of an "occupational" initiative being implemented for combined health, social, and economic benefits. Other people who are at risk of illness from occupational deprivation include disadvantaged groups within the community, such as the poor and ethnic minorities, with the WHO noting "the remarkable sensitivity of health to the social environment."[115,116]

Women, too, have generally suffered occupational deprivation for hundreds of years to a point, seen by Mackie and Pattullo, as destroying the vitality of women.[117] They have enjoyed some respite during particular eras when more equal opportunity between men and women is apparent but subject to subservience to fathers or husbands and not extending to political equality. In the medieval period, women in towns were able to engage in many trades, as the number of medieval English words ending in "ster" or "ess" attests, such as "webster" (woman weaver), "baxter" (woman baker), and "seamstress" (woman sewer).[117-121] In fact, Etienne Boileau's 13th century *Book of Trades* records that women in Paris worked in 86 of 100 trade and professional guilds.[119] Although accepted as of lesser value than the roles men undertook, women's occupations, which were often "gruelling and virtually unending," were also productive, rich in variety, self-expression, responsibility, achievement, satisfaction, and not "compartmentalized, isolated, or solitary."[117] Unmarried women from the upper and merchant classes could receive a better education and the chance to engage in a greater range of occupations by entering a nunnery.

The restricted occupational role of affluent women was hazardous to health because their physical activity was slight, the use of their mental capacities restricted, and their "social usefulness was never recognized or recompensed."[122] Florence Nightingale at the age of 26 said that she knew of some women who had gone mad for lack of things to do, observing that many "don't consider themselves as human beings at all;"[123] similarly Elizabeth Garrett Anderson suggests that "there is no tonic in the pharmacopoeia to be compared with happiness, and happiness worth calling such is not known where the days drag along filled with make-believe occupations and dreary sham amusements."[124]

The strong preference for women to follow domestic and child-raising occupations in the home in Victorian times was linked with infant health.[125] It was thought that if married women undertook paid employment outside the home, this could be at the sacrifice of infant lives.[126] Criticism of this conclusion was linked with statistics providing evidence that overcrowding and insanitary conditions were more crucial variables and that some children might benefit from better food and conditions provided by mother's wages.[127] The 1893–1894 Royal Commission on Labour, which investigated conditions of women's work, including "the effects of women's industrial employment on their health, mortality, and the home," found the association between women's employment and infantile mortality was imprecise and impressionistic.[128] Yet as recently as 1976 in the field of social health, Gordon expressed occupational gender bias:

> It is said that a man's job provides him with a means to satisfy his ego by preserving his personal integrity and by maintaining his place in the world. On average a man's occupation is more important to his mental health than is outside occupation to a woman. She gains status as a wife and mother and from her home. ... Some women need to work outside: a lot do not wish to do so. At least that is what they say.[46]

The inequality of opportunity that has characterized women's occupations for thousands of years is still evident today, particularly in developing countries, although in affluent societies it has improved greatly. Increased opportunity for women to exercise capacities and develop potentials has contributed to remarkable improvements in women's morbidity and mortality since the 19th century. However, the improvement is multifactoral, including the effects of reduced birth rate, greater understanding of obstetrics and gynecology, emancipation, and changed attitudes. The study of the relationship between women's occupations and health are limited, on the whole, to job stress,[129-132] reproductive hazards,[132-136] and the threat to family function and maternal responsibilities.[137]

Occupation evolved as people adapted to challenge, and this process is escalating. The technological possibility of more radical changes in occupation could result in serious health consequences. Dubos warned half a century ago that although humans may appear to adapt to new environments, their biological inheritance only enables adaptation up to a point and that chronic disease states can develop over time.[138] Maslow too was concerned that humankind was "at a point in history unlike anything that has ever been before" with "huge acceleration in the growth of facts, of knowledge, of techniques, of inventions, of advances in technology."[10] He suggested that the rapidity of the changing world calls for "a different kind of human being ... who is comfortable with change" because "societies that cannot turn out such people will die."[10] Because parts of the brain are rooted in earlier species' inheritance, people are only able to respond with biological reactions that are either "obsolete" or "inappropriately elicited."[23] It is recognized in the OCHP that there are health concerns associated with socioecological change in calls for a "systematic assessment of the health impact of a rapidly changing environment, particularly in areas of technology, work, energy production, and urbanization."[24]

OCCUPATIONAL ALIENATION

Alienation is used to describe a feeling of estrangement; a lack of familiarity or comfort; a separation or divorce from; and a turning away from or being set against some thought, place, person, or situation.[139] It is a concept that is not easy to understand. I found it useful to consider the analogy of an animal born in captivity—a lion, for example, who has only ever known a world of a cage, of other animals living solitary lives in their own cages, and of people who feed and care for him, but who demand particular behavior from time to time. It is possible to understand that the lion will experience needs and instincts that relate to the natural environment in which he would have lived in the wild but with no means of really appreciating or satisfying them. He is estranged or alienated from his species' nature, from his activities, and from other animals but because he has never known a natural lifestyle, he does not understand why he feels unhappy, frustrated, or the need for something different. Humans because of their occupational species' nature have constructed, over time, their own cages. The bars are the products and results of their occupations; the sociocultural values, laws, and rules; political direction; and economic structure that grew from what they do or their forebears did. Like the lion, humans are estranged from their species nature, from others, from what they do, and from the results of their activities.

Since the time when people lived in harmony with the natural environment with only the simplest of technology to assist them to meet their occupational needs, humankind has sought to challenge and master nature by developing more and more sophisticated technology to meet their occupational needs and wants, to conquer ill health, and to delay death by ever-increasingly sophisticated medical science. Such technological change can be described as potentially alienating even if at the time it seems to be a good thing. Daniel Miller suggests that the status given to the medical profession and its scientific values can be alienating factors in the way that they exert control over the procedures aimed at rapid repair of body parts, decontextualized from the recipient's mental or social needs.[140]

Alienation is a theme that surfaced as a central concept of Marx's philosophy; it is intimately connected with his views about human nature, praxis, and activity as a union of naturalism and humanism.[141-143] He regarded any productive, economic, social, or spiritual activity, as well as the products of activity such as philosophies, morals, money, commodities, laws, or social institutions, as potentially alienating.[141] Because of "cultural" and "capitalist" history, such activities and products have become estranged from the natural creativity of humans, resulting in them experiencing feelings of alienation toward themselves, others, activities, and products. These alienating activities (such as the division of labor) are "forced upon individuals by the society which they themselves create,"[144] and as long as "activity is not voluntary ... man's own deed becomes an alien power opposed to him, which enslaves him instead of being controlled by him."[145] Marx suggested a direct illness connection with the processes of industrialization because "factory work exhausts the nervous system to the uttermost, it does away with the many sided play of the muscles, and confiscates every atom of freedom, both in bodily and intellectual activity."[146]

Those conditions are now regarded as so unhealthy that it is difficult to understand why people made the mass exodus from country to town until it is appreciated that "the move from farm to factory was based on social trends that the individual could not control" and economic need.[147] Huge numbers of the population changed not only their habitats but the structure of their social networks from small, cohesive groupings, which worked and played together, to large populations in which individuals knew or were close to few people. Work separated men and women, altering the value of their occupations and experiences of social and mental well-being; it separated adults from children, altering teaching and learning roles; and children, unless engaged in child labor with their parents, no longer observed or participated with them as they engaged in the daily round of socially valued roles and skills. Instead, they learned from strangers.

Such changes to basic human relationship patterns may well have gradually impacted on some of the family loneliness and social alienation problems common in the modern world and that lead directly or indirectly to ill health. Mijuskovic puts a case that alienation and individual loneliness are more pronounced and prevalent in postindustrial "atomistic societies" than in "organic communities."[148] In the latter, natural functions, role perspectives, mutual interdependence, and intrinsic relations are stressed in contrast to individual freedom, external connections, causal and reductionistic explanations, rule orientation, and artificial frameworks of the former.[148] His view has some merit when it is observed how current postindustrial values and changing occupational structures, language, and technologies can:

* Restrict freedom of action by ever-increasing rules, regulations, and bureaucracy.

* Replace ongoing human endeavor with labor-saving technology, which often creates work of a mundane variety.

* Reduce the availability of paid employment, which has interest, meaning, or meets individual needs for growth and challenge.

* Create a materialistic way of life out of step with sustaining the natural world of which humans are a part.

All of these changes have the potential to create environments that are alienating enough to spawn discontent and disease (Figure 5-2).

Since Marcuse's renewed attention to Marx's theme of alienation in 1932, others, such as Fromm, have continued widespread and intense discussion that links the notions of alienation with sickness or ill health for individuals and for societies.[149] In numerous recent studies, alienation associated with unsatisfactory occupational factors is implicated in illness and health-risk behaviors, particularly for people already disadvantaged.[150-157] While technological change in itself (unless toxic) is unlikely to cause illness, the effects on people's engagement in occupations and their reaction to the changes can lead to illness even in high demand jobs.[158] Justice argues that when work is perceived as stressful, boring, or meaningless, the likelihood of "mass illness" is increased,[159] and this is evidenced by a review of material from 16 epidemics of illness at various workplaces and schools.[160]

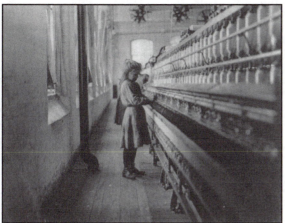

Figure 5-2. Work of a mundane variety with little interest or meaning is alienating. An example at the Carolina Cotton Mills in 1908. (Reprinted with permission of the Library of Congress, Prints & Photographs Division, National Child Labor Committee Collection.)

There is convincing evidence that the health benefits of paid employment depend on its quality,[161-165] and those who are dissatisfied with work experience numerous symptoms and stress and tend to drink or smoke more than those who are satisfied.[166] Alienation will continue to increase as production and service jobs become "deskilled" and lose their capacity to interest those doing them because "many jobs that have been transformed by new technology are characterized by high levels of boredom."[167,168] For those employed in intellectual occupations, such as educators, administrators, scientists, and health professionals, stresses caused by what Naisbit calls the "chaos of information pollution" are frequently described as overwhelming.[169]

So much respect is progress accorded in today's world that the natural health needs of people pale in significance beside the drive to create more sophisticated technology. Technological progress has altered the character of many shared social occupations, including entertainment and sport for which chemical potions as well as mechanical, biophysical, and electronic apparatus have been developed and marketed so that individuals may achieve previously unrealized feats. Such technology subtly reduces the use of human energies, creativity, and potentials; alters the elements of human toil, the pure skill, and the mental and social exercise components drawn from within any participant; and can be alienating to individual growth. Because the technology is primarily created to meet market purposes rather than human needs, it is alienating. Lorenz saw the acquisition of assets becoming a primary need, reaching a "pathological" state with the potential to cause mental and social disruption that he deemed to be symptoms of cultural ill health.[36]

Other major and potentially alienating change that goes along with rapid technological advances has been a marked increase in the urge to accumulate material goods and property without a thought for the potential of materialism to destroy the ecosystem. Many erroneously equate material wealth with happiness and health, mistaking the means for the ends. By the mid-20th century, Mumford was obviously alienated by "over-charges of empty stimuli, ... materialistic repletion, ... costly ritual of conspicuous waste, ... and highly organized purposelessness" as part of the "clinical picture of the cultural disease from which the world suffers."[170] He went as far as to assert that:

> The supernatural theology of the Middle Ages was closer to reality than the crass materialism of an age which fancies that the achievement of an 'economy of abundance' will automatically ensure a maximum of human felicity.[170]

OCCUPATIONAL IMBALANCE

The central place held by the notion of balance in Classical Greek medicine based on humoral physiology has already been discussed. A physician's job was to advise on due proportion, to "restore a healthy balance," and to aid "the natural healing powers believed to exist in every human being."[171,172] Plato, for example, espoused avoiding "exercising either body or mind without the other" in order to maintain "an equal and healthy balance between them."[173] He advised those engaged in "strenuous intellectual pursuit" to exercise the body, and those interested in physical fitness to develop "cultural and intellectual interests."[173] When the Greek citizen engaged in both or either of those pursuits he, and sometimes she, did so in the social environment of the gymnasia, so combining the 3 WHO components of physical, mental, and social well-being.

In the present day, occupational balance is more often than not thought of solely in terms of a balance between work and leisure. As Sigerist suggested, work may:

> ... be harmful to health, may become a chief cause of disease, when there is too much of it, when it is too hard, exceeding the capacity of an individual, when it is not properly balanced by rest and recreation, or when it is performed under adverse circumstances.[174]

Those are important aspects of occupational balance but so, too, is the need to consider balance such as that between physical, mental, and social capacities; intrinsic and extrinsic factors; activity and food; obligation and choice; excitement and lethargy; the Romantic and the rational; isolation and togetherness; or boredom and burnout. Heeding such aspects of healthy balance is seldom, if ever, the primary concern of medical science, political planning, or sociocultural structures. A pilot study in Australia began to explore perceptions of occupational balance and its relationship to health from the viewpoint of physical, mental, social, and rest activities. It was found that for the respondents, ideal occupational balance was approximately equal involvement in each. A significant relationship, using one-way analysis of variance ($p = 0.0001$), was found between the closeness of current occupational patterns to those perceived by the respondent to be ideal and his or her reported health. Eighteen of the respondents (12.3%) had identical current and ideal balances, and each of these reported his or her health to be fair or excellent, while none of the respondents who reported poor health rated their current balance as identical to their ideal balance.[175] A study replicating this in the United Kingdom and Europe largely supported these findings.[176]

In this text, a few of the types of balance mentioned above are considered to support the idea that imbalance involves a state that occurs because people's engagement in occupation fails to meet either their natural health requirements for physical, social, and mental exercise or rest or their unique doing, being, and becoming needs. Imbalance will differ for each individual because their capacities, interests, and responsibilities differ, and illness as a response to imbalance will differ according to physiology, environment, and occupational natures and needs. That is, physiological imbalance and illness result from individual responses to, and coping with, the vicissitudes of everyday life, which are closely tied to peoples doing, being, and becoming. The arbitrary dividing of occupation into socially discrete categories such as work and play impedes the conscious awareness of the need for occupational balance as an integral aspect of health. However, Friedman suggests that Cannon's ideas about homeostasis "may well come to dominate medical thinking in the 21st century... as the interdependence of the internal bodily systems is revealed, and as the role of harmony between the person and the environment is documented."[177] In terms of the so-called lifestyle disorders of the present day, imbalance can be a cause of the production of "excessive stress hormones—cortisol and catecholamines—which can lead to artery damage, cholesterol buildup, and heart disease."[159,178] When "our responses to problems in life are excessive or deficient, ... the balance is upset between us and our resident pathogens" because "the central nervous system and hormones act on our immune defences in such a way that the microbes aid and abet disease."[159,179]

When the natural balance between activity and rest is considered, apparent from the study of more primitive cultures, it would seem that artificial constructs, such as the 8-hour day, 5-day work week, or shift work, have little to recommend them. These are socially, economically, or politically based "temporal" constructs. Despite studies that have found that shift work, which disrupts sleep-wake patterns, can lead to irritability, malaise, fatigue, stomach complaints, diminished concentration, diminished functional capabilities, mood changes, and increased susceptibility to accidents, there remains a lack of action to alter existing work patterns to reduce the illness impact of biologically based temporal rhythms.[180-182]

In evolutionary terms, the activity-rest continuum appears to have a biological balancing function that serves a survival purpose whereby energy is conserved and stored during resting, and resting, as well as contributing to the other purposes of sleep discussed in the first chapter, provides a time for watchfulness. A state of watchfulness provides data in readiness for action should a need arise. The watchfulness remains, although its original survival function is obscured sometimes under the sociocultural guise of entertainment. Television, for example, one of the most common "resting" occupations of present times, provides a time for watchfulness, but also a time for people to learn about and reflect on their world for similar survival reasons to ages past. In contemporary Western society, the instinct for recreational inactivity as a natural means of resting or conserving energy remains although the need for it has been largely eliminated.[183] Passive activity seldom provides for being and becoming needs. It is universally reported that watching television, for example, involves practically no challenges or skills, does not provide flow experiences,[184-186] and may lead to "a progressive atrophy of the desire for new challenges."[44]

Arguing from the other extreme, it can be suggested that the amount of time people have available for restful occupations may not meet their overall needs in terms of biological balance. An example, but just one of many possibilities, is the way most people are obliged to use their mental capacities differently to earlier times. That is, there is a probable decrease of time and opportunity for intellectual or spiritual reflection and much more time required to attend to routine, but demanding, paper or electronic work. For many, this is stressful, and a common complaint is that people lack energy and are tired by the mental and social demands of their occupations. Such lack of balance can result in boredom or burnout.

Boredom is the most common emotional response to lack of occupation particularly of a being and becoming nature, and burnout is the widely reported emotional response to overstimulation, inappropriate occupation, and too much to do. Both boredom and burnout are forms of stress that have been linked with illness. Ornstein and Sobel argue there is an optimal set point for stimulation "in the middle of an organism's response level" maintained "through feedback processes similar to the homeostatic mechanisms of the body" and that when there is either "too much or too little, instability results and disease may follow."[23] While overload has received more attention than insufficient occupation as a cause of illness, if energy systems are not used they deteriorate. Both "highly conditioned endurance athletes who go through a period of detraining" and people who are bedridden experience huge "decreases in the oxygen energy system in relatively short periods of time."[187] This phenomenon can decrease immune responses and increase susceptibility to illness.[188-191] Ardell claims that "boredom is the arch-enemy of wellness" and that "it is the leading cause of low level worseness."[192] He argues that it can be held responsible for health risk behaviors, such as smoking, drug, and alcohol abuse, and "a failure to take the positive initiatives associated with potent lifestyles."[192]

Apart from individual experience of imbalance, there is an imbalance in health opportunities through occupation throughout communities according to sociocultural and spiritual values, political direction, welfare economics, and community history. This imbalance is becoming a cause for concern to the extent that it is a common topic of conversation in many community venues and is a constant theme in popular media. In terms of paid employment, for example, at one extreme are the unemployed and at the other the over-employed. Both have decreased opportunity for engagement in satisfying and valued occupation that may enable them to maximize their potential. The *Weekend Australian Review*, dated April 8–9, 1995, anticipated 21st century reality when it devoted more than a page to an article addressing the age of overwork. This article presented evidence from several major postindustrial nations to suggest that many people in paid employment are now expected to take on increased duties, to spend longer hours on work tasks without extra rewards, and that health breakdowns from this cause are increasing.[193,194] Women are particularly at risk because they often undertake a double role of domestic and paid employment occupations.[195-197] This is the case not only in postindustrial societies. Barrett and Browne assert that African women have a triple workload as biological, social, and economic producers, which is deleterious to their health,[198,199] and Ferguson found that women in a marginal area of Kenya experience stress-related illness because of the demands of their many occupations, as well as poor nutrition, high fertility rates, and limited access to health care.[200]

Another cause for concern that makes a frequent appearance in popular media of affluent countries is obesity, yet in the multitude of articles and texts about diets there is only limited reference to all the activities that people do as opposed to exercise per se. Often the small percentage of people committed to physical exercise regimens and "physical health" are very aware of how their food intake affects what they do, but many widely differing circumstances associated with occupation affect the prevalence of weight disorders. Much more could be highlighted, such as the need to vary nutritional intake when occupations change. If it does not, there is a resultant imbalance between energy input and output. For example, according to Garrow's obesity index based on the ratio W/H^2, an individual per 121 pounds of body weight will expend approximately 1.5 calories per minute employed as a typist, in contrast to 3.5 if engaged in domestic work.[201-203]

Despite affluent societies having an abundance of occupational choices that offer opportunity for the exercise and development of physical, mental, and social skills, the structures, material costs, and values placed upon different aspects of occupation may well affect how successfully individuals access these opportunities. People may also be restricted in their choice by factors as various as time, lack of resources, lack of awareness, or, perhaps, because the focus of their occupations appears irrelevant to survival, health, or well-being. Communities in the developing world who have to meet their becoming as well as their doing and being needs in industrial environments that were depriving, imbalanced, and alienating a hundred years or so ago in Europe are experiencing similar disadvantages to their health as was the case then. This is doubly so for those in absolute poverty because they face lack of opportunity to meet even the prerequisites of health. Such obstacles do cause occupational imbalance, occupational deprivation, or occupational alienation even though many live more natural lifestyles than postindustrial affluence permits.

References

1. Storr A. *Churchill's Black Dog and Other Phenomena of the Human Mind.* Glasgow: William Collins Sons & Co Ltd; 1989:168.
2. Browning R. Andrea del Sarto: lines 97-98.
3. Wilson Schaeff AA. *Meditations For Women Who Do Too Much.* San Francisco, Calif: Harper Collins; 1990.
4. Wilson Schaeff AA. *Living in Process: Basic Truths for Living the Path of the Soul.* New York: The Ballantyne Publishing Group; 1999.
5. Burnham WH. *The Wholesome Personality.* New York: Appleton-Century; 1932.
6. Fromm E. *Man for Himself.* New York: Holt, Rinehart and Winston; 1947.
7. Rogers C. *On Becoming a Person.* Boston, Mass: Houghton Mifflin; 1961.
8. Bullock A. *The Humanist Tradition in the West.* London: Norton; 1985.
9. Ingleby D. Mental health. In: Kuper A, Kuper J, eds. *The Social Science Encyclopedia.* London: Routledge; 1985.
10. Maslow A. *The Farther Reaches of Human Nature.* New York: Viking Press; 1971.
11. Maslow A. *Toward a Psychology of Being.* 2nd ed. New York: D. Van Nostrand Company; 1968:191.
12. Maslow AH. *Motivation and Personality.* New York: Harper and Row; 1954.
13. Rogers CR. Towards a theory of creativity. In: Vernon PE, ed. *Creativity.* London: Penguin Books; 1970:140.
14. Amabile TM. *The Social Psychology of Creativity.* New York: Springer Verlag; 1983.
15. Gardner H. *Creating Minds: An Anatomy of Creativity Seen Through the Lives of Freud, Einstein, Picasso, Stravinsky, Eliot, Graham, and Gandhi.* New York: Basic Books; 1993.
16. Stein MI. *Stimulating Creativity.* Vols 1 and 2. New York: Academic Press; 1974 and 1975.
17. Golann SE. Psychological study of creativity. *Psychol Bull.* 1963;60:548-565.
18. Potentiality. BrainyMedia.com; Copyright 2005.
19. Doyal L, Gough I. *A Theory of Human Need.* London: Macmillan; 1991.
20. Gecas V. Self concept. In: Kuper A, Kuper J, eds. T*he Social Science Encyclopedia.* London: Routledge; 1985:739-740.
21. Brainy Quote. Potentialities. Available at: http://www.brainyquote.com/quotes/keywords/potentialities.html. Accessed April 21, 2006.
22. McMichael T. *Human Frontiers, Environments and Disease: Past Patterns, Uncertain Futures.* Cambridge: Cambridge University Press; 2001:xiii.
23. Ornstein R, Sobel D. *The Healing Brain, A Radical New Approach to Health Care.* London: Macmillan; 1988:207,214.
24. World Health Organization, Health and Welfare Canada, Canadian Public Health Association. *Ottawa Charter for Health Promotion.* Ottawa, Canada: Author; 1986.
25. Agius T. Aboriginal health in Aboriginal hands. In: Fuller J, Barclay J, Zollo J, eds. *Multicultural Health Care in South Australia. Conference Proceedings.* Adelaide: Painters Prints; 1993:23.
26. Carrel A. *Man, the Unknown.* London: Burns and Oates; 1935:178-179.
27. Glass TA, Mendes de Leon CF, Marotolli RA, Berkman LF. Population based study of social and productive activities as predictors of survival among elderly Americans. *BMJ.* 1999;319:478-483.
28. House JS, Robbins C, Metzner HL. The association of social relationships and activities with mortality: prospective evidence from the Tecumseh community health study. *Am J Epidemiol.* 1982; 116:123-140.
29. Welin L, Larrsen B, Svardsudd K, Tibblin B, Tibblin G. Social network and activities in relation to mortality from cardiovascular diseases, cancer and other causes – a 12 year follow up of the study of men born in 1913-1923. *J Epidemiol Community Health.* 1992; 46:127-132.
30. Kannel WB, Belanger A, D'Agostino R, Israel I. Physical activity and physical demand on the job and risk of cardiovascular disease and death: The Framingham study. *Am Heart J.* 1986; 112:820-825.
31. Paffenburger RS, Hyde RT, Wing AL, Lee IM, Jung DL, Kampert JB. The association of changes in physical activity and its correlates: associations with mortality among men. *N Engl J Med.* 1993; 328:538-545.
32. Kaplan GA, Strawbridge WJ, Cohen RD, Hungerford LR. Natural history of leisure time physical activity and its correlates: associations with mortality from all causes and cardiovascular disease over 28 years. *Am J Epidemiol.* 1996;144:793-797.
33. Simonsick EM, Lafferty ME, Phillips CL, Mendes de Leon CF, Kasl FV, Seeman TE et al. Risk due to inactivity in physically capable older adults. *Am J Public Health.* 1993;83:1443-1450.
34. Watts ED. Human needs. In: Kuper A, Kuper J, eds. *The Social Science Encyclopedia.* London: Routledge; 1985:367-368.
35. Knight R, Knight M. *A Modern Introduction to Psychology.* London: University Tutorial Press Ltd; 1957:56-57.

36. Lorenz K. *Civilized Man's Eight Deadly Sins.* Latzke M, trans. London: Methuen and Co Ltd; 1974:3-5,12-13.

37. Abraham Maslow. wikipedia. Last modified November 2005. Accessed December 2005.

38. Jung CG. The development of personality. In: Clemens SM, Rothgeb, eds. *Collected Works.* Vol 17. London: Routledge and Kegan Paul; 1953-79: paragraph 289.

39. Erikson E. *Identity.* London: Faber and Faber; 1958:19.

40. Wallas G. *The Art of Thought.* London: Cape; 1926.

41. Gombrich E. *The Sense of Order: A Study in the Psychology of Decorative Art.* Oxford: Phaidon; 1979.

42 Watson L. *Neophilia: The Tradition of the New.* Great Britain: Hodder and Stoughton Ltd; 1989:13.

43. Jamison KR. Mood disorders and seasonal patterns in top British writers and artists. In: Storr A, ed. *Churchill's Black Dog and Other Phenomena of the Human Mind.* Glasgow: William Collins Sons & Co Ltd; 1989:254.

44. Csikszentmihalyi M. Activity and happiness: toward a science of occupation. *J Occup Sci. Australia.* 1993;1(1):38-42.

45. Dubos R. *Mirage of Health.* New York: Harper & Row Publishers, Inc; 1959:43.

46. Gordon D. *Health, Sickness and Society: Theoretical Concepts in Social and Preventive Medicine.* St. Lucia, Queensland: University of Queensland Press; 1976:311.

47. Mumford L. *The Culture of Cities.* New York: Harcourt, Brace; 1938.

48. Dubos R. Foreword. In: Hinrichs N, ed. *Population, Environment and People.* New York: McGraw-Hill; 1971: xi.

49. Bullock ALC. Post industrial society. In: Bullock A, Stalleybrass O, Trombley S, eds. *The Fontana Dictionary of Modern Thought.* 2nd ed. London: Fontana Press; 1988:670.

50. Bell D. *The Coming of Post Industrial Society. A Venture in Social Forecasting.* New York: Basic Books; 1973.

51. Touraine A. *Post Industrial Society.* London: Wildwood House; 1974.

52. Jones B. *Sleepers, Wake! Technology and the Future of Work.* Melbourne, Australia: Oxford University Press; 1995:43-44.

53. Toffler A. *The Eco-Spasm Report.* New York: Bantam Book Inc; 1975:3

54. Hazan H. Gerontology, social. In: Kuper A, Kuper J, eds. *The Social Science Encyclopedia.* London: Routledge; 1985:337

55. Parker S. *Leisure and Work.* London: George Allen and Unwin; 1983: 119.

56. Toynbee AJ. A study of history. Vol XII. Reconsiderations. In: Kohn H, ed. *The Modern World.* New York: Macmillan; 1963:303-304.

57. Robertson J. *Future Work.* England: Gower Publishing Co; 1985.

58. Cornaro L. A Treatise on a Sober Life. Padua; 1558. In: Sinclair J, ed. *Code of Health & Longevity.* Edingburgh: Arch Constable & Co; 1806:50-52.

59. World Health Organization. *Mental Health: Strengthening Mental Health Promotion.* Fact sheet N°220. Revised November 2001; © World Health Organization 2005.

60. Department of Public Information. *Yearbook of the United Nations 1982.* New York: United Nations; 1982:1186.

61. Flynn-Connors E, ed. *Yearbook of the United Nations 1989.* The Hague: Martinus Nijhoff Publishers; 1989:688-689.

62. Gordon K, ed. *Yearbook of the United Nations 1999.* New York: United Nations; 1999.

63. World Health Organization. *Active Aging: A Policy Framework. Second United Nations World Assembly on Aging.* Madrid, Spain: Author; 2002:13.

64. Botes A. A comparison between the ethics of justice and the ethics of care. *J Adv Nurs.* 2000;20:55-71.

65. Metz T. Arbitrariness, justice, and respect. *Social Theory and Practice.* 2000;26:24-45.

66. Marshall W, Schram M, eds. *Mandate for Change.* New York: Berkley; 1993:228.

67. Gilbert N. *Welfare Justice: Restoring Social Equity.* New Haven, Conn: Yale University Press; 1995:151.

68. Commission on Social Justice. *Social Justice: Strategies for National Renewal. The Report of the Commission on Social Justice.* London: Vintage; 1994:3.

69. Organization for Economic Cooperation and Development. The future of social protection. Paris OECD, 1988.

70. Kalisch D. The active society. *Social Security Journal.* 1991;August:3-9.

71. Wilcock AA. Older people and occupational justice. In: McIntyre A, Atwal A, eds. *Occupational Therapy and Older People.* Oxford, UK: Blackwell Publishing; 2005.

72. Comfort A. *A Good Life.* Melbourne, Australia: The Macmillan Company of Australia Pty Ltd; 1977:28.

73. Csikszentmihalyi M. *Flow: The Psychology of Optimal Experience.* New York: Harper and Row; 1990.

74. McNeill WH. *Plagues and People.* London: Penguin Books; 1979.

75. Adams JD, ed. *Understanding and Managing Stress: A Book of Readings.* San Diego, Calif: University Associates Inc; 1980.

76. Selye H. A syndrome produced by diverse nocuous agents. *Nature.* 1936;138:32.

77. Selye H. History and present status of the stress concept. In: Monat A, Lazarus RS, eds. *Stress and Coping: An Anthology.* 2nd ed. New York: Columbia University Press; 1985:25.
78. Selye H. *The Stress of Life.* New York: McGraw-Hill; 1976.
79. Kobasa SC, Maddi SR, Courington S. Personality and constitution as mediators in the stress-illness relationship. *J Health Soc Behav.* 1981;22:368-378.
80. French JRP, Caplan RD. Organizational stress and individual strain. In: Marrow AJ, ed. *The Failure of Success.* New York: Amacon; 1972:30-66.
81. McQuade W, Aikman A. *Stress.* New York: EP Dutton and Co; 1974.
82. Roskies E, Lazarus RS. Coping theory and the teaching of coping skills. In: Davidson PO, Davidson SM, eds. *Behavioural Medicine: Changing Health Lifestyles.* New York: Brunner/Mazel; 1980.
83. Moore JC. Neurosciences and Their Application to Occupational Therapy. Unpublished lecture notes. Neuroscience Conference, Adelaide, 1989:185.
84. Temoshok L. On attempting to articulate the biopsychosocial model: psychology-psychophysiological homeostasis. In: Friedman HS, ed. *Personality and Disease.* New York: John Wiley and Sons; 1990:211.
85. Smith LA, Roman A, Dollard MF, Winefield AH, Siegrist J. Effort reward imbalance at work: The effects of work stress on anger and cardiovascular disease symptoms in a community sample. *Stress and Health.* 2005; 21:113-128.
86. Dollard MF, Dormann C, Boyd CM, Winefield HR, Winefield AH. Unique aspects of stress in human service work. *Australian Psychologist.* 2003;38:84-91.
87. Winefield AH, Gillespie NA, Stough C, Dua J, Hapuarachchi J, Boyd C. Occupational stress in Australian university staff: Results from a national survey. *International Journal of Stress Management.* 2003;10:51-63.
88. Dollard MF, Winefield AH, Winefield HR, eds. *Occupational Stress in the Service Professions.* London: Taylor and Francis; 2003.
89. Winwood PC, Winefield AH, Lushington K. The role of occupational stress in the maladaptive use of alcohol by dentists: A study of South Australian general dental practitioners. *Austr Dent J.* 2003: 48:102-109.
90. *Funk & Wagnall's Standard Desk Dictionary.* Vol 1 A-M. New York: Harper and Row; 1984:172.
91. Whiteford G. Occupational deprivation and incarceration. *J Occup Sci.* 1997; 4:126-130.
92. Whiteford G. Occupational deprivation: global challenge in the new millennium. *Br J Occup Ther.* 2000;63:200-204.
93. Whiteford G. (2004) When people cannot participate: occupational deprivation. In: Christiansen C, Townsend E, eds. *Occupation: The Art and Science of Living.* Upper Saddle River, NJ: Prentice Hall; 2004:221-242.
94. Whiteford GE. Understanding the occupational deprivation of refugees: a case study from Kosova. *Can J Occup Ther.* 2005;72(2):78-88.
95. Mackie A. Social deprivation and the role of psychological services. *Educational and Child Psychology.* 1992;9(3):84-89.
96. Townsend P, Simpson D, Tibbs N. Inequalities in health in the city of Bristol: a preliminary review of statistical evidence. *Int J Health Serv.* 1985;15(4):637-663.
97. Mechanic D. Adolescents at risk: new directions. *J Adolesc Health.* 1991;12(8):638-643.
98. Gilfoyle EM, Grady AP, Moore JC. *Children Adapt.* Thorofare, NJ: SLACK Incorporated; 1981.
99. Short MA. Vestibular stimulation as early experience: historical perspective and research implications. *Phys Occup Ther Pediatr.* 1985;5:135-152
100. Drotar D. Failure to thrive and preventive mental health: knowledge gaps and research needs. In: Drotar D, ed. *New Directions in Failure to Thrive.* New York: Plenum Press; 1985:27-44.
101. Provence S, Lipton RC. *Infants in Institutions.* New York: International Universities Press; 1962.
102. Day S. Mother-infant activities as providers of sensory stimulation. *Am J Occup Ther.* 1982;36:579-589.
103. Itard J. The wild boy of Aveyron. In: Malson L, ed. *Wolf Children and the Problem of Human Nature.* New York: Monthly Review Press; 1972
104. Bascom B. Program summary, projects and descriptions. In: *Brooke Foundation Annual Report.* Washington, DC: Brooke Foundation; 1993:12.
105. DeGangi GA, Greenspan SI. *Test of Sensory Functions in Infants (TSFI) Manual.* Los Angeles, Calif: Western Psychological Services; 1989.
106. Haradon G, Bascom B, Dragomir C, Scipcaru V. Sensory functions of institutionalized Romanian infants: a pilot study. *Occup Ther Int.* 1994;1:250-260.
107. Dimsdale, JE. The coping behavior of Nazi concentration camp survivors. *Am J Psychiatr.* 1974;131(7):795.
108. Frankl VE. *Man's Search for Meaning.* Boston, Mass: Beacon Press; 1962.
109. Bomfim V. Once a street kid, now a citizen of the world. In: Kronenberg F, Pollard N, eds. *Occupational Therapy Without Borders: Learning From the Spirit of Survivors.* London: Elsevier Ltd; 2005.
110. Useem B. Disorganization and the New Mexico prison riot of 1980. *Am Sociol Rev.* 1985;50(5):677-688.
111. Liebling A. Suicides in young prisoners: a summary. *Death Studies.* 1993;17(5):381-409.

112. Zamble E. Behavior and adaptation in long term prison inmates: descriptive longitudinal results. *Criminal Justice and Behavior.* 1992;19(4):409-425.

113. Jensen H. What it means to get off sit-down money: Community Development Employment Projects (CDEP). *J Occup Sci. Australia.* 1993;1(2):12-19.

114. Aboriginal and Torres Strait Islander Commission. No Reverse Gear: A National Review of the Community Development Projects Scheme. 1993.

115. Marmott M, Wilkinson RG, eds. *Social Determinants of Health.* Oxford, UK: Oxford University Press; 1999.

116. International Centre for Health and Society Social Determinants of Health: The Solid Facts. World Health Organization, Europe. 2003.

117. Mackie L, Pattullo P. *Women at Work.* London: Tavistock Publications; 1977:10.

118. Stavrianos LS. *The World to 1500: A Global History.* 4th ed. Englewood Cliffs, NJ: Prentice Hall; 1988:273-275.

119. Boileau E. *Livre de Metiers* (Book of Trades). 13th century.

120. Power E. The position of women. In: Crump CG, Jacob EF, eds. *The Legacy of the Middle Ages.* Oxford, UK: Clarendon Press; 1926:401-434.

121. Gross SH, Bingham MW. *Women in Medieval-Renaissance Europe.* St. Louis Park, Minn: Glenhurst; 1983.

122. Rowbotham S. *Hidden from History.* London: Pluto Press; 1973:58.

123. Woodham-Smith C. *Florence Nightingale.* London: The Reprint Society; 1952:71.

124. Anderson EG. Sex in mind and education: a reply. *Fortnightly Review.* The Fortnightly Review. 1874;21:582-594.

125. Jones H. The perils and protection of infant life. *Journal of the Royal Statistical Society.* 1894;1(vii):1-98.

126. Hewitt M. *Wives and Mothers in Victorian Industry.* London: Rockcliff; 1958.

127. Dyhouse C. Working class mothers and infant mortality in England, 1895-1914. *Journal of Social History.* 1978;xii:248-267.

128. Collett CE. The collection and utilization of official statistics bearing on the extent and effects of the industrial employment of women. *Journal of the Royal Statistical Society.* 1898;219-261.

129. Waldron I. The coronary-prone behavior pattern, blood pressure, employment and socio-economic status in women. *J Psychosom Res.* 1978;22:79-87.

130. Lemkau JP. Women and employment: some emotional hazards. In: Beckerman CL, ed. *The Evolving Female.* New York: Human Sciences Press; 1980.

131. Haw MA. Women, work and stress: a review and agenda for the future. *J Health Soc Behav.* 1982;23:132-144.

132. Lewin E, Olesen V. Occupational health and women: the case of clerical work. In: Lewin E, Olesen V, eds. *Women, Health and Healing: Toward a New Perspective.* New York: Tavistock Publications; 1985.

133. Bell C. Implementing safety and health regulations for women in the workplace. *Feminist Studies.* 1979;5(2):286-301.

134. Hunt VR. A brief history of women workers and hazards in the workplace. *Feminist Studies.* 1979;5(2):274-285.

135. Petcheky R. Workers, reproductive hazards, and the politics of protection: an introduction. *Feminist Studies.* 1979;5:233-245.

136. Wright MJ. Reproductive hazards and "protective" discrimination. *Feminist Studies.* 1979;5(2):302-309.

137. Fogarty MP, Rapoport R, Rapoport RN. *Sex, Career, and Family.* Beverly Hills, Calif: Sage Publications; 1971.

138. Dubos R. Changing patterns of disease. In: Brown RG, Whyte HM, eds. *Medical Practice and the Community: Proceedings of a Conference Convened by the Australian National University, Canberra.* Canberra: Australian National University Press; 1968:59.

139. Alienate. Editors of Readers Digest Services Pty Ltd in association with Gordon IA, Wilkes GA. *Word Finder: A Dictionary of Synonyms and Antonyms.* Sydney, Australia: Readers Digest Services Pty Ltd; 1983:24.

140. Miller D. Dissociation in medical practice: social distress and the health care system. *Journal of Social Distress and the Homeless.* 1993;2(4):243-267.

141. Marx K. Economic and philosophical manuscripts. In: Livingstone R, Benton G, trans. *Karl Marx: Early Writings.* New York: Penguin Classics; 1992.

142. Marx K. *Grundisse.* London: Penguin Classics; 1970.

143. Petrovic G. Alienation. In: Bottomore T, ed. *A Dictionary of Marxist Thought.* 2nd ed. Oxford, UK: Blackwell; 1991:11-16.

144. Mohun S. Division of labour. In: Bottomore T, ed. *A Dictionary of Marxist Thought.* 2nd ed. Oxford, UK: Blackwell; 1991:155.

145. Marx K, Engels F. *The German Ideology..* London: Lawrence and Wishart; 1964.

146. Fischer E. *Marx in His Own Words.* London: Allen Lane, The Penguin Press; 1970:43-44.

147. Triplett T. Hebrides women: a philosopher's view of technology and cultural change. In: Wright BD, Ferree MM, Mellow GO, et al, eds. *Women, Work and Technology*. Ann Arbor, Mich: The University of Michigan Press; 1987:147.

148. Mijuskovic B. Organic communities, atomistic societies, and loneliness. *Journal of Sociology and Social Welfare*. 1992;19(2):147-164.

149. Fromm E. *The Sane Society*. New York: Rinehart; 1955.

150. Burke RJ. Career stages, satisfaction, and well-being among police officers. *Psychol Rep*. 1989;65(1):3-12.

151. Winefield HR, Winefield AH, Tiggemann M, Goldney RD. Psychological concomitants of tobacco and alcohol use in young Australian adults. *British Journal of Addiction*. 1989;84(9):1067-1073.

152. Nutbeam D, Aaro LE. Smoking and pupil attitudes toward school: the implications for health education with young people: results from the WHO study of health behaviour among schoolchildren. *Health Education Research*. 1991;6(4):415-421.

153. Mosher A, Pearl M, Allard MJ. Problems facing chronically mentally ill elders receiving community based psychiatric services: need for residential services. *Adult Residential Care Journal*. 1993;7(1):23-30.

154. Nah KH. Perceived problems and service delivery for Korean immigrants. *Social Work*. 1993;38(3):289-296.

155. Semyonova ND. Psychotherapy during social upheaval in the USSR. Special section: in times of national crisis. *Group Analysis*. 1993;26(91):91-95.

156. Hammarstrom A. Health consequences of youth unemployment: review from a gender perspective. *Soc Sci Med*. 1994;38(5):699-709.

157. Rodenhauser P. Cultural barriers to mental health care delivery in Alaska. *Journal of Mental Health Administration*. 1994;21(1):60-70.

158. Haynes SG. Type A behavior, employment status, and coronary heart disease in women. *Behavioural Medicine Update*. 1984;6(4):11-15.

159. Justice B. *Who Gets Sick: Thinking and Health*. Houston, Tex: Peak Press; 1987:179.

160. Colligan MJ, Murphy LR. Mass psychogenic illness in organizations: an overview. *J Occup Psychol*. 1979;52:77-90.

161. Warr P. Twelve questions about unemployment and health. In: Roberts R, Finnegan R, Gallie D, eds. *New Approaches to Economic Life*. Manchester: Manchester University Press; 1985.

162. Warr P. *Work, Unemployment and Mental Health*. Oxford, UK: Oxford Science Publications; 1987.

163. Winefield A, Tiggerman M. A longitudinal study of the psychological effects of unemployment and unsatisfactory employment on young adults. *J App Psychol*. 1991;76(3):424-431.

164. Winefield A, Tiggerman M, Winefield H. Unemployment distress, reasons for job loss and causal attributions for unemployment in young people. *Journal of Occupational and Organizational Psychology*. 1992;65:213-218.

165. Winefield A, Tiggerman M, Winefield H, Goldney R. *Growing Up with Unemployment*. London: Routledge; 1993.

166. Verbrugge LM. Work satisfaction and physical health. *J Community Health*. 1982;7(4):162-283.

167. Farnworth L. An exploration of skill as an issue in unemployment and employment. *J Occup Sci. Australia*. 1995;2(1):22-29.

168. Adler P. Technology and us. *Socialist Review*. 1986;85:67-96.

169. Naisbitt J. *Megatrends; Ten New Directions Transforming Our Lives*. New York: Warner Books; 1982:24.

170. Mumford L. *The Condition of Man*. London: Heinemann; 1963:380.

171. Risse GB. History of Western medicine from Hippocrates to germ theory. In: Kiple KF, ed. *The Cambridge World History of Human Disease*. New York: Cambridge University Press; 1993:11.

172. Hippocrates. Regimen. In: Hutchins RM, ed. *Hippocratic Writings: On Ancient Medicine*. Chicago, Ill: William Benton; 1952.

173. Plato. *Timaeus*. Lee HDP, trans. New York: Penguin Classics; 1965:116-117.

174. Sigerist HE. *A History of Medicine. Vol 1. Primitive and Archaic Medicine*. New York: Oxford University Press; 1955:254-255.

175. Wilcock AA, Hall M, Hambley N, et al. The relationship between occupational balance and health: a pilot study. *Occup Ther Int*. 1997;4(1):17-30.

176. Lovelock L, Bentley J, Wallenbert I. Occupational balance and perceived health: a study of occupational therapists. Conference Abstracts, World Federation of Occupational Therapists' Congress. Stockholm: WFOT; 2002

177. Friedman HS, ed. *Personality and Disease*. New York: John Wiley and Sons; 1990:7,11.

178. Price VA. *Type A Behaviour Pattern: A Model for Research and Practice*. New York: Academic Press; 1982.

179. Wolf S, Goodell H. *Behavioural Science in Clinical Medicine*. Springfield, Ill: Charles C Thomas; 1976.

180. Monk T. Coping with the stress of shift work. *Work and Stress*. 1988;2:169-172.

181. Dinges D, Whitehouse W, Carota-Orne E, Orne M. The benefits of a nap during prolonged work and wakefulness. *Work and Stress*. 1988;2:139-153.

182. Rosa R, Colligan M. Long workdays versus restdays: assessing fatigue and alertness with a portable performance battery. *Human Factors.* 1988;5:87-98.
183. Hetzel BS, McMichael *T. L S Factor: Lifestyle and Health.* Ringwood, Victoria: Penguin; 1987:186-187.
184. Kubey R, Csikszentmihalyi M. *Television and the Quality of Life.* Hillsdale, NJ: Erlbaum; 1990.
185. Csikszentmihalyi M, Larson R, Prescott S. The ecology of adolescent activity and experience. *Journal of Youth and Adolescence.* 1977;6:281-294.
186. Larson R, Kubey R. Television and music: contrasting media in adolescent life. *Youth and Society.* 1983;15:13-31
187. Williams MH. *Lifetime Fitness and Wellness: A Personal Choice.* 2nd ed. Dubuque, Iowa: Wm. C. Brown Publishers; 1990:9,27.
188. Geschwind N, Galaburda A, eds. *Biological Foundations of Cerebral Dominance.* Cambridge, Mass: Harvard University Press; 1984.
189. Andervont HB. Influence of environment on mammary cancer in mice. *Journal of National Cancer Institute.* 1944;4:579-581.
190. Achterberg J, Collerrain I, Craig P. A possible relationship between cancer, mental retardation and mental disorder. *Soc Sci Med.* 1978;12:135-139.
191. de la Pena A. *The Psychobiology of Cancer.* New York: Praeger Publishers; 1983.
192. Ardell DB. *High Level Wellness.* 2nd ed. Berkeley, Calif: Ten Speed Press; 1986.
193. Gare S. The age of overwork. *The Weekend Australian Review.* 1995;April 8-9:2-3.
194. Schor J. *The Overworked American: The Unexpected Decline of Leisure.* New York: Basic Books; 1991.
195. Cox, R. (1997). Invisible labour: perceptions of paid domestic work in London. *J Occup Sci Australia.* 4(2):62-68.
196. Primeau LA. Household work: when gender ideologies and practices interact. *J Occup Sci.* 2000;7(3):118-127.
197. Zuzanek J, Mannell R. Gender variations in the weekly rhythms of daily behaviour and experiences. *J Occup Sci. Australia.* 1993;1(1):25-37.
198. Barrett HR, Browne A. Workloads of rural African women: the impact of economic adjustment in Sub-Saharan Africa. *J Occup Sci Australia.* 1993;2:3-11.
199. Barrett HR. Women, occupation and health in rural Africa: Adaptation to a changing socioeconomic climate. *J Occup Sci. Australia.* 1997;4(3):93-105.
200. Ferguson A. Women's health in a marginal area of Kenya. *Soc Sci Med.* 1986;23:17-29.
201. Passmore R, Eastwood MA. *Davidson and Passmore, Human Nutrition and Dietetics.* Edinburgh: Churchill Livingstone; 1986.
202. Garrow JS. *Treat Obesity Seriously.* Edinburgh: Churchill Livingstone; 1981.
203. Hafen BQ, ed. *Overweight and Obesity: Causes, Fallacies, Treatment.* Provo, Utah: Brigham Young University Press; 1975.

Suggested Reading

Barrett HR. Women, occupation and health in rural Africa: Adaptation to a changing socioeconomic climate. *J Occup Sci. Australia.* 1997;4(3):93-105.
Kronenberg F, Pollard N, eds. *Occupational Therapy Without Borders: Learning From the Spirit of Survivors.* London: Elsevier Ltd; 2005.
Maslow A. *The Farther Reaches of Human Nature.* Viking Press; 1971
Mumford L. *The Condition of Man.* London: Heinemann; 1963.
Ornstein R, Sobel D. *The Healing Brain, A Radical New Approach to Health Care.* London: Macmillan; 1988.
Storr A. *Churchill's Black Dog and Other Phenomena of the Human Mind.* Glasgow: William Collins Sons & Co Ltd; 1989
Whiteford G. Occupational deprivation: global challenge in the new millennium. *Br J Occup Ther.* 2000;63:200-204.
Winefield A, Tiggerman M, Winefield H, Goldney R. *Growing Up With Unemployment.* London: Routledge; 1993.
World Health Organization. *Active Aging: A Policy Framework.* Second United Nations World Assembly on Aging. Madrid, Spain: Author; 2002.
Wilcock AA. Older people and occupational justice. In: McIntyre A, Atwal A, eds. *Occupational Therapy and Older People.* Oxford, UK: Blackwell Publishing; 2005.

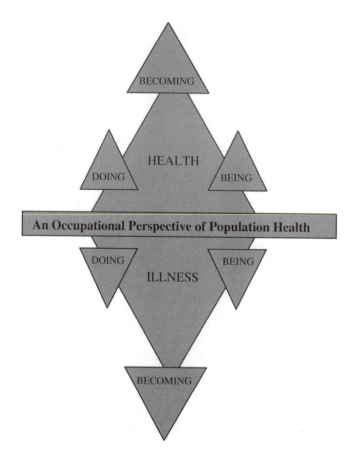

BECOMING

HEALTH

DOING   BEING

An Occupational Perspective of Population Health

DOING   BEING

ILLNESS

BECOMING

OCCUPATION AS AN
AGENT OF PUBLIC HEALTH

Theme 6:
  "Health is created and lived by people within the settings of their everyday life;
  where they learn, work, play and love."
  WHO, *Ottawa Charter for Health Promotion,* 1986

The chapter summarizes and presents:
* An occupational perspective of natural health and biological needs
* Public health through doing, being, and becoming
* Occupation-focused directives for health
* An "occupation for population health pyramid"

It is in this chapter that the ideas that have emerged in the previous ones will be drawn together to offer a particular view of health from the perspective of people as occupational beings and of occupation as a potential agent of public health. The summation of the ideas about natural health and biological needs that have come to light are combined into an occupational perspective. The focus will be on the positive and the negative; people doing, being, and becoming well or doing, being, and becoming ill. The chapter then links these perspectives to useful directions that have surfaced from both the ancient and modern rules about creating or maintaining health. Because we live in the present, those are, of course, in line with WHO directives that have provided chapter themes and the source of ideas for this text. The chapter concludes with an introduction to an "occupation for population health pyramid." I suggest that a device such as this is required to assist with increasing understanding concerning the poorly understood facts about the relationship of occupation to health. The discussion about this leads naturally to the second section of the book that suggests 4 occupation-focused approaches to improvement in population health.

An Occupational Perspective of
Natural Health and Biological Needs

From "ancient times, the theory that most of the ills of mankind arise from failure to follow the laws of nature" has been reasserted time and time again.[1] Ideas and health practices purported to be based on natural lifestyles resurfaced with the countercultural movements of the 1960s, the growth of holistic and natural health approaches, and the green movement of the present time. It is beyond the bounds of practicability to suggest that modern populations should return to a "natural" lifestyle based on hunter-gatherer occupations in the cause of health and happiness. However, the repeated interest in the topic suggests that keeping in touch with innate needs is important in refocusing attention on matters relating to healthy survival of the species.

Despite such interest, it is perhaps medicine's overwhelming attention to healing that may account for the current fascination with the reversal of illness rather than natural health. In fact, whether people can achieve health through meeting natural laws that ensure health of mind, body, and spirit is, in many respects, socioculturally determined. Cultures and communities provide the structure and value systems that determine which, how, and why particular needs can be met and what, how, and why people get to do, be, and become.

The exploration detailed in previous chapters leads to the proposition that people need to make use of their biological capacities if they are to enjoy health and well-being. For people to flourish, they not only need to meet the prerequisites of health but also an apparent need for meaning, purpose, and self-actualization. It is the total range of people's obligatory, meaningful, and fulfilling doings that can maintain homeostasis, ensure social connectedness, and provide sufficient exercise to keep body, mind, and spirit functioning efficiently. Studies have demonstrated that even older people who lead active lives following a wide range of occupations tend to feel better and to require less medical attention than those who are isolated and sedentary.[2,3] "The best sort of exercise in terms of retaining one's powers is the kind you don't call exercise."[4] Doing a multitude of occupations can enhance or, at the very least, maintain, joint stability and range, muscle tone, cardiovascular fitness, and respiratory capacity without undue consideration of body functioning; provide balance between physical and mental challenges and relaxation; and provide a vehicle that enables effective use of mental and social characteristics.

It was proposed in Chapter 2 that there is a 3-way link between survival, health, and occupation. This proposal has been supported by the wide-ranging exploration undertaken in search of an occupational perspective of health reported in this text. Throughout time, occupation has provided the mechanism for people to fulfil biological needs essential for survival, to adapt to environmental changes, to develop and exercise genetic capacities in order to maintain health, and for some populations, communities, and individuals to flourish. However, a downside to the mechanism has also been uncovered: it has the capacity to lead to the creation of societies and ways of life that are far from health-maintaining, that increase the health divide between "the haves and the have nots"; and that is so powerful that it could result in the demise of the world as we know it because of failure to halt occupation that leads to potentially irreversible ecological degradation that will be discussed further in the next chapter.

Biological needs were described well by Wolman in the 1970s as "a force in the brain which directs and organizes the individual's perception, thinking, and action, so as to change an existing, unsatisfying situation."[5] From my reading of the ideas that have been unearthed, it is also possible to propose that needs, from a homeostatic perspective, have a 3-way role in maintaining the stability and health of the organism through occupation prompted by a specific feeling experienced. Three categories of needs provide both motivation and feedback: they serve to warn when a problem occurs, to protect and prevent potential disorder, and to prompt and reward use of capacities so that the organism will flourish and reach potential (Figure 6-1).

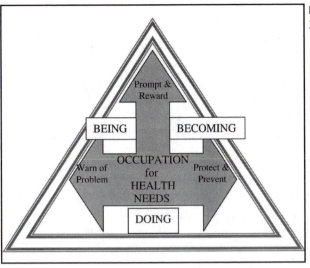

Figure 6-1. Occupation prompting needs: 3-way role in health.

1. To warn and protect, "primary doing needs" are experienced as a form of discomfort that calls for some kind of action to satisfy or assuage the need. Examples of these experiences are cold, hunger, pain, fatigue, fear, boredom, tension, depression, anxiety, anger, or loneliness. In psychology texts contemporary with those discussing biological needs and drives, there is general acceptance of the notion of activities that do not involve purposive "foresight" or "distant ends," that incline humans to act or to experience an impulse toward action that is conducive to biological well-being.[6,7] Many studies have researched these experiences as separate emotions.[8-11] Csikszentmihalyi uses the term *psychic entropy* to describe these states.[12] He sees them as an "integrated response to the self system," with a main goal to "ensure its own survival," a view that is compatible with this study.

2. To prevent disorder and prompt the use of capacities, "doing needs" are experienced in a positive sense, such as a need to spend extra energy, walk, explore, create, understand or make sense of, use ideas, express thoughts, talk, listen, look, meditate or worship, spend time alone or with others, and so on. This mechanism, in interaction with the first, acts to balance over- or underuse. If capacities are overused, people feel fatigue, stress, and burnout, which can lead to increased susceptibility to accident and illness. If capacities are underused, they will atrophy, cause disturbance to equilibrium, and produce stress and a decline in health. The balanced exercise of personal capacities to enable maintenance and development of the organism is perhaps the most primary and least appreciated function of people's occupations, except in terms of physical/aerobic exercise. Some authorities throughout the 20th century have been exceptions. Meyer considered "it is the use that we make of ourselves that gives the ultimate stamp to our every organ."[13] In similar spirit, Sigerist proposed that occupation is essential to the maintenance of health "… because it determines the chief rhythm of our life, balances it, and gives meaning and significance. An organ that does not work atrophies and the mind that does not work becomes dumb."[14]

3. To reward the use of capacities, there are "being and becoming needs" such as for meaning, purpose, satisfaction, fulfillment, happiness, and pleasure. Happiness has been recognized as a powerful human need by many writers, from Aristotle

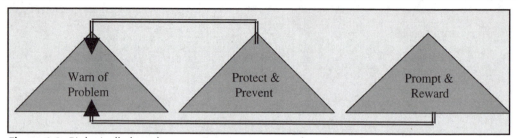

Figure 6-2. Biologically based occupation prompting needs' 3-way role in maintaining stability and health through feedback loop reverting to "warning" if other needs are not met.

over 2000 years ago, to public health pioneers like Southwood-Smith,[15] to current researchers who maintain that pleasure is biologically related to health-promoting activity[12,16-22] that is biologically triggered in areas of the limbic system.[23] This does not mean that pleasure is the ultimate drive of humans but rather that it forms an integral part of health maintenance.[11]

Together, the second and the third categories of needs serve to establish a sense of identity and autonomy, the latter being recognized by Doyal and Gough as 1 of 2 universal needs, the other being physical health. In the negative terms of their concept, physical health is the "minimization of death, disability and disease," and autonomy includes minimization of "mental illness, cognitive deprivation, and restricted opportunities."[24]

The proposal that biologically based occupation needs have this 3-way role in maintaining stability and health was tested in a survey of 150 subjects with ages ranging from 6 to 98 years (mean: 35 years).[25] Asked if they had experienced such needs, 99% admitted they had experienced all 3 types and had acted upon them. Failure to do so resulted in up to 99% of respondents experiencing the type of discomfort described in the first category. The majority of those surveyed reported that they consider the satisfaction of the 3 categories of needs affected their mental, physical, and social health in a positive way (Figure 6-2).

People's intellectual and cognitive capacity, freed by the mechanism of choice, has enabled satisfaction of those needs despite diverse challenges that have been addressed over time. In affluent nations, action to satisfy or assuage discomfort, such as the regulation of temperature, the acquisition of food and water, or measures to reduce pain, have reached a level of sophistication far beyond the simple methods used by early humans living in natural habitats. To prevent disorder, people have developed ways of using their capacities in adaptive, inventive, and exploratory fashions to the extent that they can provide meaning and purpose as well as prompt the pursuit of potential and reward with happiness, self-esteem, and belonging. In fact, these needs have focused human energies toward developing both occupations and sociocultural structures to meet them. Because of this, humans have been successful survivors—to the point of overpopulation. There are downsides to the mechanism of choice in that humans can "act in ways that [go] against the millennial wisdom that natural selection had built into the biological fabric of the species."[11] The capacity to ignore biological needs in either a general or a particular way enables people to sanction the development of sociopolitical structures or make lifestyle choices that result in detrimental health consequences for all or only limited members of the population. Recall a prime example: occupational restrictions were the common lot of women until recently. Then, consider the related gender injustices concerned with government until early in the 20th century and of the starvation diets aimed at women's suffrage. Alternatively, consider choosing not to eat in order to achieve a fashionable appearance and then being unable to accept the illness that is anorexia nervosa to the point of untimely death.

People are not usually conscious of survival and health-maintaining functions. These, rather like the autonomic nervous system, are built into the organism to go on working. Because of this, people are able to use their capacities for their own purposes, to explain the purpose of life in abstract rather than biological ways, and to attribute meaning to activity based on sociocultural influences. It follows that, in present circumstances, many people are not able to distinguish biological needs from socioeconomically determined wants or preferences that ultimately impact on their health.[26] "Even phylogenetically evolved programs of ... behavior are adjusted to the presence of a culture."[27] Needs and wants work in partnership; needs identifying biological requirements, and wants, in many instances, formulating ways that individual biological or socioeconomically determined requirements can be achieved.

Being responsive to biologically driven needs and using capacities has been, in the past, central to maintaining homeostasis and promoting physical, mental, and social well-being. Indeed, there is a pleasure response from "restoring a homeostatic balance of bodily needs ... that leads to the mastery of new challenges."[28] Because biological mechanisms are informed, stimulated, influenced, and adapted by conscious social processes, these too become very influential determinants of occupation and of health. For health and well-being to be experienced by individuals and communities, engagement in occupation needs to provide the prerequisites, balanced use of capacities, meaning, optimal opportunity for desired growth toward potential, and flexibility to develop and change according to context and choice. Such engagement, if it is in accord with sociocultural values and ecological sustainability, will enable populations, communities, families, and individuals to flourish and the species to survive. However, because needs are not omnipotent, lack of awareness about health's dependence on engagement in balanced and satisfying occupation can lead to unhealthy consequences because of the complexity of the interaction with sociocultural and economic processes.

Some of the features of natural health and biological needs as they relate to what people do, be, and strive to become that have surfaced are provided below as an overview.

The links between human biology, human need, the natural environment, social and occupational behaviors, health and illness are dynamic.

The encounters of human communities with new environmental hazards have led to changes in occupational form and performance and subsequent experience of health and illness.

There is a recurring tension between biological needs and changes in living conditions that is manifest in both occupation and health and illness.

The impact of changes from natural, to rural, to urban living along with population ageing is manifest in occupational structures, performance and technology, and patterns of health and illness.

Health and illness are products of biological variability and the meeting of biological needs, social and occupational behaviors and relationships, and environmental possibilities or constraints.

(continued)

Adaptiveness provides more chance (relative to others) of some individuals or communities surviving and reproducing in given social, occupational, and environmental situations.

Health and illness affect the chances of individuals to survive and reproduce. Those who do are able to extend the social and occupational environment best suited to their needs into the future. In turn, this affects the health and survival of future humans.

Participation in occupations directly related to the health and maintenance of the organism and survival can be in tune with the natural world, and must be so in terms of long-term species survival.

Occupational behavior that fails to meet biological, social, and environmental needs can result in failure to flourish because of a reduction of physical mental, or social well-being, the occurrence of illness, and possibly premature death.

The exploration of the evolution of the species in the previous chapters has established the force of the idea that the biological need to engage in occupation is a major characteristic of humans aimed at enabling survival and natural health. Three major functions of occupation have been identified and described in terms of doing, being, and becoming:

1. Doing to provide the prerequisites of health—for immediate bodily needs of sustenance, self-care, and shelter and to develop skills, social structures, and technology aimed at safety and superiority over predators and the maintenance of a supportive environment.

2. Being to maintain health by balanced exercise of personal capacities that provide meaning, purpose, satisfaction, and belonging.

3. Becoming toward potential to enable population, social, and individual development so that each person and the species will flourish.

Public health practitioners are addressing some, but not all, of those occupational needs. They evince particular interest in paid employment, the negative consequences of doing, being, and becoming and some of the prerequisites of health more than others, such as food, income, and social justice and equity. They demonstrate less interest in research or programs aimed at meaning, satisfaction, purpose, and belonging and advocate for physical activity, community development, and sociopolitical changes to promote better health for populations as a whole. Occupational therapists, too, are addressing some but not all of those doing, being, or becoming needs. They evince interest in the occupational nature of humans as a whole, but demonstrate more concern for the substrata of people who are disadvantaged by physical or mental disability that leaves the great majority of people without access to information that might assist understanding of the health impact of their occupations. Their practice within the doing and being categories is limited to pockets of interest according to the availability of their own employment opportunities and directives for practice largely being according to medical or other senior health personnel's ideas. In the last decades, that has led to more concentration on purposeful activities of self-care, productivity, and leisure rather than in people finding meaning through what they do. Hammell addresses these issues in a recent paper, suggesting that:

Although espousing the importance of meaning in occupation, occupational therapy theory has been primarily preoccupied with purposeful occupations and thus appears inadequate to address issues of meaning within people's lives. This paper proposes that the fundamental orientation of occupational therapy should be the contributions that occupation makes to meaning in people's lives, furthering the suggestion that occupation might be viewed as comprising dimensions of meaning: doing, being, belonging and becoming.[29]

The becoming aspect of the trilogy is seldom addressed by occupational therapists in current times except in rhetoric, although it was at the forefront of earlier approaches. Hammell believes that greater focus on meaning will more closely align occupational therapists with an "espoused aspiration to enable the enhancement of quality of life."[29] This coincides with Hocking's call for occupational therapists to revisit in practice their earlier focus on Romantic as opposed to rational ideologies:

Most pertinent here is the Romantics' belief in self-creation, that each man could invent himself, fashion his own character, or by heroic effort, transform himself. This is achieved, in part, by construing one's world of desires, values, meanings and physical circumstances.[30]

More attention to, or advocacy for, population health approaches to embrace "becoming" within health promotion schemes is called for. This also requires advocacy to acquire adequate resources to fund such programs. In current socioeconomic climates, that would necessitate attention to how the economic benefits would outweigh the costs of establishing programs.

For either profession, the teasing out of positive or negative health attributes of occupation is difficult, even though it is relatively easy to see that there is a correlation between health and obvious survival occupations concerned with shelter, food, clean air, and water. Indeed, these have been well-researched. The correlation between health and the biological need of humans to engage in other types of occupations tends to be obscure, complex, and poorly researched. However, because of the variety and complexity of the occupational needs that are prerequisite to meeting the 3 functions listed previously, alienation, imbalance, and deprivation are possible. This may differ for particular groupings within any given population. Additionally, if the needs are not recognized for what they are, political will could establish occupational expectations of a population that are counter to long-term survival of the species and the health of people over a lifetime.

Public Health Through Doing, Being, and Becoming

To increase the health of populations throughout the world, public health has embraced the ideas of the WHO that are the result of the combined wisdom of experts from around the globe. Both WHO and public health practitioners attend to the health and illness experiences of communities as a whole, often by recognizing and advising public agencies on manifestations of the experiences. The advice given is, largely, according to the directives drawn up by world health experts, and this is provided to political bodies, social planners, and the like to assist them to recognize overall trends and problems relating to physical, mental, and social health apparent in every sphere of life. The advice is aimed at enabling future policy to address the reduction of illness and premature death more effectively and at increasing the experience of social, physical, and mental well-being in a way that is just for people everywhere.

When illness occurs, the usual course of action, at least for people in advanced societies, is to seek medical explanation. Thagard contends that within medicine there are 2 kinds of important explanations. The first of these is a physician's explanation of the presenting symptoms: a diagnosis. The second is usually the job of medical researchers. They seek explanations for the reasons behind the illness.[31] In the field of public health, it is mainly the role of epidemiologists to find medical explanations for illness. Over recent years, though, public health explanations have expanded with WHO directives to include environmental and sociopolitical causes of illness in line with the increasing understanding of external determinants of health and illness. The determinants now embrace broad-ranging causal factors. It is within all parts of this expanded field of causal factors that occupation as a determinant of illness or of well-being can be explored more fully and inclusively. The 13-year longitudinal Harvard public health study of mortality published in the *BMJ* in 1999 of older Americans with regard to their social and productive activities is one that clearly shows the long-term positive and protective impact of doing more than physical exercise.[2] Glass argues "while physical fitness itself is important and clearly related to health and survival, the exclusive focus on physical activity obscures the health benefits that may be associated with other, non-physical activities...."[2] Another study of note is a randomized controlled trial conducted by occupational scientists and therapists at the University of Southern California to evaluate the effectiveness of preventive occupational therapy services for 361 multiethnic, independent older adults. This study found significant benefits for the occupational therapist administered intervention group in various health, function, and quality of life domains, while these tended to decline over the study period for members of the 2 control groups.[32]

Contemporary occupational structures and the social environment and political agendas that support these structures may not provide people with opportunities for health enhancing, balanced yet stimulating, and challenging use of capacities because occupational value in both postindustrial cultures and many others striving to emulate postindustrialism usually centers around paid employment. Within paid employment, there is little commonality in the range and extent of physical, mental, and social doing. Obligatory requirements or opportunities for choice also differ so it is necessary to engage in other forms of doing to ensure that all capacities are exercised and healthily balanced. These can be associated with domestic or leisure pursuits. However, a limited understanding of the need for exercise of people's total range of capacities suggests that it is chance, rather than design, that leads to lifestyles that provide physical, mental, and social well-being. Physiological imbalance and illness can result from individual responses to, and coping with, the vicissitudes of everyday life, which are closely tied to what people do or do not do and how they feel about such doings. They relate to people's different natures and needs being met through what they do; simply recommending an exercise regime that meets predetermined health criteria, for example, is not effective for everybody. Activity in the past met many occupational needs and societal values; what is recommended to replace "superseded" physically, mentally, and socially demanding occupations in the present age has got to meet similar basic needs and values. This requires vigilance in terms of health requirements and research because societal values will continue to alter with the impact of future environmental change.

Present research is vigilant, but because of the dominance of quantitative methodology, holistic and complex mechanisms are often reduced in ways that make it hard for people to consider total lifestyle effects. While the research is valuable, the concentration on the benefits of physical exercise, for example, in both professional and popular media leads to the assumption that other types of doing are of less value. It is hardly surprising that people hearing this type of rhetoric do not equate their health status with their everyday doings as a small retrospective study found. One hundred people over 60 years of age were sampled, and the majority did not associate their life's occupations with their health.[33] This finding appears to be indicative of a "medicalized" understanding of health by the general public that is, perhaps inadvertently, being reinforced by health education strategies, the limited direction of occupation-focused research, and the media.[2]

Modern reductionism contrasts with the holistic nature of earlier lifestyles in which active or restful doing often associated with nutrition was part of an ecological healthy whole.[34] In the present day, many widely differing circumstances associated with what people do, as well as what they eat, have led to a prevalence of weight disorders. Even those committed to physical excellence are subject to breakdown of health because of insufficient understanding of the complexities of its relationship to occupation. For example, although athletes generally experience a high level of physical fitness, they frequently suffer some form of breakdown of health at the time of major competition. Evidence about the cause of pathophysiology of such overtraining syndrome is limited, but it has been suggested that the stress of training can cause depression and decreased immune function.[35] This gives rise to the notion that too much exercise, taken to reach peak performance in this case, is detrimental to health as is too little exercise, which can lead to atrophy of body tissue and organs, as well as obesity. Kenneth Cooper, who is credited with coining the term *aerobics*, suggests that overexercising can trigger the overproduction of free radicals, which could be linked with many lifestyle disorders and even death.[36] Indeed, from a study of cases of sudden death during exercise, Siscovick et al found that the risks of death during exercise are increased by 700%, despite men who exercise having half the death rate of those who do not exercise.[37]

Closely associated with the nutrition-activity nexus, the activity-rest continuum is another aspect of occupation that is not given sufficient attention despite it being one of the ancient rules of health and despite substantial exploration of sleep patterns over the past 40 years. Sleep provides the natural mechanism to prevent activity overuse and a time for repair. Emerging theories point to a complex relationship between it and what people do during waking states, suggesting that recuperation, information processing, energy conservation, and self-preservation are important aspects of the relationship. Kleitman saw sleep as complementary to wakefulness as he explored and then described the day/night sequence as the "basic rest activity cycle."[38,39] Because sleep deprivation results in symptoms such as decreased coordination and reaction times, irritability, and blurred vision,[40] sleep appears to be necessary to effective doing, being, and becoming. Leger suggests that "just as musicians' pauses are a component of the performance, pauses from the stream of behavior are a component of the repertoire. The organism 'doing nothing' is doing something."[39]

Many authorities fail to consider adequately the impact of the activity-rest continuum on health. Even some occupational therapists, with their holistic view, do not consider sleep as part of occupation. Add to that arbitrary dividing of occupation other common forms like the socially determined categories of paid or unpaid employment and leisure or play, and it is possible to appreciate some of the impediments to understanding the need to balance mental, physical, social, solitary, spiritual, rest, chosen, and obligatory occupations as integral aspects of health.

This results in societal pressure to pursue particular types of work that may impose upon communities or individuals the apparent need to do more than they are capable of or to do less than they can achieve meaning or satisfaction from. It also results in social welfare programs that provide money rather than opportunities for involvement, that put risk elimination before reasonable challenge to capacities, and that favor keeping people breathing rather than living in a way that promotes what limited capacities they may have. Consider the rows of older well-rugged and drugged people in some nursing homes seated day after day in warm and sanitary conditions but without stimulation to enable continued achievement, however small that may be.

Table 6-1

Comparison of World Health Organization Directives for Well-Being With "Doing, Being, and Becoming"

WHO Directives for Well-Being	Doing, Being, and Becoming
Capacity to change or cope with the environment	Doing to satisfy the prerequisites of health
Capacity to satisfy needs	Being satisfied and finding meaning and purpose through use of capacities
Capacity to identify and to realize aspirations	Becoming according to potential

---

Such modern ways of going about things are a far cry from some valuable, but half forgotten ways of less than a century ago. The "mental hygiene movement" is a case in point. This was influential in the growth and development of mental health services of the first half of the 20th century and was another factor in the formal birth of occupational therapy.[13] Adolph Meyer, a "leader of the advanced guard in American Psychiatry,"[41] held a then-radical viewpoint that life experiences play an important role in the etiology of mental disease.[42] His fundamental psychobiological approach conceptualized whole people in action, which includes society as part of the whole.[43] Repudiating reductionist, analytical, and mechanistic views, Meyer took a holistic standpoint influenced by William James' pragmatism[44] and John Dewey's functionalism.[41,45] He made use of their "concept of habit," arguing that the "cumulative effect of early faulty habit patterns was to produce abnormal or inefficient behavior in later life."[41] Meyer embraced the revolutionary view that the chief purpose of the mind "is to enable individuals ... to pursue specific interests and achieve specific goals" and that its study should consider "the ordinary, practical situations of everyday life."[41] He professed that "doing, action, and experience are being" and that the activities expressed in living demonstrate mind-body synthesis.[46,47]

Gaining an increased understanding of an occupational perspective of natural health and biological needs as Meyer attempted to do is worthy of further extensive inquiry because it appears appropriate to many of the problems the world faces today and in the future. It has the potential to provide direction on how to maintain health and ensure human survival in economic and self-sustaining ways that meet the biological and socio-cultural needs of people, as well as redressing ecological degradation.

For those committed to understanding people as occupational beings and who recognize the health and illness impact of what people do, be, and become, the challenge is to increase awareness of the connection. Especially in recent times, it has been overlooked as a holistic phenomenon despite the fact that the WHO and public health practitioners do recognize limited aspects of it as particularly problematic and that the WHO rhetoric appears to embrace the whole. The theme of this chapter—"health is created and lived by people within the settings of their everyday life; where they learn, work, play and love"—is an example of the latter thought. The theme is about what people need to be able to do to reach a state of complete physical, mental, and social well-being while the theme of the last chapter offers 3 occupational directives to achieve this.[48] These are very similar to how the terms of doing, being, and becoming are addressed in the previous chapters (Table 6-1).

There are very few venues where all 3 happen effectively for all members of a community despite many obvious attempts. It may be a Utopian vision, but radical improvement

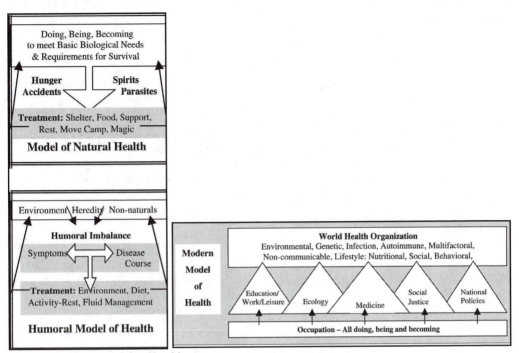

Figure 6-3. Three models of health.

requires Utopian thought. How health is achieved through what people do, be, and strive to become requires spelling out in practical ways by people who understand the power of occupation and the critical need for inclusive health and social policies to that end.

In this text, understanding has been sought by an exploration throughout human evolution. During that long period, different models to explain health have surfaced according to lifestyle, cultural beliefs, and scientific expertise at the time. Three very different models have emerged, and it is appropriate at this point to reflect briefly on the nature of these. A diagrammatic representation of each indicates how aspects of doing, being, and becoming mesh with the core ideas of each model (Figure 6-3).

The first model was that of natural health and biological need that probably coexisted with concepts of spirit or magic for millennia. It was dependent of what and how people went about their lives, what they did, how they felt about what they did, and continual exploration to improve their experiences. In terms of illness, a seeking out of shelter, food, or environment that appeared to reduce both symptoms and course of illness is likely along with rest, support from community members, and possibly advice from spiritual leaders or those seen to have special healing skills.

The second of these, the humoral model, arose in ancient Greece, and this model was accepted throughout Arabia and Europe for the next 2000 years. Based on naturalistic observation, it has already been observed that the 4 elements of air, fire, water, and earth that are the foundation stone of the model bear remarkable similarities to the 4 basic human needs that are a requirement of life itself: oxygen, warmth, water, and food. Health, according to humoral physiology, is the first known scientific explanation, the 4 humors being determined as "the things that make up its (the human body) constitution and causes its pains and health."[31] Imbalance of the humors was thought to be the cause of illness and could be the result of behavior as well as heredity or environmental factors. Treatment was aimed at correcting humoral imbalance (the doing, being, and becoming elements are included within "non-naturals").

The third model is that of the present day. It began with germ theories that arose in the 19th century but is now multifactoral because health is understood to be more complex than the absence of disease. The WHO offers the overarching picture that is inclusive of physical, mental, and social well-being as well as medical explanations of infectious, autoimmune, genetic, noncommunicable, nutritional, social, and behavioral disease.[31] Lifestyle factors based on what people do in their daily lives that are determinants of positive or negative health experiences are easily overlooked in favor of economic gains in sociopolitical or environmental planning and resource allocation. The call for policy makers of all kinds to recognize the health consequences of their decisions remains elusive.

At this point, it is possible to summarize what is meant by health through occupation to indicate the approaches that could be taken to improve population health:

* Healthy life expectancy and a reduced experience of illness or disability.

   Research, publish, and advocate for increased understanding of a holistic appreciation of occupation, and how all doing, being, and becoming impacts on morbidity, mortality, and well-being. Seek powerful allies and media support to spread the facts about the occupation/health relationship.

* Requirements for the sustenance of life are attainable through participation in range of socially acceptable and ecologically sustainable activities.

   Occupation-based programs need to be at the forefront of intervention in countries that are striving to meet the fundamental prerequisites for life so that ongoing health benefits accumulate. The provision of social welfare should be tied to an occupational requirement whenever possible to reduce the illness-producing ennui that results from lack of purpose and meaning.

* Physical, mental, and social well-being attained through occupation that is socially valued, sufficiently challenging, and meaningful.

   Increase of community and political awareness that meaningful and challenging doing, being, and becoming are integral to the absence of illness and experience of well-being.

* A balance of active and rest occupations that maintains physical, mental, and social fitness.

   Increase awareness of the holistic physical, mental, and social fitness effects of balancing active and rest occupations, food, and activity, advocating for and enabling practical education programs to suit personal and community interests.

* Availability of opportunity for enhancement of capacities, individual potential, spiritual contentment, and quality of life.

   Actively advocate for public policies that enable rather than restrict a wide range of occupations as many of the risk-reducing litigation-scared policies do.

* Occupationally-just social policies enable and encourage active participation in wide-ranging occupations for people of all ages without discrimination.

   Do not necessarily accept the policies or social conventions of the time if people of any age, in any situation, or walk of life are occupationally deprived, alienated, or lacking occupational balance. Increase awareness of occupational injustices in the community and at policy level, research the causes and effects, and actively advocate for change, mediating on behalf of those less able.

* Community cohesion, support, and opportunity.

   Learn to recognize the positive and negative impact of supportive and cohesive or fragmented and isolating communities and take an enabling approach appropriate to its particular needs and potential, encouraging local participation and leadership and being ready to advocate and mediate for improvement of occupation for health opportunities.

* Occupations are encouraged that are compatible with a sustainable ecology.

Recognize that people are an active part of ecosystems and as such, their needs are as important but not more so as those of any other animate or inanimate species. With that in mind, support occupations that are compatible with ecological sustainability. Seek and advocate for alternative occupational opportunities through legitimate "sought" comment on policies particularly when communities and political determination appear tied to unsustainable and damaging practices.

Throughout the text, it has been suggested that because of the complexity of occupation it has rarely been considered as a holistic entity even though segments of occupation such as "learning, loving, work and play" are mentioned in the WHO directives.[48] Segmentation fails to acknowledge the interactive nature of the brain-body-environment occupation-health nexus. This results in inadequate recognition or understanding of the total picture of what people do, be, and strive to become in terms of health effects. It is for that reason that occupational science (ie, the study of humans as occupational beings) seeks to be multidisciplinary.

The study of population health is also multidisciplinary as it too becomes more holistic. Ironically, wholeness is a synonym of health, the word being derived from Old English.[49,50] The need to talk about holistic health is perhaps evidence of the term *health* having come to mean "something less than wholeness."[51] Smuts, in 1928, was the first to use the word *holism* (from the Greek "holos" meaning whole) to describe philosophies that consider whole systems rather than parts of systems (reductionism).[47,52] He observed "a basic tendency of nature and evolution to produce novel, irreducible wholes" and that living systems are more than the sum of their parts.[53] Also subscribing to this view, von Bertalanffy developed "general systems theory" in the 1950s that proved to be a major "impetus toward a more holistic approach" in the biological sciences and health care.[54-56] In some ways, this may be considered a return to older values but with an added bonus of recent evidence (provided by reductionist research) of the holistic nature of living systems that are central in the OCHP and other WHO directives. Disappointingly, it can be argued that few health services or health resource allocations have been shifted in a holistic direction as a consequence. The apparent difficulty of actioning holistic health approaches is also true of actioning holistic occupational approaches. The combination of the complexity of both occupation and health appears to render action impossible, but bearing both in mind and working toward such approaches is vital for the future. Without a more complete and holistic understanding of the integral place of occupation within natural health and biological needs, it is difficult to achieve human rights in terms of healthy lifestyles even though the *Jakarta Declaration* attested that the social and occupational health concern—poverty—is the greatest threat to health at the present time.[57] There are some places in the world where the situation is desperate. The UN's *Declaration of Human Rights* provides a way forward in terms of research, diagnosis, prescription, and action. However, the implementation of those rights is highly dependent on political will.

Occupation-Focused Directives for Health

In preceding chapters, both ancient rules and modern directives for health have been explored. In this section of the chapter, these will be used in tandem to establish occupation-focused directives toward population health. The directives require ongoing exploration of their effectiveness as they are acted upon by occupational therapists and public health practitioners. In considering the history that preceded the formal separate establishment of both those health professions, many connecting and founding ideas can be found. This suggests a coming together at this point in terms of occupation-focused population health initiatives that might prove advantageous in terms of public health in the foreseeable future. To consider 21st century directions that address issues of occupation and public health concern, it is necessary to recognize the part played by changing global and national politics, spiritual beliefs and philosophical mores, sociocultural contexts, and changing technologies. A brief look at the occupation-focused founding ideas will set the scene.

Histories that consider the evolution of public health[31,58-60] and occupational therapy[61-64] have traced developments from the earliest times. These tell of how early humans survived and thrived naturally as they met their innate biological needs through what they did within communities as an integral part of their ecosystem. This provides the foundation for understanding both health and occupation. It also suggests the intimacy of this relationship. For millennia, self-health practices such as rest; familial/tribal care such as provision of shelter, food, and water; and community action such as moving camp provided the basis for population health. What was originally based on trial and error and what appeared to be common sense gradually became part of folklore and, later, the basis of rules of health formulated in the classical Greek period that were transmitted across the centuries until very recently. Within those, occupation was recognized for its potential as exercise and interwoven with ideas about healthy rest, nutrition, personality type, environment, and emotional tone as related to everyday aspects of life. The notion of exercise meshed well with the "physical" perfection orientation of ancient Greece but was less valued as Christian beliefs became dominant. For many centuries, spiritual matters reigned supreme but even so, the rules of health formulated in Greco-Roman times remained the basis of public health. St. Benedict's 6th century rule that labor was necessary for a healthy soul and that a healthy soul was essential for a healthy body and mind was particularly useful in an age when medicine had no sophisticated tools to aid recovery. Occupation such as prayer, pilgrimages, and physical labor was used for illness prevention, curative medicine, therapy, or health promotion purposes.[61] Even after the demise of monasteries in Britain these health ideals continued. Young King Edward VI's agreement to establish a Hospital of Occupation to overcome the social illness largely caused by closure of the monasteries mentioned earlier is a case in point. Modern research has upheld earlier beliefs that body, mind, and spirit connect with and influence each other.[65]

The importance of the 6 rules of humoral physiology (and the *Regimen* and *Tacuinum Sanitatis*) to this occupation-focused population health perspective is 2-fold. First, it lies in the fact that the notion of occupation for health can be encompassed as a preventive mechanism within a primary system of medical care. The extent of medical knowledge during the long period of time the rules were used meant that preventive medicine was paramount because even the most minor illnesses or disorders were potentially life threatening or could become ongoing impediments to normal living. Second, the inclusion of occupation as a curative agent was embedded in medical practice for centuries. Despite the physiology on which it is based being outdated, the formula still makes remarkably good sense. No clear-cut difference was made between social, mental, and physical health. People were much more holistic in their views enmeshing "body and soul, flesh and spirit, mind and matter," and bodily condition and the fluctuations between health and sickness interlocked with social ideas about identity, destiny, and moral and spiritual well-being.[66]

The rules also make remarkably good sense in terms of a current occupational perspective of natural health and biological needs and in terms of the more recent directives of the WHO. They require reconsideration against modern day understanding of physiology and terminology. Air and environment, for example, anticipate the importance of the ecology to matters of healthy populations and public health interest in healthy cities; motion, rest, sleep, and waking might be considered in terms of daily life-balance, of exercise regimes, and of active aging; food and drink are easily allied to the current concern about nutrition; evacuation and repletion might point attention to overindulgence, famine, self-care activities; and affections of the soul appear closely related to mental and spiritual health and notions of people needing to find meaning, satisfaction, purpose, belonging, and self-actualization through what they do.

The new public health ambitions to create healthy cities reflect the idea of a golden age in times past. Both are Utopian.[67] Utopia was the name given by Sir Thomas More to his vision of an ideal environment in which all people lived free, simple, and natural lives without the excesses of affluence on the one hand or deprivation, alienation, or imbalance on the other.[68] At an international conference on Utopian thought and communal experience, Hardy and Davidson recognized "the idea of contemplating the perfect society and of seeking to create it in practice has roots that run deep in human history."[69] It is apparent in work of philosophers like John Locke who anticipated the need for a science of occupation,[70] and philanthropists like John Howard who recognized that people were turned out of hospital "unfit to work, or the common mode of living."[71] It is manifest in the works of physicians such as Pare's and Mercurialis' therapeutic and preventive approach to using occupation as exercise,[72,73] Ramazzini's recognition of the need to include occupational reform to prevent disease,[74] and in moral treatment.[75-77] It is also plain in the work of a large group of Utopian social activists during the late 18th and 19th centuries. This group includes Robert Owe, who is considered the father of British Socialism; Karl Marx; Edwin Chapman; Thomas Southwood-Smith; Octavia Hill; Henrietta and Samuel Barnett; John Ruskin; William Morris; and Jane Addams, whose work has been noted in earlier chapters.[61,62] All have contributed in some way to the ideologies of either or both disciplines of public health and occupational therapy (Table 6-2).

Over the last half century, the WHO has provided many directives for righting what they have identified as problems preventing the attainment of health for all the peoples of the world. Implementing those directives appears to be extremely difficult despite them making good sense and being paid lip service by many. Public health is the major force to uphold the directives and to have them put into practice, but it is a small force when compared with clinical and individually based medical practice in terms of resources, and the mammoth number of tasks before it. It is hardly surprising, therefore, that the importance of a holistic understanding of occupation based on all that people do, be, and strive to become has not been addressed in relation to population health. Despite the overload, public health practitioners need to be open to the integrative nature and potential health or illness outcomes of occupational determinants of health that relate to more than paid employment or physical exercise. Occupational therapists, on the other hand, have recently begun to appreciate the importance of a holistic view of both occupation and health. They are in a prime position to work with the WHO directives, to explore them further, to enact them with population groups as well as individuals, and to bring them to the attention of sociopolitical planners. The WFOT's 2004 definition of occupational therapy that is provided in the scroll in the section openers demonstrates their interest. However, because of the strength of their commitment to people with disability and individuals treated within the medical health context, there remains a general lack of attention to the broader notion of population health and social, occupational, and ecological

Table 6-2

Abbreviated History of the Use of Occupation for Physical, Social, and Mental Well-Being During the Term of the Ancient Rules of the Non-Naturals and the Transition to Current Ideologies

Director	Links	Physical WB	Mental WB	Social WB
Hippocrates and Galen, physicians	OT PHP		Application of the non-naturals	
St. Benedict and monastic rule	OT PHP		Spiritual health through labor, prayer, good works, and pilgrimage	
Thomas More, philosopher/statesman	OT PHP		Utopianism	
Ambrose Pare, physician	OT PHP	Occupation as exercise		
Hieronymous Mercuriali, physician	OT PHP	Occupation as exercise		
John Locke, philosopher	OT PHP		Scientific theory	
Bernadino Ramazzini, physician	OT PHP		Occupational health and safety	
John Howard, philanthropist	OT PHP		Hospital and prison research Environmental and social conditions	
P. Pinel, W. Tuke, et al, moral treatment	OT		Justice, benevolence, and occupation	
Robert Owen, industrialist/socialist	OT PHP		Education, community development, housing, industrial reform	
Karl Marx, philosopher	OT PHP		Nature of doing, occupational health and safety Social and communal reform	
John Ruskin and William Morris, Arts and Crafts movement	OT		Nature of doing Social and communal reform	
Edwin Chadwick, lawyer/politician	PHP			Industry, sanitation

(continued)

Table 6-2

Abbreviated History of the Use of Occupation for Physical, Social, and Mental Well-Being During the Term of the Ancient Rules of the Non-Naturals and the Transition to Current Ideologies (continued)

Director	Links	Physical WB	Mental WB	Social WB
T. Southwood-Smith, physician/reformer	OT PHP	Happiness and longevity		Housing, mines, industry
Octavia Hill, social environmentalist	OT		Housing, environment, doing	
H. & S. Barnett, social settlements	OT PHP			Community development
Jane Addams, social settlements	OT PHP			Community development

OT: occupational therapy
PHP: public health practice

illness outside the medical field. This is evident in the wording of the second paragraph of the definition provided by the WFOT that, disappointingly in this regard, is not clear of a broad population intent:

> *Occupational therapists have a broad education that equips them with skills and knowledge to work collaboratively with individuals or groups of people who have an impairment of body structure or function due to a health condition, and who experience barriers to participation.*[78]

For occupational therapists to become recognized as practitioners in public health, they will need to broaden either their thinking or, if they have already done so, ensure that their terminology demonstrates their interest in the health of all people. That it is occurring in some places and some documentation is evident. The British College of Occupational Therapist's 2002 strategy *From Interface to Integration*, which embraces the directives of both the WHO ICF and the OCHP, is a case in point (Figure 6-4).

The American Occupational Therapy Foundation, too, expresses interest in the broader terms of public health. On their Website, among a range of articles on population health issues, they draw attention to papers such as the UN "Millennium Development Goals" agreed on at the Millennium Summit in September 2000 by world leaders to:

* Eradicate extreme poverty and hunger.

* Achieve universal primary education.

* Promote gender equality and empower women.

* Reduce child mortality.

* Improve maternal health.

Figure 6-4. COT Strategy 2002: A mix of the WHO OCHP and ICF. (Reproduced by kind permission of the British Association and College of Occupational Therapists.)

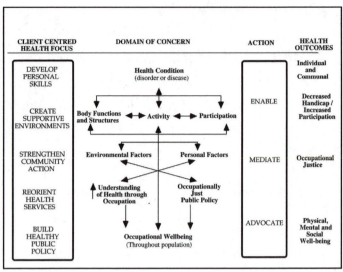

* Combat HIV/AIDS, malaria, and other diseases.
* Ensure environmental sustainability.
* Advance a global partnership for development.

To assist with the task of reorientation for public health practitioners to a holistic occupation-focused perspective and for occupational therapists toward a population health focus, a collection of occupation-focused directives toward the absence of illness and physical, mental, and social well-being has been listed in Table 6-3. This will also summarize what is discussed throughout the text. The collection has been selected from various WHO publications, namely its *Global Strategy on Diet, Physical Activity and Health*,[79] its *Mental Health Fact Sheet 220*,[80] its *Active Ageing Policy*,[81] the *Jakarta Declaration*,[57] but mainly, in the spirit of the text as a whole, from the OCHP.[48] The table does not include all the relevant directives that could be in such a listing. The fact is that despite being incomplete, it is extensive and does more than suggest the importance of actively seeking to extend its implementation.

The lack of implementation of the WHO ideas by health professionals, governments, and the wider community perhaps illustrates a lack of understanding, lack of agreement, or the difficulty of appropriate action. It might also indicate a lack of dissemination of the WHO directives among the wider population. When I recently introduced some of the ideas to a group of participants of the University of the Third Age (U3A) in my local rural community, they were receptive, intrigued, and accepting. They had not been aware of them before. It can be queried why this is so. Lack of awareness of WHO directives and initiatives seems common. This effectively negates the work of many thoughtful leaders in the field of health. More worrisome is the lack of awareness of the WHO directives seeming also to apply to many workers in health services. They may be in the position where they are constrained to take their direction from local sources, and these directions may be largely economically driven, often according to higher political decisions. It may also be that the WHO directives are not given sufficient emphasis in the education process of health professionals or that their importance is lost in the acquisition of particular skills for daily practice. It is a matter of great concern that there is a lack of awareness and/or implementation of WHO directives in terms of health workers in the field of occupation

Table 6-3

World Health Organization Occupation-Focused Directives Toward the Absence of Illness and Physical, Mental, and Social Well-Being

WHO Occupation-Focused Directives	*Possible Occupation-Focused Action for PHPs and OTs*
OCHP: An individual or group must be able to identify and realize aspirations, to satisfy needs, and to change or cope with the environment.	Review Ch 2 and 5 See Ch 8 and 10: Occupational Justice, Health Promotion and Well-Being
OCHP: Improvement in health requires a secure foundation in the basic prerequisites.	Review Ch 3 See Ch 10: Health Promotion and Well-Being
OCHP: Good health is a major resource for social, economic, and personal development.	Review Ch 1 See Ch 10: Health Promotion and Well-Being
OCHP: Changing patterns of life, work, and leisure have a significant impact on health.	Review Ch 3 and 4 See Ch 8, 9, and 10: Occupational Justice; Prevention; Health Promotion and Well-Being
OCHP: Work and leisure should be a source of health for people.	Review Ch 3, 4, and 5 See Ch 10: Health Promotion and Well-Being
OCHP: Health promotion generates living and working conditions that are safe, stimulating, satisfying, and enjoyable.	See Ch 10: Health Promotion and Well-Being
OCHP: Systematic assessment of the health impact of rapidly changing environments is essential particularly in technology, work, energy production, and urbanization.	See Ch 7: Eco-Sustainable Community Development
OCHP: Protection of natural and built environments and conservation of natural resources must be addressed in any health promotion program.	See Ch 7: Eco-Sustainable Community Development
OCHP: Community development based on self-help, social support, local resources, and access to funding are required to encourage effective community action.	See Ch 7: Eco-Sustainable Community Development
OCHP: Provision of information, health education, and enhancement of life skills to increase healthy options.	See Ch 9 and 10: Prevention; Health Promotion and Well-Being
OCHP: Enabling life-long learning facilitated in school, home, work, and community settings.	See Ch 7 and 8: Eco-Sustainable Community Development; Occupational Justice *(continued)*

Table 6-3

World Health Organization Occupation-Focused Directives Toward the Absence of Illness and Physical, Mental, and Social Well-Being (continued)

WHO Occupation-Focused Directives	Possible Occupation Focused Action for PHPs and OTs
OCHP: Reorientation of health services beyond the clinical and curative toward health promotion—opening channels to broad social, political, economic, and environmental components.	Review Ch 1 and 3 See Ch 7 and 8: Eco-Sustainable Community Development; Occupational Justice
OCHP: Health is created and lived by people within the settings of their everyday life; where they learn, work, play, and live.	Review Intro to Section 1, Ch 2 See Ch 8 and 10: Occupational Justice; Health Promotion and Well-Being
OCHP: Health is created by caring for one's self and others by being able to take decisions and have control over one's life circumstances.	Review Ch 2, 3, 4, and 5 See Ch 8, 9, and 10: Occupational Justice; Prevention; Health Promotion and Well-Being
OCHP: Focus attention on public health issues such as pollution, occupational hazards, housing, and settlements.	See Ch 7 and 9: Eco-Sustainable Community Development; Prevention
AAPF: Optimizing opportunities for health, participation, and security to enhance quality of life for individuals and populations.	Review Ch 1 and 5 See Ch 8, 9, and 10: Occupational Justice; Prevention; Health Promotion
AAPF: Recognition of the UN principles of independence, participation, dignity, care, and self-fulfillment, allowing people to realize their potential for physical, mental, and social well-being throughout the life course and to participate in society according to their needs, desires, and capacities.	Review Ch 1 and 5 See Ch 8, 9, and 10: Occupational Justice; Prevention; Health Promotion
AAPF: Increase number of people actively participating as they age in the social, cultural, economic, and political aspects of society in paid and unpaid roles and in domestic, family, and community life.	Review Ch 1 and 5 See Ch 8, 9, and 10: Occupational Justice; Prevention; Health Promotion
AAPF: Encourage and balance personal responsibility (self-care), age-friendly environments, and intergenerational solidarity.	Review Ch 1 and 5 See Ch 8, 9, and 10: Occupational Justice; Prevention; Health Promotion

(continued)

Table 6-3

World Health Organization Occupation-Focused Directives Toward the Absence of Illness and Physical, Mental, and Social Well-Being (continued)

WHO Occupation-Focused Directives	Possible Occupation Focused Action for PHPs and OTs
MHFS: Enable people to realize abilities, cope with the normal stresses of life, work productively and fruitfully, and make a contribution to the community.	Review Ch 2, 3, 4, and 5 See Ch 8, 9, and 10: Occupational Justice; Prevention; Health Promotion and Wellness

MHFS: World Health Organization. *Mental Health Fact Sheet 220*. Geneva: WHO; 2001. OCHP: World Health Organization. *Ottawa Charter for Health Promotion*. Geneva: WHO; 1986. AAPF: World Health Organization. *Active Ageing: A Policy Framework. Second United Nations World Assembly on Ageing*. Madrid, Spain: WHO; 2002:12,13.

and health. Perhaps a more rigorous campaign is called for to increase awareness of the WHO's broader understanding of health.

AN "OCCUPATION FOR PUBLIC HEALTH PYRAMID"

The question arises as to whether such messages as the WHO directives could be disseminated to both people in positions of influence and to the population at large, by a modern equivalent of the 3 methods employed to propagate the *Regimen Sanitatis*. Mass media should make the task easier than in the 2000 years of the "non-naturals" primacy, even though handing down of traditional understandings by word of mouth was valued more than it is today. In present day terms, the 3 methods that proved effective over the years can be equated to the literature and media of professional education, personal trainers or life-style counsellors, and using cutting-edge technology and popular media more effectively and creatively. The latter might include getting the occupation for health message onto the World Wide Web as part of popular sites and within computer and Internet games, as well as being integrated into children's stories, novels, and films or featured in popular magazines. The population at large needs the information, but there is also a requirement to ensure that the occupation for health needs of all people are adequately recognized in social, political, and health planning. This may be by making sure that material about the topic is available in health and wellness centers, that those with interest in disseminating the ideas become occupation for health consultants, motivational speakers or media personalities, or political advisers, as well as occupation for health researchers. A 3-fold strategy like those of the ancient rules of health would be useful to get the message across to all sectors of the population.

A simple but effective method of education is being used to spread the word about healthy nutrition. A poster (or illustration in magazines or newspapers) of a colored triangle depicting the necessary food groups and indicating advisability of greater to lesser consumption is to be found everywhere in affluent countries. Even if obesity is increasing as a problem for many living in such countries, the constant reminders do not allow

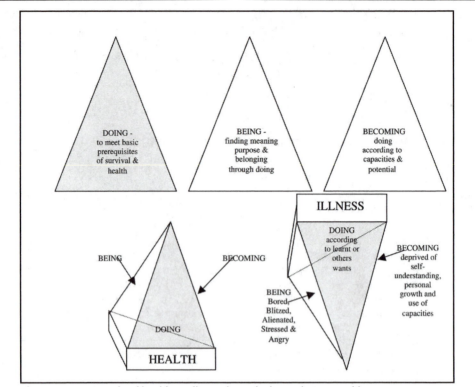

Figure 6-5. Pyramids of health or illness through doing, being, and becoming.

the right information to be entirely cast aside and eventually may cause changes in habit in the right directions. It is effective "reminder advertising." A similar population health device based on the concepts of "doing, being, and becoming" would be useful to get the message across to many people that it is all the things that people do that affect health and not simply paid employment or physical exercise. I presented the idea of a "Daily Occupation for Health Triangle" in *Willard and Spackman's Occupational Therapy*[82] and planned to develop it further in this text. However, as the chapters developed, it became clear that doing, being, and becoming were all requirements for physical, mental, and social well-being and that a depiction that suggested a hierarchy was inappropriate.

Instead of a triangle, 2 3-sided (plus base) pyramids emerged from the exploration as a possible tool toward the same ends. The base triangle of each pyramid represents either health or illness, and the 3 sides represent doing, being, or becoming well or alternatively, doing, being, or becoming ill. A depiction of the words used on these pyramids has gradually built up as the chapters unfolded. Their final form is shown as Figure 6-5. Displayed in poster or solid form as a paperweight, mobile, or desk device, if this pictorial representation of occupation for health could become as common as the healthy nutrition posters, a large step in public health promotion direction would have been taken. Such a poster or device provides a focus for discussion and a reminder whenever they are seen.

The worldwide exploration of population health from the perspective of people's occupational nature and needs has foundered and is in danger of sinking out of sight forever. Despite enormous energy and commitment of strong leaders in both the public health and occupation fields, understanding of the occupational nature of people and its intimate relationship to health remains poorly understood. Occupational therapists have been largely restricted to working in the illness industry rather than the wellness industry. Both illness and wellness are important but have different orientations and language. It is difficult to cross the divide because of lack of holistic understanding about occupation. Public health practitioners have been restricted in their appreciation of occupation as a holistic notion because the work and teaching of occupational therapists with this understanding is largely confined to fellow therapists with a disability focus within the medical field. As part of this process, the burgeoning occupational therapy that grew from humanist and socialist ideas about health became bound to medical and individualist models becoming disconnected from what appear to be ideologically compatible health workers. That has restricted others' understanding about occupation and what could be offered in the way of useful programs for physical, mental, and social well-being. As the WHO explains about just one aspect of occupation, "Appropriate regular physical activity is a major component in preventing the growing global burden of chronic disease."[79] Increasing "physical activity is a societal, not just an individual problem, and demands a population-based, multi-sectoral, multidisciplinary, and culturally relevant approach," and "inactivity greatly contributes to medical costs—by an estimated \$75 billion in the USA in 2000 alone."[79] Imagine the impact of a mix of appropriate physical, mental, and social activity initiatives at public policy level down.

Summary

Health; absence of illness; and physical, mental, and social well-being result naturally from "doing, being and becoming" in tune with our "'occupational" species' nature. It will not prevent every illness or disability, but it will be protective and it will provide advantages to the promotion of health even for those who experience poor health. This is well recognized in WHO directives for people all around the world and at any age. Being responsive to biological needs that are, in part, stimulated, influenced, and adapted by conscious social processes and making use of capacities remains central to maintaining homeostasis, promoting positive health and physical, mental, and social well-being. This can be provided, in large part, through engagement in occupation to obtain the prerequisites of survival and health; those that provide meaning, purpose, and belonging; and those that meet the need for optimal opportunity toward desired outcomes. If this can be achieved, individuals, families, and communities will flourish but not all illness or disability will be avoided. On the downside, if sociocultural and political processes continue the track to economic wealth for a minority, even with apparently generous handouts to the majority who live in poverty, it is doubtful whether health and well-being can be sustained in the long term or that the species and planet will survive. The complexity of the interaction of sociocultural processes with biological needs and lack of awareness about health's dependence on engagement in balanced and satisfying occupation rather than wealth for its own sake can, and does, lead to unhealthy consequences for the majority of the world's human population, animal, and plant species and ecological health (Figure 6-6).

This text continues by presenting some ideas about different approaches that could increase awareness and alleviate difficulties that many people are experiencing in attaining improved health through what they do, be, and strive to become. For public health to accept the conceptualization of occupation as a powerful influence on health, it is necessary to suggest a direction that occupationally based public health can espouse. Articulation of this direction forms the main thrust of future chapters. I propose an action-research approach that grew from the exploration of ideas presented in this text.

Figure 6-6. Factors underlying illness, health, and well-being from an occupational perspective.

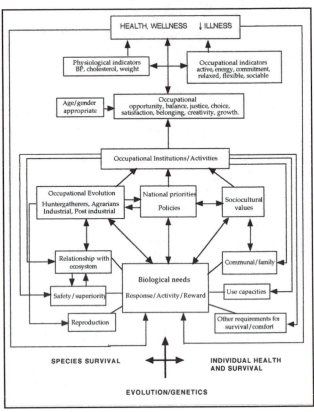

It requires acceptance of occupation's fundamental relationship to health, a change of attitudes, an extension of domains of concern to include all people, and a commitment to action-research that is applied to individuals, groups, communities, and the global population.

References

1. Dubos R, ed. *Mirage of Health: Utopias, Progress and Biological Change.* New York: Harper and Row; 1959:9,.
2. Glass TA, Mendes de Leon CF, Marottoli RA, Berkman LF. Population based study of social and productive activities as predictors of survival among elderly Americans. *BMJ.* 1999:319:478-483.
3. Corbin HD. Brighter vistas for senior citizens: salient thoughts. *Journal of Physical Education and Recreation.* 1977;October:52-53.
4. Comfort A. *A Good Age.* Melbourne, Australia: Macmillan Co Pty Ltd; 1977:82.
5. Wolman B, ed. *Dictionary of Behavioral Science.* New York: Van Nostand, Reinold Co; 1973:250.
6. Knight R, Knight M. *A Modern Introduction to Psychology.* London: University Tutorial Press Ltd; 1957;56-57,177.
7. McDougall W. *Social Psychology.* 23rd rev ed. London: Methuen; 1936.
8. Izard CE. *Human Emotions.* New York: Plenum; 1977.
9. Izard CE, Kagan J, Zajonc RB. *Emotions, Cognition, and Behavior.* New York: Cambridge University Press; 1984.
10. Frijda NH. *The Emotions.* New York: Cambridge University Press; 1986.
11. Csikszentmihalyi M, Csikszentmihalyi I, eds. *Optimal Experience: Psychological Studies of Flow in Consciousness.* New York: Cambridge University Press; 1988:20-25.

12. Csikszentmihalyi M. Activity and happiness: toward a science of occupation. *J Occup Sci: Australia.* 1993;1(1):38-42.
13. Meyer A. The philosophy of occupational therapy. *Archives of Occupational Therapy.* 1922;1:1-10.
14. Sigerist HE. *A History of Medicine. Vol 1. Primitive and Archaic Medicine.* New York: Oxford University Press; 1955:254-255.
15. Southwood-Smith T. *The Philosophy of Health; or an Exposition of the Physical and Mental Constitution of Man, with a View to the Promotion of Human Longevity and Happiness.* Vol 1. London: Charles Knight; 1836.
16. Argyle M. *The Psychology of Happiness.* New York: Methuen and Co; 1987.
17. Leone RE. Life after laughter: one perspective. *Elementary School Guidance and Counselling.* 1986;21(2):139-142.
18. Ornstein R, Sobel D. *Healthy Pleasures.* Reading, Mass: Addison-Wesley Publishing Co Inc; 1989.
19. Simon JM. Humor and its relationship to percieved health, life satisfaction, and moral in older adults. *Issues in Mental Health Nursing.* 1990;11(1):17-31.
20. Southam M, Cummings M. The use of humour as a technique for modulating pain. *Occupational Therapy Practice.* 1990;1(3):77-84.
21. Buxman K. Make room for laughter. *Am J Nurs.* 1991;91(12):46-51.
22. Mallett J. Use of humour and laughter in patient care. *Br J Nurs.* 1993;2(93):172-175.
23. Rose S. *The Conscious Brain.* Rev ed. Harmondsworth, England: Penguin Books; 1976:39,292-293.
24. Doyal L, Gough I. *A Theory of Human Need.* Houndmills, Hampshire: Macmillan; 1991:172.
25. Unpublished Survey. University of South Australia; 1993.
26. Fitzgerald R, ed. *Human Needs and Politics.* Sydney, Australia: Permagon; 1977:153.
27. Lorenz K. *The Waning of Humaneness.* Munich, Germany: R Piper and Co Verlag; 1983:124.
28. Csikszentmihalyi M, Jackson S. *Flow in Sports.* Champaign, Ill: Human Kinetics; 1999:167.
29. Hammell KW. Dimensions of meaning in the occupations of daily life. *Can J Occup Ther.* 2004;71:5:296-305.
30. Hocking C. The Relationship Between Objects and Identity in Occupational Therapy: A Dynamic Balance of Rationalism and Romanticism. Unpublished PhD thesis. Auckland University of Technology; 2004:171.
31. Thagard P. *How Scientists Explain Disease.* Princeton, NJ: Princeton University Press; 1999.
32. Clark F, Azen SP, Zemke R, et al. Occupational therapy for independent older adults: A randomised controlled trial. *JAMA.* 1997;Oct 22/29:1321-1326.
33. Wilcock AA, et al. Retrospective Study of Elderly Peoples' Perceptions of the Relationship Between Their Lifes' Occupations and Health. Unpublished material, University of South Australia, 1990.
34. King-Boyes MJE. *Patterns of Aboriginal Culture: Then and Now.* Sydney, Australia: McGraw-Hill Book Co; 1977:17,155.
35. Budgett R. Overtraining syndrome. *Br J Sports Med.* 1990;24(4):231-236.
36. Cooper K. *Dr Kenneth Cooper's Antioxidant Revolution.* Melbourne, Australia: Bookman; 1994.
37. Siscovick DS, Weiss NS, Fletcher RH, Lasky T. The incidence of primary cardiac arrest during vigorous exercise. *N Engl J Med.* 1984;311:874-877.
38. Kleitman N. *Sleep and Wakefulness.* Chicago, Ill: University of Chicago Press; 1963:188.
39. Leger DW. *Biological Foundations for Behavior: An Integrative Approach.* New York: Harper Collins Publishers; 1992:374.
40. Horne JA. A review of the biological effects of total sleep deprivation in man. *Biol Psychol.* 1978;(7):55-102.
41. Leys R, Evans R, Evans B, eds. *Defining American Psychology: The Correspondence Between Adolph Meyer and Edward Bradford Titchener.* Baltimore, Md: The Johns Hopkins University Press; 1990:43-46,59,162.
42. Meyer A. The problems of mental reaction types, mental causes and diseases. In: Winters EE, ed. *The Collected Papers of Adolph Meyer.* Vol 2. Baltimore, Md: The Johns Hopkins Press; 1951:598.
43. Muncie W. The psychobiological approach. In: Arieti S, ed. *American Handbook of Psychiatry.* Vol 2. New York: Basic Books, Inc; 1959.
44. James W. *Pragmatism: A New Name for Some Old Ways of Thinking.* New York: Longmans, Green and Co; 1907.
45. Dewey J. *Democracy and Education: An Introduction to the Philosophy of Education.* Toronto, Canada: Collier-MacMillan; 1916.
46. Breines E. *Origins and Adaptations: A Philosophy of Practice.* Lebanon, NJ: Geri-Rehab, Inc; 1986:46.
47. Golley FB. *A History of the Ecosystem Concept in Ecology.* New Haven, Conn: Yale University Press; 1993.
48. World Health Organization, Health and Welfare Canada, Canadian Public Health Association. *Ottawa Charter for Health Promotion.* Ottawa, Canada: Author; 1986.
49. Turner GW, ed. *The Australian Concise Oxford Dictionary of Current English.* Melbourne, NY: Oxford University Press; 1987.
50. *Funk & Wagnall's Standard Desk Dictionary.* Vol 1. New York: Harper and Row; 1984:296.

51. Boddy J, ed. *Health: Perspectives and Practices.* Auckland, New Zealand: The Dunmore Press; 1985:113.
52. Smuts JC. *Holism and Evolution.* London: Macmillan and Co Ltd; 1926.
53. Kopelman L, Moskop J. The holistic health movement: a survey and critique. *J Med Philos.* 1981;6(2):209-235.
54. von Bertalanffy L. *Problems of Life.* New York: Wiley; 1952.
55. Wilkinson P. General systems theory. In: Bullock A, Stalleybrass O, Trombley S, eds. *The Fontana Dictionary of Modern Thought.* 2nd ed. London: Fontana Press; 1988.
56. Pietroni PC. Holistic medicine. In: Bullock A, Stalleybrass O, Trombley S, eds. *The Fontana Dictionary of Modern Thought.* 2nd ed. London: Fontana Press; 1988.
57. World Health Organization. *Jakarta Declaration on Leading Health Promotion Into the 21st Century.* Geneva: Author; 1998.
58. McMichael T. *Human Frontiers, Environments and Disease: Past Patterns, Uncertain Futures.* Cambridge: Cambridge University Press; 2001
59. Porter R. *The Greatest Benefit to Mankind: A Medical History of Humanity.* London: Harper Collins; 1997.
60. McKeown T. *The Origins of Disease.* Oxford, UK: Basil Blackwell; 1988.
61. Wilcock AA. *Occupation for Health. Vol. 1. A Journey from Self-Health to Prescription.* London: British College of Occupational Therapists; 2001.
62. Wilcock AA. *Occupation for Health. Vol. 2. A Journey from Prescription to Self-Health.* London: British College of Occupational Therapists; 2002.
63. Bing RK. The evolution of occupation. In: Christiansen CH, Baum CM, eds. *Occupational Therapy: Performance, Participation, and Well-Being.* Thorofare, NJ: SLACK Incorporated; 2005.
64. Christiansen CH, Townsend EA, eds. *Introduction to Occupation: The Art and Science of Living.* Upper Saddle River, NJ: Prentice Hall; 2004.
65. Ornstein R, Sobel D. The Healing Brain: A Radical New Approach to Health Care. London, England: MacMillan; 1988.
66. Porter R. *Disease, Medicine and Society in England 1550-1860.* London: MacMillan Education; 1987.
67. Wilcock AA. Occupational utopias: back to the future. *J Occup Sci.* 2001;1(1):6-13
68. More T. *Utopia.* Abridged edition. London: Phoenix; 1996.
69. Hardy L, Davidson L, eds. *Utopian Thought and Communal Experience.* Middlesex University, UK: Geography and Management Paper No 24; 1989:Introduction.
70. Locke J. *An Essay Concerning Humane Understanding.* London: Tho. Basset; 1690.
71. Howard J. An Account of the Principle Lazarettos in Europe; With Varios Papers Relative to the Plague: Together with further Observations on some Foreign Prisons and Hospitals; And Additional Remarks on the Present State of those in Great Britain and Ireland. Warrington, UK: Printed by William Eyres; 1789:140-142.
72. Pare A. The Authors dedication to Henry the third, the Most Christian King of France and Poland. 1579. In: Johnson T. The Workes of that Famous Chirurgion Ambroise Parey. Translated out of Latin and compared with the French. Printed by Th Cotes and R Young; 1634.
73. Blundell JWF. The Muscles and their Story from the Earliest Times (an Adaptation of the 'Ars Gymnastica') including the Whole Text of Mercurialis, and the Opinions of other Writers Ancient and Modern on Mental and Bodily Development. London: Chapman & Hall; 1864.
74. Ramazzini B. Of The Diseases Of Tradesmen, Shewing The Various Influence Of Particular Trades Upon The State Of Health; With The Best Methods To Avoid or Correct It,...London: Printed for Andrew Bell et al.; 1705
75. Pinel P. A *Treatise on Insanity.* Birmingham, Ala: Classics of Medicine Library; 1983.
76. Tuke S. *Description of the Retreat.* York: Alexander; 1813:141,156.
77. Browne WAF. What asylums were, are and ought to be. In: Carlson ET, advisory ed. *Classics in Psychiatry: Arno Press Collection.* North Stratford, UK: Ayer Company Publishers Inc; 2001:177.
78. World Federation of Occupational Therapists. Definition. 2004. Accessed February 2006.
79. World Health Organization. *Global Strategy on Diet, Physical Activity and Health. Chronic Disease Information Sheets.* World Health Organization Documents and Publications: 2004. Accessed WWW, December 2005.
80. World Health Organization. *Mental Health Fact Sheet 220*; 2001. Accessed November 2005.
81. World Health Organization. *Active Ageing: A Policy Framework. Second United Nations World Assembly on Ageing.* Madrid, Spain: Author; 2002:12,13.
82. Crepeau AB, Cohn ES, Boyt Schell BA, eds. *Willard and Spackman's Occupational Therapy.* Philadelphia: Lippincott, Williams & Wilkins; 2003:42

Suggested Reading

Browne WAF. What Asylums Were, Are and Ought to Be. Edinburgh: A. & C. Black; 1837. Reprinted: *Classics in Psychiatry: Arno Press Collection.* North Stratford, UK: Ayer Company Publishers Inc; 2001.

Doyal L, Gough I. *A Theory of Human Need.* Houndmills, Hampshire: Macmillan; 1991.

Locke J. An Essay Concerning Humane Understanding. London: Printed for Tho. Basset, and sold by Edw. Mory at the sign of the Three Bibles in St Paul's Church-Yard; 1690.

Ornstein R, Sobel D. *Healthy Pleasures.* Reading, Mass: Addison-Wesley Publishing Co Inc; 1989.

Pinel P. A *Treatise on Insanity.* Translated from the French by D. D. Davis, MD. Sheffield: Printed by W. Todd, for Messrs Cadell and Davies, Strand London: 1806. Reprinted: Birmingham, Alabama: Classics of Medicine Library, 1983.

Tuke S. *Description of the Retreat.* York: Alexander; 1813.

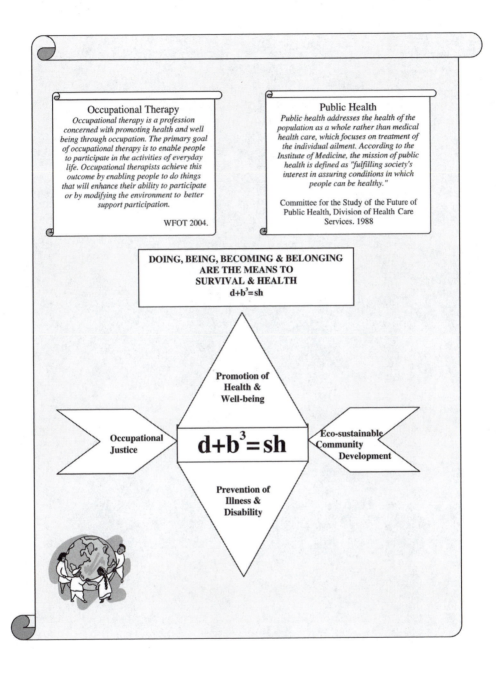

Occupational Therapy

Occupational therapy is a profession concerned with promoting health and well being through occupation. The primary goal of occupational therapy is to enable people to participate in the activities of everyday life. Occupational therapists achieve this outcome by enabling people to do things that will enhance their ability to participate or by modifying the environment to better support participation.

WFOT 2004.

Public Health

Public health addresses the health of the population as a whole rather than medical health care, which focuses on treatment of the individual ailment. According to the Institute of Medicine, the mission of public health is defined as "fulfilling society's interest in assuring conditions in which people can be healthy."

Committee for the Study of the Future of Public Health, Division of Health Care Services. 1988

DOING, BEING, BECOMING & BELONGING ARE THE MEANS TO SURVIVAL & HEALTH
$d+b^3=sh$

Promotion of Health & Well-being

Occupational Justice

$$d+b^3=sh$$

Eco-sustainable Community Development

Prevention of Illness & Disability

SECTION II
AN ACTION-RESEARCH APPROACH

INTRODUCTION TO SECTION II

Action-Research in Population Health

The final chapters bring together the major ideas that have emerged from the explorations presented in this text to suggest 4 different approaches to population health that are all based on participatory action research. Previous chapters have explored ideas about health; an occupational theory of human nature; population health experiences, views, and rules throughout time in terms of people as occupational beings; of occupation as doing, being, and becoming; of the instrumental part these have played in illness, health, and well-being throughout evolution; and of current initiatives and directives from the WHO that encompass the relationship between occupation and health. The exploration so far has suggested that public health practitioners and occupational therapists could and should be primary sources of expertise for research and development of population health approaches that take an occupational perspective. Together they might form a new and useful partnership in the spirit of the *Jakarta Declaration*. To do so, each would require a well-developed and holistic concept of the relationship between people's engagement in occupation and population health.

Public health practitioners have a wide understanding of population health from a social perspective, but this has not embraced, in any depth, the notion of people's occupational natures and needs and the closeness of those to natural health. This is despite the obvious goodness of fit with many of its principles. Many occupational therapists consider their role to extend beyond the amelioration of illness to the promotion of optimal states of health in line with WHO philosophies, but remain trapped within conventional medical and disability services and one-to-one practice. They could play an important role in public health as it is currently conceived; however, if they are to deliver the promise of the understanding of humans as occupational beings as part of the total picture of an evolving ecology, they should not conform to the present biases of public health as they have to conventional medicine. They must bring to public health their concept of the "occupational human" and be prepared to challenge and analyze socioeconomic policies and public health research directions and strategies from this perspective. At present, because the distinct contribution occupational therapists could bring to health promotion is barely recognized by governments and other public health workers, the understanding of the complex interaction between occupation and health is largely lost. Bockhoven, a psychiatrist taking a multidisciplinary look at community mental health in the 1970s, considered that:

> *Acknowledgment of the critical moral importance of occupation in human life demands*
> *an in-depth review by the health professions of their own value judgments and prac-*

tices with respect to identifying which are the means and which are the ends of our endeavors.[1]

He argued that occupational therapy is "a neglected source of community rehumanization" that is:

> ... *blocked from perceiving either the depth or the breadth of its role as a moral and scientific force. This role has even more central importance to future human development than could possibly be claimed by any existing scientific specialty which neither has nor claims a moral basis.*[1]

He considered that occupational therapists are the health professionals most skilled to advance this concept because they have "acquired a body of moral perspectives and occupational lore of unique value to society" that "can be more effectively utilized if it is not limited to being a service solely for sick people."[1]

The starting point for any health professional planning to work in the area of occupation-focused population health is a clear description of the key features and factors to be incorporated. These are:

* Understanding that action to obtain the prerequisites for healthy survival is a basic human need that cannot be met fully by welfare handouts alone.

* Aiming for a balance of physical, mental, and social well-being attained through valued occupation that does more than meet the prerequisites of health.

* Enhancement of species' common and individually unique natures, needs, capacities, and potential.

* Occupational and social justice and support for all people and communities upheld and encouraged by political advocacy.

* Community cohesion through politically supported and socially valued, well-balanced, occupational opportunity that again might require political lobbying.

* Research and action aimed at enabling, mediating, and advocating for healthy public policy that is responsive to human needs rather than materialistic wants all within, and as part of, a sustainable ecology.

* Health care aimed at the maintenance and enhancement of physical, psychological, spiritual, and social functioning of individuals and communities toward maximum potential and quality in everyday living, in interaction with the natural world that sustains all creatures and on which everything depends, and in a way that ensures its healthy survival.

These 7 points are inclusive of WHO directives that have been discussed in previous chapters, and particularly of the 5 strategies within the OCHP as ratified by the *Jakarta Declaration* and of the latter's priorities for health promotion in the 21st century.[2]

While different types of research will be valuable and necessary to explore aspects of occupation-focused approaches and are mentioned or suggested in the text of the following chapters, in the main, it is participatory action-research (PAR) that will be most appropriate to enable change for a participatory action view of health. A PAR approach is advocated in line with critical social science, which recognizes people as "participants in the sociohistorical development of human action and understanding,"[3] Trentham and Cockburn suggest that:

> *Generally speaking, PAR practitioners embrace a critical social science perspective in their acknowledgement that existing social structures are unjust, benefiting privileged groups over marginalized groups, and are therefore in need of change.*[4]

Action-research aims at facilitating social change through self-reflective inquiry and consciousness raising, which enlightens participants about equity and hegemony issues, collective sharing of critical self-reflections, dialogue, and questions, leading to collective planning and action.[5] Action-research is a collaborative process that is participatory, practical, emancipatory, critical, and recursive. It is a social process in which people are enabled to understand the social forces working on them and how they and the processes might be changed. This is achieved through participation with others learning and doing together to review social relationships of power, and reconstruct communities so that they are not alienating but more natural, productive, just, and satisfying.[6] It can meet the needs of large groups of people, although not the needs of all types of research or inquiry.[7]

Comstock suggests that such research includes "repeated movement" through several phases—the interpretive, the empirical-analytical, the critical-dialectical, and the practical-educational and political-action phases—in its progress toward increased understanding and social action.[3] This approach is suggested because critical social science has beliefs in common with this occupational perspective of health, specifically the assumption that "humans are active creatures"[8] and that people shape both natural and social environments through their activity. Because people are largely unaware of themselves or their cultures as "the 'objects' they have created," their activity "is carried out in a disorganized and often self-defeating way," which can result in less than optimum conditions or opportunities.[9] To overcome the problems associated with this lack of awareness, it is essential to use approaches that raise consciousness, as well as provide support for reflection and informed action. Environments and health services can be shaped through participatory action-research. If such an approach is adopted, it would enable the communities involved to create a way of life, in balance with the ecology, in which individuals as well as the population at large are able to meet the prerequisites of health and their need for occupational meaning, belonging, satisfaction, increased well-being, and health.

Action-research is participatory in that it is the community that identifies the issues to be explored and these are context specific rather than generic aimed toward improving particular situations, so sharing between the community of researchers is central to the process.[4] The PAR model espoused includes 4 interlinking phases:

1. Research centers on exploring issues about doing, being, and becoming; biological nature and needs; meeting the prerequisites of health, capacities, meaning, balance, satisfaction, and potentials; activity-rest continuums; activity-nutrition factors; occupational deprivation, alienation, and imbalance at individual, community, national, global, and ecological levels; using quantitative or qualitative methodologies.

2. Awareness and education involves a multilevel educational strategy to raise consciousness of a holistic occupational perspective of viewing health, technology, societies, population, and global activities.

3. Activism aims at gradual social change toward individual and population occupation (on a global scale), which is in line with biological needs, social justice, intraspecies flourishing, and a sustainable ecology.

4. Analysis of occupational change at personal and population levels as well as at socio-techno-political levels through socio-techno-political response to the global and local needs of people as part of the natural world rather than materialistic and power-based wants.

These phases are never complete, each one leading to the next, but available to be revisited to check or alter as new evidence suggests new possibilities. The interlinking involves ongoing research and exploration to monitor the effects, to feed back into education, activism, socio-techno-political change, and so on in a continuous spiral. The components of the approach are not compartmentalized, and interaction between them is ongoing, reflective, and dynamic in order to investigate and act according to multiple truths in a way that is flexible and able to anticipate needs or meet them as they occur and that can take corrective action when required. The research and awareness-raising phases will now be introduced. The action and occupational change phases, which are dependent on the occupation for health issue, will be considered within the next 4 chapters about approaches.

RESEARCH PHASE

The research phase would make use of existing studies that inform the problems being addressed. Public health has always favored an epidemiological approach, and this remains an approach of choice for clinically based aspects of occupation studies. Such empirical studies can be used to inform the action-research participants and the public at large, and so can be used in combination with other types of exploration. Occupational scientists, in contrast to public health epidemiologists, have favored qualitative approaches in order to explore the complexities of humans as occupational beings, their experiences, and the individual meaning given to engagement in occupation.[8] This preference is strong because of the fear that reductionist study will remain predominant to the detriment of in-depth work on the complexities of people interacting with their environment (Yerxa, personal communication, 1990). Indeed, the preference for qualitative research has arisen because of concern that occupational therapists have been overly influenced by the positivistic assumption that "all true knowledge is scientific, in the sense of describing the coexistence and succession of observable phenomena"[10] and that philosophical and theoretical observations are only significant if they are constructed from empirical, preferably numerical, data. This has limited occupational therapists' research, in the past, to explorations such as surveys or clinical trials in the medical science tradition; as a result, many questions of a holistic nature, important from the profession's philosophical foundations, and the health approaches discussed here remain unanswered. Qualitative approaches have the potential to answer some of these questions because they "extend traditional views of 'truth' to include multiple realities, values, and meanings"[11] from participants' points of view. Such research can be part of participatory action research. Data can be collected by participants, for example, by interviews, storytelling, time-diaries, experience sampling, observation, documenting conversations, interactions and activities, focus groups, searching out, and reviewing records and written documentation as in this history of ideas approach,[11] all of which can "produce meaningful descriptions and interpretations of social processes," "offer explanations of how certain conditions came into existence and persist," and provide "the basis for realistic proposals" for improving social environments.[12,13]

In the proposed PAR approach, no one methodology is favored; rather, appropriate combinations of research methods would allow for the research to be exploratory, descriptive, or explanatory and for analysis to be empirical, interpretative, or critical.[12] Qualitative researchers, particularly, recognize the complementary value of quantitative and qualitative approaches rather than their incompatibility. In combination, they can add rigor and breadth and provide a more complete picture than either approach used alone.[14-16] Different blends will lead to new ways of knowing about humans as occupational beings and will help to provide different perspectives of people's experience of engagement in occupation, of the organization and balance of occupations in lifestyle throughout lifespan, and the relationship of each to acquiring the prerequisites of healthy survival, adaptation, social expectations, life satisfaction, and health.[8] Accessing extended methods of inquiry will inform the study of underlying factors that prompt people to do the things they do, day by day, often or occasionally; why different social groups, cultures, and populations use time differently; and whether current sociocultural structures and institutions are based on values that will enable humans to continue evolving in directions that are appropriate and necessary to the ecology and our species' survival and well-being.

While occupational science should provide one of the major research bases of occupation-focused health approaches, it will need to draw upon the expanding knowledge of the medical, social, and behavioral sciences, as well as the natural and biological sciences. Human occupation crosses all boundaries from genetic codes, cellular system formation, biological capacity, and personal ideas, through family, community, social, and political domains to have effects upon the world ecology. Within all these domains, there is a need for research to begin to understand and influence occupation choices toward healthier bodies, minds, lifestyles, environments, national and international policies, and ecological sustainability. While many may not be part of PAR, they will—from time to time—be mentioned in the ensuing chapters so that the base for PAR is expanded.

EDUCATION-AWARENESS PHASE

Findings from this diverse research need to be accessible to the public at large. In action-research terms, they must lead to an education-awareness phase. This includes increasing understanding of how doing, being, and becoming can prevent illness and promote health and well-being, and how political, social, and technological structures facilitate or inhibit achievement of occupational meaning, satisfaction, and potential. Strategies that could be used to increase political, population, community, or individual awareness include social planning, which, in turn, includes problem-solving based on data gathering and goal setting; social action, such as rallies and boycotts, conferences, workshops, seminars, in-service training, health fairs, brochures, and circulars in libraries; and group discussion and individual counseling in community agencies, health centers, schools, and the workplace, as well as in routine health provider-consumer interactions.

Behavior modification or mass propaganda principles that provide information about healthy living, such as health warnings on cigarette packs, assume that at least some people accessing the information will adjust behaviors as a result of the message. The effects of such programs can usually only be expected in the long-term and are difficult to measure, and, indeed, there are some who would deny this as a health education approach. Green et al suggest that health education requires voluntary participation of the consumer,[17] and for individuals to change habitual patterns of behavior this is probably the most effective approach. Unless information is specifically sought by people motivated to use it, learning, which is cumulative, can only occur after repeated exposure to an idea. However, in the case of increasing awareness about the relationship between occupation and health, it may be necessary to use mass propaganda approaches because the basic relationship is so little understood. For example, awareness can be raised following mass media exposure of the ideas in topical programs, in documentaries, as themes in soap operas, and using posters and desk devices such as the "occupation for health pyramid" in much the same way as other health messages, such as about nutrition or abortion, have been conveyed to the public.

Public health practitioners appear more skillful than occupational therapists at accessing the media in part because their health message may appear closer to a medical science "illness" approach to health. If occupational therapists do take up the challenge of population health practice, they will need to develop advocacy and public relations skills to ensure that their health education messages are accessible. Alternatively, their public health partners, more experienced in disseminating information, could become their advocates. However, even these health professionals have less success in accessing the media than conventional medicine in terms of spectacular cure rather than preventive approach.

A greater emphasis on individual and group education and teaching skills is also required. Jungfer, a medical practitioner who pioneered an integrated health service in South Australia, believed that every member of the health care team "must seize every teachable moment to explain fully to the patient the part he must play in maintaining his health" because reinforcement from many sources facilitates increased awareness.[18] Increased awareness enables people to decide for themselves the most appropriate action to promote healthy living, to understand and define their own health problems and needs, and to understand what action they can take using their own resources.

The education-awareness phase of this public health action-research model requires more than providing information and more than participants engaging in a change-growth experience, important though these may be. It should link structuralism and individualism, broader social processes with the problems people face in their daily lives, issues about doing, being, becoming, and health outcomes and should be viewed as an agent of sociopolitical structural change that can empower and enhance awareness of optimum physiological functioning, role performance, and potential.[19,20] It should, for example, encompass the occupational determinants that can contribute to health and well-being or contribute to the preclinical health disorders and ultimately to disease, disability, or death as discussed in earlier chapters.

The action phase of the approach will vary according to the problem but will be based on issues concerning doing, being, and becoming and on developing techniques and strategies that may facilitate improved health though occupation for individuals and community, national, and international populations.

Four approaches to promoting better population health are discussed in the next chapters. These are not mutually exclusive. The following table provides an overview. The approaches are all occupation-focused and address eco-sustaining community development, matters of justice, prevention of illness, and health promotion and well-being. An overview of the differing ideologies of each reveals how they might be integrated and what direction an action-research approach could take from an occupational perspective. This method of dividing out differing aspects of services aiming at health promotion provides us with ways of seeing (understanding), organizing (setting objectives and deploying resources), and doing (research, strategies, and programs). All are important and need not be separated in practice.

In order to realize the implications of the ideas raised in this text, it will be necessary to challenge many ideas that are central to political, social, and health ideologies. This is particularly so because in postindustrial societies with an economic-technological-power focus, rather than one aimed primarily at meeting the needs of humans in a way that recognizes ecological strengths and constraints, highly technical, illness-based health services are fostered and applauded. This type of service encourages people to continue stressful, regulated, time-dictated, and unnatural lifestyles because it offers to undo many of the obvious effects of consumer societies with spare parts and chemical remedies; it is essentially antidotal. The whole societal configuration inhibits, by default, the establishment of alternative systems that may help prevent illness and promote improved health. This implies that the theoretical foundations of these action-research approaches must address structural, environmental, and population issues as well as individual health needs.

Overview of Occupation-Focused Approaches to Population Health

Occupation-Focused Approaches	Definition
Ecologically sustainable community development	The promotion of ecologically sustainable policies and community-wide action to maintain or re-establish healthy relationships between people, human societies, other living organisms, their environments, habits, and modes of life through community consultation, deliberation, resource management, development, and participation in health-giving and ecologically sustaining occupations.
Justice	The promotion of just socioeconomic and political conditions to increase individual, population, and political awareness, resources, and opportunity for people to participate in doing, being, and becoming healthily through engagement in occupations that meet the prerequisites of health and every person's different natures, capacities, and needs.
Prevention of illness and disability	The application of medical, behavioral, social, and occupational science to prevent physiological, psychological, social, and occupational illness, accidents, and disability and prolong quality of life for all people through advocacy and mediation and through occupation-focused programs aimed at enabling people to do, be, and become according to their natural health needs.
Health promotion	"Health promotion is the process of enabling people to increase control over and to improve their health. To reach a state of complete physical, mental, and social well-being, an individual or group must be able to identify and realize aspirations, to satisfy needs, and to change or cope with the environment. Health is, therefore, seen as a resource for everyday life, not the objective of living. Health is a positive concept emphasizing social and personal resources as well as physical capacities. Therefore, health promotion is not just the responsibility of the health sector, but goes beyond healthy lifestyles to well-being."[21]

References

1. Bockhoven JS. *Moral Treatment in Community Mental Health.* New York: Springer Publishing Co, Inc; 1972:219.
2. World Health Organization. *Jakarta Declaration on Leading Health Promotion Into the 21st Century.* Geneva: Author; 1998.
3. Comstock D. A method for critical research. In: Bredo E, Feinberg W, eds. *Knowledge and Values in Social and Educational Research.* Philadelphia: Temple University Press; 1982:377.
4. Trentham B, Cockburn L. Participatory action research: creating new knowledge and opportunities for occupational engagement. In: Kronenberg F, Simo Algado S, Pollard N, eds. *Occupational Therapy Without Borders: Learning from the Spirit of Survivors.* London: Elsevier Ltd; 2005:442.
5. McCutcheon G, Jung B. Alternative perspectives on action research. *Theory Into Practice.* 1990;29(3):147.
6. Kemmis S, Wilkinson M. Participatory action and the study of practice. In: Atweh B, Kemmis S, Weeks P, eds. *Action Research in Practice: Partnership for Social Justice and Education.* London: Routledge; 1998.

7. Letts L. Occupational therapy and participatory research: a partnership worth pursuing. *Am J Occup Ther.* 2003;57:577-587.
8. Yerxa EJ, Clark F, Frank G, et al. An introduction to occupational science: a foundation for occupational therapy in the 21st century. *Occupational Therapy in Health Care.* 1989;6(4):1–17.
9. Fay B. *Critical Social Science: Liberation and Its Limits.* Ithaca, NY: Cornell University Press; 1987:47-53.
10. Quinton A. Positivism. In: Bullock A, Stalleybrass O, Trombley S, eds. *The Fontana Dictionary of Modern Thought.* 2nd ed. London, England: Fontana Press; 1988:669.
11. Wilcock AA. Biological and socio-cultural perspectives on time-use studies. In: Pentland WE, Harvey A, Lawton MP, McColl MA, eds. *Time Use Research in the Social Sciences.* New York: Kluwer Academic/Plenum Press; 1999.
12. Denzin NK. *Interpretive Interactionism: Applied Social Research Methods Series.* Vol 16. Newberry Park, Calif: Sage Publications; 1989:23.
13. Becker HS, Horowitz IL. Radical politics and sociological observation: observations on methodology and ideology. In: Becker HS, ed. *Doing Things Together: Selected Papers.* Evanston, Ill: Northwestern University Press; 1986:83-102.
14. Tripp-Reimer T. Combining qualitative and quantitative methodologies. In: Leininger M, ed. *Qualitative Research Methods in Nursing.* Orlando, Fla: Grune and Stratton; 1985:179.
15. Silverman D. *Qualitative Methodology and Sociology.* Brookfield, Vt: Gower Publishing Co Ltd; 1985:17.
16. De Landsheere G. History of educational research. In: Keeves JP, ed. *Educational Research, Methodology and Measurement.* Oxford, UK: Permagon Press; 1988:10.
17. Green L, Kreuter M, Deeds S, Partridge K. *Health Education Planning: A Diagnostic Approach.* Palo Alto, Calif: Mayfield Publishing Co; 1980:8.
18. Jungfer C. Prevention—an attitude of mind. *Australian Family Physician.* 1979;8:219-221.
19. French J, Adams L. From analysis to synthesis: theories of health education. *Health Education Journal.* 1986;45(2):71-74.
20. Colquhoun D. *Health Education Politics and Practice.* Geelong, Victoria: Deakin University; 1992.
21. World Health Organization, Health and Welfare Canada. Canadian Public health Association. *Ottawa Charter for Health Promotion.* Ottawa, Canada: Author; 1986:2.

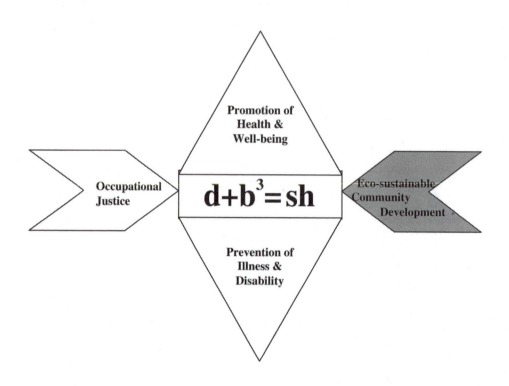

Occupational Justice

Promotion of
Health &
Well-being

$d+b^3=sh$

Prevention of
Illness &
Disability

Eco-sustainable
Community
Development

OCCUPATION-FOCUSED ECO-SUSTAINABLE COMMUNITY DEVELOPMENT APPROACH

Theme 7:

"To accept the community as the essential voice in matters of its health, living conditions and well-being."
"To recognize health and its maintenance as a major social investment and challenge: and to address the overall ecological issue of our ways of living."
WHO, *Ottawa Charter for Health Promotion*, 1986

The chapter addresses:

* The concepts of occupation-focused eco-sustainable community development approach
  * Ecological sustainability
  * Community development
  * An amalgamation and an occupation focus
* An occupation-focused eco-sustainable community development approach to health
* Why an occupation-focused eco-sustainable community development approach is necessary
* An action-research approach to health through occupation-focused eco-sustainable community development

The first of 4 approaches to be considered in the final chapters is occupation-focused eco-sustainable community development (OESCD). It combines the concept of community development with that of ecological sustainability; the latter aspect is, perhaps, the least understood health approach and the most vital in terms of the health of all people in the long term. The combination of these concepts is useful so that the lesser known concept becomes an accepted part of community development initiatives in all parts of the world. In the last chapter of the first edition of this book, I discussed separately a community development approach and a sustainable ecological approach. In this edition I decided to combine them, as have others in the field, so that readers are more able to recognize how an ecological approach could be incorporated into practice. Another reason is that if and when issues of the environment are fought without putting people into context, conflict that already exists between, for example, humanist and naturalist proponents will continue. People are integral to ecosystems and without that being taken into consideration, methods to sustain the ecology are doomed in the longer term. I also decided to place this combined approach at the start of the second section to point to the importance of all people taking such approaches very seriously at all times, which is in line with directives from the UN and WHO with regard to the promotion of health. The approaches in the following chapters could all equally be linked with either community development or ecological sustainability.

The Concepts of Occupation-Focused Eco-Sustainable Community Development Approach

ECOLOGICAL SUSTAINABILITY

"The idea of ecology remains a relatively novel perspective."[1] Responsible, to some extent, for growing concern about it was James Lovelock, an atmospheric chemist who formulated the Gaia Hypothesis in the mid-1960s.[2] He proposed that the Earth is a single living organism that maintains its own conditions necessary for its survival. Not substantiated but much expanded, the hypothesis provides a basis for considering the interaction of the Earth's biosphere, atmosphere, oceans, soil, climate, rocks, and all living things as part of a self-regulating process that constitutes a feedback system seeking an optimal physical and chemical environment for life on the planet. Lovelock's hypothesis stimulated a new awareness of the connectedness of all things on earth and the impact people have on global processes such as the deforestation or reforestation of trees, the removal or planting of crops, or the increase or decrease of emissions of carbon dioxide. While not necessarily accepting all of the Gaia postulates, scientists today generally support the idea that life has a substantial effect on abiotic processes.[3] Campbell, mirroring Lovelock's viewpoint, provides a simple but cogent pointer to the foundation of the concept in this approach, "... the components of the natural world are myriad but they constitute a single living system. There is no escape from our interdependence nature ..."[4]
So does David Suzuki:

> ... *you and I do not end at our fingertips or skin—we are connected through air, water and soil; we are animated by the same energy from the same source in the sky above. We are quite literally air, water, soil, energy and other living creatures.*[5]

The science of ecology is broad, covering:

* "Individual organisms (eg, behavioral ecology, feeding strategies)."
* "Populations (eg, population dynamics)."
* "Entire communities (eg, competition between species for access to resources in an ecosystem or predator-prey relationships)."[6]

Ernest Haekel coined the word *ecology* in 1866 to refer to the interdependency between plants, animals, and their natural environments[6]; however, it was not until the 1992 UN Conference on Environment and Development in Rio de Janeiro that world attention was directed to the issue of ecological sustainability as a matter for everyone. Since that time the sustainable development lobby has made clear that the necessary transformational changes are far from being achieved.[7] The lobby argues that the policy prescriptions of a market industrial system based on economic rationalism are unable to deal with emerging world complexity and that such systems lead to a continuation of environmental degradation and an ever-widening gap between the "haves and the have nots."[8,9] Only 20% of humanity accounts for an estimated 80% of the humans who burden the earth's ecology but enjoy its material rewards. The 20% of humanity who live in a state of absolute deprivation and a further 60% whose traditional lifestyles are disrupted by the promise of "economic growth" experience ongoing social and occupational injustice. Indeed, "those who control accumulated financial credits seek out ecological stocks wherever environmental frontiers remain"[7] and affect the resubordination of countries that appear to be breaking through to developed status.[10] Such actions support the myth that human survival is an "economic and political science problem" that "assumes that man is free or could be free from the forces of nature."[11]

That is far from the case, as recognized, to some extent by the first professorial appointment of human ecology in the latter half of the 20th century. Paul Shepard, the appointee in question, explained that because "there is only one ecology; not a human ecology on one hand and another for the subhuman," it needs to be considered with "an element of humility" and not "human superiority."[1] At that time, it was challenging to consider that people were "subject to ecological interdependence and that there were limits to the ecosphere's capacity to supply, replenish, and absorb, particularly under the weight of human numbers and economic activities."[1] The way that people fit into ecology highlights the connectedness and interdependence of human groups, societies, and the natural world. It is, however, only recently that scientists have become serious about understanding "human biology, culture, social relationships, health and disease within an ecological framework,"[1] McMichael arguing that the criteria relating to ecosystem health include "diversity, vigor, internal organization and resilience."[1] It is also only recently that occupational science emerged and the human need to do, be, and become has become part of that interconnection for its scientists. The concept of ecology provides the means to think broadly and in an integrative way about the complexities of the natural world and the place of people within it and dependence on it. Its breadth and holistic vision, in ways similar to occupational science, "is a world of contingent probabilities" that lack specificity, precision of measurement, crispness of definition, and causal inference, so that McMichael claims it is unsettling and threatening to many scientists and research funding bodies.[1] He asserts that such big questions are not deliberately ignored but are often side-stepped or not asked because they do not fit the accepted template of Western science. In line with Lander and Weinberg, he calls for a "more integrative systems type of science,"[12] and in tune with Shepard, that:

> Earth is too small. If we do not respond constructively to the ideas of ecology, then we can hardly avoid living in a world of declining natural capital, of persistent poverty for many people, of increasing political tensions, and of increased risks to our health and survival.[1]

The WHO recognizes:

> ... the need to encourage reciprocal maintenance—to take care of each other, our communities and our natural environment. The conservation of natural resources throughout the world should be emphasized as a global responsibility.[13]

Further than that, "the inextricable links between people and their environment constitutes the basis for a socio-ecological approach to health."[13]

COMMUNITY DEVELOPMENT

The idea of community development draws on the appreciation that people are social creatures living and doing in the company of others with survival itself dependent on cooperation or competition within populations. It is difficult to assess the health of individuals without also understanding the health of others within a community.[14] The concept of community development grew in the 20th century with the social model of health, and it addresses social determinants of health as the primary concern. The WHO recognizes that these are responsible for many of the worst health concerns of the present time as they have been in the past.

The advancement of human progress throughout time has not always been for the betterment of a great number of communities. The United Kingdom in the late 18th and 19th centuries is a case in point. It was discussed earlier that the change from agriculture to industry resulted in large populations leaving their former places of abode and livelihood and resettling en-masse into towns not ready for such immigration and that issued forth smoke and fumes damaging to human and ecological health. While most industrialists, who were the financial beneficiaries of this occupational change, did not consider community or environmental health as their concern, there were exceptions. Welsh-born Robert Owen (1771–1858) perhaps is the prime example. (Interestingly, in terms of the thrust of this text, his vision of Utopian communities and experiments in reforming society can be traced forward to the early days of occupational therapy through the work of Octavia Hill.[15]) Expanding the ideas of European communalism that rejected and condemned the dehumanizing effects of industry and capitalism,[16-19] Owen advocated for

> *... a society in which individuals shall acquire increased health, strength and intelligence—in which their labor shall be always advantageously directed—and in which they will possess every rational enjoyment.*[20]

A brief description is provided below.

Robert Owen's mill at New Lanark in Scotland was set in the idyllic Clyde Valley where many find solace today as "the wild wood" is once more beginning to flourish on the banks of the river. Although an outstanding theorist, Owen was, essentially, a practical man who put thought into action. He addressed many occupational health issues such as occupational alienation, deprivation, and imbalance by, for example, providing education for his workers, their families and children and by shortening working hours. He improved the worker's immediate environment by adding extra rooms to their one-roomed homes, establishing cooperative buying to reduce costs and improve the range of goods available, and by cleaning and paving the streets.

Believing that the essence of communities was created by the nature of their institutions and practices, Owen built a school for the children to attend from the day they could walk by themselves until they started work and for employees and housewives to attend evening classes. He also built a community center for his workers to take part in discussion, entertainment, enjoyment and leisure. He named it the Institute for the Formation of Character.

Many similar "Villages of Cooperation" known more commonly as Owenite Communities were established throughout the UK, and further afield. At least sixteen were established in America including New Harmony, a "Community of Equality," which Owen established personally.[1]

Although his approach was basically apolitical, Owen recognized the need to publicize his ideas for the benefit of other communities suffering similar social ills to those addressed in New Lanark and to stimulate reform about issues such as child labor and inequities of the poor law.[1,2] In doing so he provides an excellent role model for current day population health community developers. His life and work demonstrates the benefits of action to address immediate problems and advocacy to promote socio-political understanding and change as well as the necessity of raising awareness of social health problems within the population at large.   *(continued)*

As part of his concept of community development, health and well-being, Owen argued that exercise and growth of an individual's "entire faculties, senses and propensities" was beneficial "for the general advantage of all thus linking community and individual approaches.[3] Anticipating the environmental lobby, he was vehement about coming to understand "ourselves, society and nature."[3]

1. Harrison J. Robert Owen and the communities. In: Cole M, ed. *Robert Owen: Industrialist Reformer, Visionary, 1771-1858*. London, UK: Robert Owen Bicentenary Association; 1971:27.
2. Owen R. Report to the Committee of the Association for the Relief of the Manufacturing and Labouring Poor. 1817.
3. Owen R. *Works of Robert Owen: Volume 3: Book of the new moral world*. London: Pickering & Chatto (Publishers Ltd.); 1993:156,157.

As Owen recognized 2 centuries ago, communities depend upon interaction despite an apparently inevitable process of forming, disbanding, and reforming.[21] That factor, in part, may be blamed for decisions, policies, and programs frequently being formulated outside communities with little regard for local social, economic, or environmental consequences. As a result, many communities have become pawns in a global economy as their environments become production sites for multinational corporations until no longer profitable.[22] Community developers seek to reverse the ill-effect of community roller coaster rides by reinstating local control over development decisions, increasing self-reliance and economic opportunity.

In terms of community development, WHO recognizes the need to "enhance self help and social support, and for developing flexible systems for strengthening public participation and direction in health matters" by drawing on "existing human and material resources" at the heart of the health promoting process.[13] To do this calls for "empowerment of communities, their ownership and control of their own endeavours and destinies."[13] The popular phrase "think globally, act locally" fits this approach perfectly.

AN AMALGAMATION AND AN OCCUPATION FOCUS

The OESCD approach concerns 2 complex sets of ideas:
1. The conceptual recognition of the need to sustain the ecology through healthy relationships between humans, other living organisms, their environments, habits, and modes of life, and the powerful effects of people's occupational nature and needs on this process.
2. The need for community involvement, exploration, consultation, deliberation, and action to promote self-sustaining occupational development, health, and well-being.

Similar to the biocultural approach described by Bush and Zvelebil that recognizes "the dynamic interaction between the environment, human populations and culture,"[14] the WHO sees matters of community and the ecology as fundamental to the health and well-being of all people. This is clear within their calls for "Health for All" as 2 of the 5 directives for action refer to these concepts specifically. The emergence of the concepts of both economic sustainability and community development in the 20th century is hardly surprising because of the breakdown of fundamental ecological and communal relationships. The lack of recognition of the occupational nature of humans is in some measure to blame because economic development that emanated from that has led in large part to current environmental concerns and loss of community values and voice. That was not the case when populations were smaller and when their occupations were in line with the natural world. Indeed, many consider that the occupational pursuits of early hunter-gatherers generally would not have disturbed the environmental balance. At least, as Lorenz suggests, such cultures "influence their biotope in a way no different from that of animal populations."[23] In a similar vein, Stephenson found that Australian hunter-gatherer societies produced "a stable relationship between man and his resources," perhaps because of their long, isolated occupancy of Australia.[24] King-Boyes agrees: "In full tribal life, the Aborigines presented an excellent example of a society working in rhythm with its environment."[25] Such indigenous communities are rapidly becoming extinct, not least because they are dependent on declining natural environments. Natural environments depend upon the species that inhabit them, but it has been estimated that more than 50,000 are made extinct each year. Wilson suggests that if "exploitative human activities continue to expand at the current rates, at least 20% of the earth's species will disappear within 30 years."[26] The hunter-gatherer lifestyle, which was followed in many parts of the world for several million years, provided a real test of the potential for engagement in occupations to effectively sustain health and well-being of people, communities, and the ecology. Unfortunately, the advancement of affluent economies is based on an "unchallenged traditional assumption that the loss is inevitable in the context of advancement of human progress."[27]

Sustainable community development fits well into a framework provided by an ecological approach because it aims at balancing development objectives with environmental concerns while enabling social relationships and humane local societies to flourish. The World Commission on Environment and Development defines it in simple terms as "...development that meets the needs of the present without compromising the ability of future generations to meet their own needs."[28] Both environmental and community development issues have escalated since the concept emerged as a popular solution to address growing concerns over the negative consequences of human activities,[22] so that sustainability has become a legitimate component of development rhetoric in various interactive fields.[29-38]

An Occupation-Focused Eco-Sustainable Community Development Approach to Health

In line with the WHO directives, I define an OESCD approach to health as the promotion of ecologically sustainable policies and community-wide action to maintain or re-establish healthy relationships between people, human societies, other living organisms, and their environments, habits, and modes of life through community consultation, deliberation, resource management, development, and participation in health-giving and ecologically sustaining occupations.

It is a holistic, participatory, diverse, and proactive approach that is self-sustaining, based on ecological, biological, natural, social, political, and occupational sciences that marry environment, human occupation, and relationships in the most generic form. It is aimed at promoting global and community health and well-being by reducing disempowerment of communities and ecological degradation and by encouraging socioeconomic development in a way that facilitates healthy natural environments and social relations globally. As Wylie maintained over 30 years ago, health "is the perfect continuing adjustment of an organism(s) to its (their) environment."[39] The approach is inclusive of all levels of the population, being applicable to policy makers, populations, communities, and individuals. It is community centered, enabling and empowering development that uses local resources that are ecologically sustaining and accepting that people are part of the natural environment, global economies, and communities.

Because it is based on environmental and community analysis, use of local resources, and self-sustaining programs, the approach is in line with new models of public health that have emerged to address health concerns about both people and their environments. Labonte, an international leader of the health promotion movement, for example, uses "econology" to describe a union between economy and ecology in theories that integrate health and sustainable development.[40,41] David Werner, a leading population health expert, links ecological and community development when he points out:

> If we are ever to approach "Health for All"—or indeed, to prevent an eco-disaster leading to "Health for No One" we must embark very soon on a radically different model of social development.[42]

He argues that the pursuit of world health cannot be separated from "global economics, preservation of ecosystems, and social justice."[42] However, although science, technology, and wisdom have developed sufficiently to permit the development of a more "healthy, humane, and sustainable paradigm," it cannot progress because political will is absent.[42] The importance of understanding the socioeconomic and political factors at work in this, as in each of the approaches presented, cannot be overstated. Enhancement and improvement of population health requires advocacy and mediation skills as well as those that enable participation.

Similar views are emerging within occupational therapy. Simo Algado, for example, uses the term *occupational ecology*. He describes this as "awareness of the occupational genocide we are confronting, along with proactive measures, through human occupation, to restore the balance with the natural environment."[43] In arguing the need to develop the idea of occupational ecology, he suggests that occupation can be regarded as the "dialogue" between people and their environment.[43] Iwami claims that much can be learned from indigenous cultures and different cosmovisions such as that held in East Asia. He describes this as "arranging deities, nature and humans as inseparable parts of a singular entity, where one's existence is no more important or meaningful than the next entity—be it a tree, a stone, a bird, or another person."[43,44]

The OESCD approach to health holds as its beliefs that people, who are occupational and social beings, are an integral part of the natural world and that the well-being of both ecology and communities is central to ongoing health for all. Communities in diverse socioeconomic systems need to participate in occupations in a manner that sustains the ecology and each other. Community action can lead to healthy socioeconomic policies fostering occupations that sustain the ecology and maintain diversity. This might require devolution of decision making to enable communities to develop in ways that enhance social and environmental health using local resources. Acceptance of these beliefs requires the provision of environments in which health-giving, safe, satisfying, stimulating, and enjoyable occupational conditions pertain across the globe.

The principles of this approach to health maintain that participation in diverse ecologically friendly and community-developing occupations promotes health and well-being for both environment and people so that health-giving occupational policy and action is integral to community development and ecological sustainability. They hold that policy makers, populations, communities, and individuals can act in ways that sustain the ecology while meeting occupational needs and that ecological degradation and community disempowerment can be reduced. In line with WHO health promotion directives, the

Table 7-1

Foundations of an Occupation-Focused Eco-Sustainable Community Development Approach to Health

Basis of Approach	Underlying Beliefs	Underlying Principles
Based on ecological, bio-logical, natural, social, politi-cal, and occupational science	Humans as an integral part of the natural world are occupa-tional and social beings	Health-giving occupational policy and action is integral to community development and ecological sustainability
Aimed at increasing global and community health and well-being by reducing eco-logical degradation and disem-powerment of communities	The health and well-being of the ecology and communities is central to ongoing health for all	Ecological degradation and community disempowerment can be reduced
Applicable to policy makers, populations, communities, and individuals	Community action can lead to healthy socioeconomic policies fostering occupations that sustain the ecology and maintain diversity	Policy makers, populations, communities, and individuals can act in ways that sustain the ecology while meeting occupational needs
Holistic ecological concept of people as part of the natural environment, global econo-mies, and supportive commu-nities	Communities in diverse socio-economic systems need to participate in occupations in a manner that sustains the ecology and each other	Enablement of occupational diversity through ecologically sustainable community action
Is community centered, enabling and empowering development that uses local resources and is ecologically sustaining	Devolution of decision making will enable communities to develop in ways that enhance social and environmental health using local resources	Empowerment through com-munity support and relevant occupation is essential to strengthen environmental, community, and social health
Is participatory, diverse, self-sustaining, and inclusive of all levels of the population	Health-giving, safe, satisfying, stimulating, and enjoyable occupational conditions are a global responsibility	Participation in diverse envi-ronmentally friendly and com-munity developing occupa-tions promotes health

principles embrace the notions of enablement and empowerment: enablement of occupa-tional diversity through ecologically sustainable community action, and empowerment through community support and relevant occupation to strengthen environmental, com-munity, and social health (Table 7-1).

An ecological approach is not restricted to the natural environment. It is often con-cerned with the minimalization or eradication of problems associated with human made environments that cause ill health to both the natural world and people. Public health has long recognized that the health and well-being of people cannot be divorced from the environment. Its greatest triumphs were the identification and virtual eradication of some diseases that emanated from "sick environments." The sick environments were, on the whole, the result of human activity, the most obvious of which were the living and working conditions imposed by widespread industrialization. Improvement in these environments led to improved physical, mental, and social health for the people living in them, and briefly, to improvement in environments surrounding the polluting industrial complexes spewing out noxious gasses. Industrial complexes, somewhat improved, but still injurious to natural and human health have moved location to continue their deadly practices for the purpose of "head in the sand" economic policies and gain.

Community development workers, who often have a public health background but increasingly may come from other allied health professions such as occupational therapy, are recognizing the urgency of including ecological sustainability as part of just, people-centered initiatives that focus on what they do or strive to be and become.[45-49] For example, Atkinson and Vorratnchaiphan argued that to redress the socioeconomic and ecological imbalance caused in Thailand by development evolving from European priorities, it is necessary to decentralize power and resources to local authorities and communities and for them to undertake action planning that focuses on improved management of the environment for the benefit of local people.[50]

Using local resources and self-sustaining programs, community development was widely used in African and Asian colonial administrations after World War II to stimulate local leadership, to facilitate a community's social and economic development, and later in rural programs aimed at mass literacy and education.[51] Found to be useful in other than hunter-gatherer or agrarian cultures, community development strategies were adopted in the 1960s in the United States and the United Kingdom for use in socially disadvantaged urban areas to stimulate self-help and innovative solutions that were cost-efficient.[52,53] (In the United States, community development became national policy under Title II of the Economic Opportunity Act of 1964.) The move toward more community-based health care in Australia can be seen as a response aimed at the social and environmental origins of much ill health and, also, at meeting the growing interest in health issues by large sections of the community. In the 1970s, Australia introduced a Community Health Program that offered a framework for funding public and private group projects for community-based preventive, diagnostic, therapeutic, and rehabilitation services based in local centers and complemented by home care, day care, health education, mental health, and alcohol and drug abuse programs.[54] This resulted in a great variety of community-based services, some, like domiciliary care, with traditional health values and others that tended to challenge vigorously conventional health ideologies, as some women's health groups did. Perhaps because of these wide-ranging community initiatives, it is common to confuse "health services based in the community" with "community development."

Health services in the community can adopt a community development approach by encouraging community consultation as the basis of the service and by being responsive to underlying social factors that affect health in the long term. Such an approach is a means of enabling all people to become involved in planning, implementing, questioning, and changing circumstances within their own communities so that they are economically and socially advantaged. It is believed that this leads to improved health and to improved community health care provisions. For this reason, the strengthening of community action is one of the 5 strategies for health promotion prescribed in the OCHP, which "accepts the community as the essential voice in matters of its health, living conditions, and well-being" and asserts that "empowerment of communities, their ownership, and control of their own endeavours and destinies" are "at the heart" of the community development process.[13] It is often the restrictions imposed by government-funding bodies that inhibit the use of community development approaches and maintain a "top down" delivery of services.

Why an Occupation-Focused Eco-Sustainable Community Development Approach Is Necessary

An ecosystem comprises a community of organisms living in an integrated way within a particular environment. The relationships between the components of the system are often complex, interactive, and difficult to appreciate without serious study. The fine balance between components is crucial to its health and survival in the long term and a change in numbers of any one or of activity can be disastrous.[6] In earlier chapters, 4 basic needs for human (and other) survival were identified. McKeown explained that without oxygen, warmth, water, and food, human life is impossible but that in the present time lack of the first 3 of these is only an infrequent cause of sickness or death.[55] Ecological scientists, however, have for decades been warning of oxygen depletion that goes along with global warming that has been recognized as a current trend. Some 245 million years ago, global warming as a probable result of massive and prolonged volcanic activity resulted in the extinction of between 70% and 96% of land and ocean species. The release of huge amounts of carbon dioxide led to a greenhouse effect that depleted oxygen levels, warmed the earth, caused environmental deterioration, sterilized the oceans, destroyed marine life, and allowed the release of hydrogen sulfide to poison the air.[56,57] The greenhouse effect is a naturally occurring process that predates human existence. Atmospheric carbon dioxide concentrations have altered throughout time. However, they can be affected by human activity; for example, there has been an exponential increase since the mid 18th century as a result of deforestation and the burning of fossil fuels such as coal, natural gas, and petroleum with a subsequent increase of mean global temperature that is occurring faster than in past geological history.[58,59] If this cannot be halted, the 4 basic needs of human life that McKeown identifies will become more and more difficult to meet.

Present day ecological degradation is being worsened by increasingly large numbers of people using too many resources and inappropriate technologies; creating too much waste; and changing the balance between species, activity, and environment within an ecosystem.[60] Many of these changes can be laid at the door of the current market-based economies of affluent countries that are driven by profit. That, plus the associated multinational corporate influence over national governments, is responsible in large part for the rapid destruction of natural resources such as air, water, soil, plants, forests, other animals, and mineral deposits on which people's existence and health depends. Most of this destruction has occurred since industrialization although, arguably, it started with agricultural deforestation. Together, both occupational eras of agriculture and industry have resulted in the loss of over 75% of the Earth's original forests and damage to its atmosphere. In terms of communities, the result has been a greater divide between rich and poor people and countries, with poverty and lack of opportunity for the majority creating a vicious cycle of social illness that includes violence, racism, social and occupational apartheid, and addiction. Indeed, it can be said that in most places the democratic process is a mockery with political campaigns supported by big business. "To make the rich richer, humanity has been thrust into a developmental paradigm that not only perpetuates poverty, but places all life on this planet at risk."[42] The accumulation of monetary wealth is a major factor in alienating individuals from a sense of community and place, in the "homogenization of cultures and of unsustainability."[7] Sustainability requires decentralization, which "distributes and roots economic power in place and community."[7]

What is called for is a reduction of population growth, lowering consumption, recycling waste, and using greener technologies as well as a restructuring of economic goals

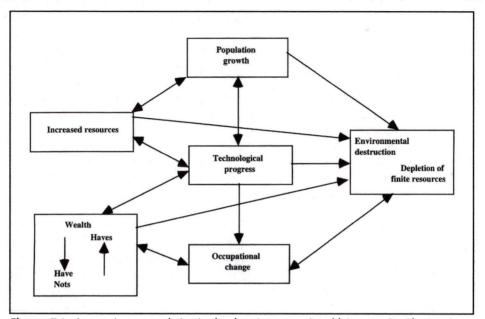

Figure 7-1. Interaction: population/technology/resources/wealth/occupation/the environment.

and societal values, reformation of resource policies to reflect community interests, a merging of the economic and biological in ecological decision making, and changes to make human activity more sustainable.[9,11,61,62] That must include recognition of people's basic occupational nature to meet their needs, interests, and personal growth. However, the problem of maintaining a sustainable ecology against global population growth, technological progress, and resource depletion is increasing (Figure 7-1). Curbing those 3 processes will require fundamental change to assumptions and values about wealth that are at the heart of business relationships. Raising awareness and understanding about those relationships in terms of people's personal health, that of communities, and that of the natural environment is a fundamental and necessary first step.[63]

Some hope for the future is provided by the growth of alternative political parties in Western countries with platforms based on ecological and community needs. While their policies may not meet with universal approval, their presence at least points to an awakening interest in issues that urgently require consideration. A case in point is provided by "The Greens/Green Party USA," which holds ecology, social justice, grassroots democracy, and nonviolence as its political values. Since 1984 it has been aiming toward "an America where decisions are made by the people and not by a few giant corporations. Our environmental goal is a sustainable world where nature and human society co-exist in harmony."[64] The growth of such parties around the world provides a pointer to other political parties about growing concern over environmental and community health issues. Yet the contrast between those values and the ones central within mainstream liberal-democratic policies is great despite a growing trend to acknowledge concern. They favor instead policies that uphold individual opportunity over community or environmental issues. This view is seductive to many. It promotes "opportunities of individuals... [so that they] gain rewards from working hard" within "a system of incentives for merit, productivity and accomplishment."[64] This platform addresses "dire need" "by providing a minimal floor of compassion" for those unable to take advantage of such opportunities, and there are many. However, to date, ecological sustainability, while given lip service, is not at the forefront of policies, and failure to sufficiently address destruction of communities as a result of multinational corporate activity is common.[65] Pelton suggests "the ultimate test of any policies and programs must be demonstration of improved outcomes ... [such as] reduced violence, drug abuse, mortality rates, child placement rates, child abuse, and homelessness."[65] Add to that improved environmental outcomes instead of continued degradation of the ecology for corporate gain. Most of those unhealthy outcomes have increased in the majority of affluent societies over past decades.

In terms of the necessity for an occupational focus within this debate, it is important to recognize that what people have done or not done for their own ends has been a primary force in ecological degradation. Although occupational development has protected people from the discomfort and unhealthy effects of natural phenomena,[66] many of those who live in cities and spend their days "doing" in the "technosphere of human creation"[67] have a loss of connection with ecological reality. For example, other animals and plants have become regarded and treated as if their only purpose were to serve humans. The widespread practices of replacing natural plants with exotics, hunting and fishing for sport rather than need, and the killing of any animal that dares to attack a human demonstrate this propensity. In addition, the very successful public health initiatives that condemned animals as the carriers of disease, linked with the hygienic "domesticity cult," separated humans still further from other species. It maintained the human superiority argument and gave permission for material wants to be considered more important than an ecological way of life in which all are dependent on each other. Darwinian theories failed to halt the segregation of people from other species, and even today, when researchers are demonstrating substantial health benefits of pets to humans, there remain many rules that restrict human-animal partnerships.[68-73]

The philosophy of humanism is in question here. The drive to "rearrange both the world of Nature and the affairs of men and women so that human life will prosper" despite nature is humanism gone awry.[66] Spiritual and occupational alienation and consequent loss of well-being are largely unrecognized sequelae. Both human doings and the natural world in combination urgently require ecological and attitudinal rehabilitation. Many believe that, in the short-term, an ecological sustainable community development approach is essential to decrease widespread spiritual alienation resulting from people's loss of contact with the natural world and each other, which, it is supposed, may account for increasing levels of stress and violence, the use of drugs, and addictive responsiveness to marketing strategies.[74]

Well-known botanist David Bellamy has suggested that one answer to many of the questions posed in this chapter is an occupation-focused approach to ecological sustainability. He envisages this through environmentally benign tourism, compulsory National Heritage Service between school and job, and immediately post retirement (ie, work in "environmental, wildlife, or artefact conservation and social services)" "labor intensive land management and redevelopment programs."[75] His explanation of the occupational base of his suggested approach:

> For 99% of our existence as a distinct species, the work ethic and everything that went with it held human society together... the answer is simple, the work ethic must be rekindled by putting people back into the economics of life.[75]

As tourism is now the world's biggest industry, he suggests as a way forward environmentally benign tourism (a term he considers preferable to ecotourism) according to 7 criteria[75]:

1. Putting more money into the local economy than offshore.

2. Creating local jobs and providing training.

3. Showing real green gain through recreation of local plant and animal habitats.

4. Minimizing adverse ecosystem effects.

5. Developing soft tourism in areas already changed by misuse such as agriculture with profits going to maintain indigenous populations continuing their local customs and land management skills.

6. Providing many jobs in large scale resorts built in areas already degraded by other use.

7. Environmental education of local people.

In the long term, an ecological sustainability model is necessary to maintain the requirements for basic sustenance of life.

An Action-Research Approach to Health Through Occupation-Focused Eco-Sustainable Community Development

The action-research taken in this approach follows the steps outlined in the introduction to Section II. It is a participatory form of critical social science research that aims to systematically examine issues of importance to particular communities and to further sustainable development from a community and environmental perspective. Such research and action must be grounded in each community's lived experience, socially constructed, and of importance to them. Each environment, community, and situation will be different, so these forms of critical inquiry and subsequent action are unlikely to generate empirical data of the type sought by health research-funding bodies because they are likely to be context specific. Trentham and Cockburn argue that despite challenges and possible limitations, PAR can be a powerful tool for empowering people "who are marginalized due to social, structural, or environmental barriers."[78]

Action-research starts by identifying and exploring matters of concern to a community bearing in mind the ecological issues that could be raised by the subsequent actions. It does so with a view to improving an unsatisfactory situation or with the aim of assisting development of some kind to occur for the community's future benefit. Occupational therapists, public health practitioners, or community development officers might act as facilitators, singly or as part of a team that recognizes and values each person's particular strengths. Alternatively, and if at all possible, an able community member should lead the community with outside enablers acting in a collaborative way as co-researchers or as part of the community group. Letting the others know of useful skills that could be utilized by them is important. Additionally identifying the skills of others that may be unrecognized because of proximity, previous obstructions, or inhibiting factors is useful. This will enable as many of the community as possible to feel that they are valued members of the action-research with the capacity to shape the action and the outcomes.

The kinds of concerns will of course differ from community to community, but bearing in mind the nature of the approach they should embrace occupational issues. OESCD within affluent nations might be useful with communities of older people who feel marginalized and subsequently restricted in what they are able to do, be, or become. It might be equally useful with communities of parents whose children are autistic, difficult, extremely clever, or dysfunctional in some way. Street kids becoming involved in community development programs might result in helping them to re-establish in mainstream

societies. Migrant groups might comprise another community that could benefit by identification of issues about their circumstances, the restrictions on what they are able to do,
or the occupational expectations of their new country. Within developing countries, concerns are often about the future of the children and about educational and employment
opportunities. They might also, on many occasions, be about other health prerequisites as
outlined by the WHO, such as food and nutrition, shelter, and social justice. These are all
about doing, being, and becoming; actually doing whatever is required to provide, build,
or advocate to meet primary health and survival needs; being energized by the doing and
finding meaning, purpose, satisfaction, and belonging through meeting personal, family,
community, and environmental needs; and becoming aware of the growth and development of the community and opportunities for its members and the renewed health of
their ecosystem in a sustainable and valued enterprise.

Initiatives aimed at helping communities develop systems of primary health care that
cater to their specific needs, use available resources, and are sustainable are more common in economically disadvantaged countries with poorly developed health services.
Such programs may use various approaches, such as the prevention and control of diseases. While medical personnel might concentrate on interventions such as immunization,
others in the community health team might focus on enabling the development of skills
to make the most use of available resources, to improve environmental conditions, and to
train local health workers. Examples are provided by a couple of schemes, in the second of
which Western-trained therapists were engaged. The first though was a reportedly very
successful action-research project in 2 Egyptian villages that took place between 1986 and
1990. Community members, and especially the women, learned to work within and as
part of the organizational structure of their local government as they participated in the
construction and improvement of local sanitation facilities. At the same time, they took
part in health education concerned with the need for proper sanitation.[77] McDonough
and several other therapists worked in Ethiopia in the late 1980s and 1990s when it was
ravaged by civil wars and famine that had devastated an economy based on subsistence
farming. An experienced Angolan paramedic explained to them that how and what therapists from outside the area do is critical.[78] He advised that initially it is important to find
out about the environment and situations people face on a daily basis, how they cope, and
what they do. The people are resourceful, willing, and able to help themselves but they
need support and resources. Such an approach demands that therapists reflect on their
own beliefs, attitudes, and assumptions about life and health or they may be ineffective
or even harmful. In small care centers, this group of therapists found a great need for
rehabilitation services that address the long-term future and the means of providing a
livelihood as well as shorter-term intervention that can be shared with family members.
They put their efforts into training the surprisingly energetic and young disabled people
as rehabilitation workers. In the spirit of action-research and sustainable community
development, success is more assured if it is founded on the strengths of the local people
and self-help groups.[78,79]

The exploration can take many forms and be multiple in order to inform the action in
a critical way. It can make use of findings from quantitative and/or qualitative research.
Community members, while probably not experts in action-research, can be encouraged
to become so or, alternatively, to recognize their particular role in shaping the direction
throughout the process of the development project. To enhance the continuing research
process, individual expertise and local knowledge need to be respected, appreciated, and
drawn upon. Community members should be enabled to act in flexible, systematic, and
critical ways that draw on actual experiences in the community and environment. It is
from the total community resource that the exploratory questions emerge or are gener-

ated. The health practitioner can add to the process through knowledge of pertinent literature especially from other community development action-research, can assist in focusing the objectives and questions, and recognize variables that lie outside the project or that cannot be controlled. As the process evolves, initial planning might undergo change according to decisions made by the community collectively and contextually.[80]

Considerable time and commitment may be required apart from the actual action-research process. This may be for community building through socialization processes; for development of understanding about power relationships; for uncovering abilities, skills, capacities, and talents; and to enable participants to appreciate issues about purpose, process, and action; differences between individual and social analysis; about group process; and about the political nature of social change.[80] It has been recognized that "purposive actions to build the community field involve the development of relationships across interest lines."[81] These lead to new sources of information to inform the community action and also to "reciprocal obligations and expectations, increased trust, and perhaps shared norms."[81] This will "enhance the likelihood that communities will develop innovative approaches to development."[82]

Raising the awareness of the community about doing, being, and becoming healthy through what they do could start by using the "Occupation for Public Health Pyramid" with particular reference to a specific community, the relationship between the people, and between them and the natural environment. This pictorial device sets out aspects of occupation for health in terms of doing to meet basic health and survival requirements; being and becoming healthier and experiencing physical, mental, and social well-being through how they feel about what they do, how it meets community and environmental needs, and how it enables them to develop. The "Occupation for Public Health Pyramid" emphasizes that doing, being, and becoming are all necessary and should be attainable if the criteria for health recognized by WHO are to be experienced across the globe. Education to increase understanding of ecological sustainability (one of the "doing" prerequisites) and how it can be addressed within community development programs would be part of this process whether the particular exploration and action are aimed at issues of occupational injustice, the prevention of illness, or to increase the well-being of particular groups of people.

The occupational action-research approach should, as soon as possible, focus on how people in partnership can meet their creative potentials without damaging the environment so that future health and well-being are ensured. Action plans devised by the community in response to their needs and in line with available expertise and resources can then be developed. These should also be aimed at enabling communities to advance toward doing, being, and becoming well in an environmentally sustaining way. The community may detail the health practitioners working with them to mediate or advocate on their behalf or they may call upon advisors for that purpose, to seek out extra resources and support or to assist in negotiating change that appears necessary as a result of the action-research.

The stages are not linear; they may interconnect, may overlap, may be repeated, or may be reordered according to community needs and development, contextual events, and changes within the sociopolitical or natural environment. Reaching a negotiated change or a desired outcome does not necessarily signal an end to the project because the community may seek to continue action toward even better outcomes and opportunities for its members and others.

Figure 7-2. An action-research approach to OESCD.

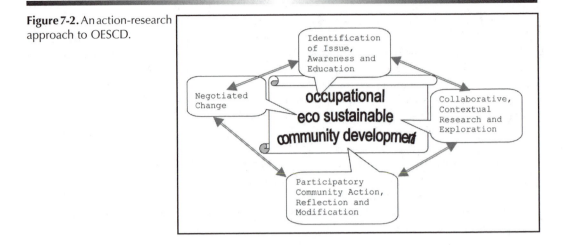

Expected outcomes of community-based action-research must be meaningful to the community, be of practical value, and result in social change of direct benefit.[80] Sometimes this may be difficult to discover because the action-research may be embedded in other community initiatives. It is worth the effort, however, because results clearly set out and articulated for all community members as well as external groups, organizations, socio-political agencies, or media will have long-term if not immediate consequences. It may also be empowering for the community to recognize what they have done and what they have achieved, empowering them to continue the development of issues that emerged from the particular action-research or becoming involved in another project (Figure 7-2).

Potential sustainable community development action-research could focus on discovering the natural balance of occupation in daily life; of the richness and wisdom of indigenous people with regard to occupation, communities, and the ecology; or of natural ontogenetic timing of occupational drives and needs including what promotes or is destructive to the health and potential of other species and ecosystems. The former World Bank economist Herman Daly, who espouses an eco-economics approach, argues that "seekers of world health need to enter into a serious dialogue with the leading advocates of healthier paradigms for development."[83] These include a growing number of, perhaps, unexpected "bed-fellows" in the corporate sector who are beginning to respond to growing community dissatisfaction and concern about the state of the ecology.

Finding out more about the health benefits of communities per se might be another line of legitimate and useful inquiry. Local communities are increasingly becoming engulfed by larger societies as technological advances in communications and transport encourage interest in happenings beyond them, less involvement in local affairs, and more frequent and distant travel.[84] It has been suggested that people such as those in America have largely "lost their sense of place and the social relationships that depended on the common experience of living and working together."[85] If that is so, aiming for local decision-making power within sustainable, self-sufficient community development could be an outdated ideal at least in terms of affluent economic rationalist societies.[86] Particularly in terms of long-term health and well-being, there is a clear need to assess contemporary communities critically and realistically.[21] When doing so, it must be borne in mind that communities are fragile, variable, and characterized by power struggles. Not uncommonly, these may be generated by "those who seek to maximize growth and profits generated through economic development activities" that are often counter to self-sufficient communities in balance with the local ecosystem.[22]

While critical social science such as described here has been acknowledged as 1 of 3 main research paradigms by the Canadian Association of Occupational Therapists,[87] to many this approach may appear outside the realm of traditional occupational therapy practice because of its concentration on social, public, and environmental health as well as or rather than physical or mental dysfunction within a medical science paradigm. Additionally, taking a political stance has been counter to the ethos of occupational therapy, and an ecological stance has been of interest to but a few. One example is provided by Loretta do Rozario who, as a group leader in a Health Promotion Workshop,[88] developed with her group the following ecological vision for occupational therapists:

> *Occupational therapists will work towards the harmonious relationship of people with their environment, by empowering individuals and communities toward health, well-being, and sustainability through the use of interaction, occupation, and socio-political action.*[89]

Times are changing. WFOT "approved their first ever position paper on community based rehabilitation (CBR 12) at the council meeting in Cape Town, South Africa in 2004."[92] They acknowledge

> *... the world wide existence of an estimated 600 million people with disabilities, predominantly in the (but not limited to) "developing countries," who with their families and communities are restricted in or denied access to dignified and meaningful participation in daily life. The council recognized the need to develop critical awareness and understanding about these realities, and in response accepted the new and emerging notions of occupational apartheid, occupational deprivation, and occupational justice to guide and inform occupational therapy thinking and action.*[90]

In 2005, the WFOT stated its belief that occupational therapy "can positively influence health, welfare, education and vocation at an international level."[91] An example of its commitment to do so is provided by its response to the tsunami disaster. In collaboration with other international organizations and key stakeholders, WFOT is developing both short- and long-term strategies to support occupational therapists to enable people and communities to rebuild their lives and help them to re-engage in meaningful occupation. WFOT describes its role as enabling and facilitating redevelopment as part of aid programs with a 10-year time frame while at the same time developing ongoing global-capacity building to enable immediate response to any future disaster. A 2-person appraisal team visited countries affected by the tsunami to meet with occupational therapists, relevant government officials, disaster relief organizations, local nongovernmental organizations (NGOs), or community-based rehabilitation (CBR) officers. The team was comprised of he President of WFOT and Kerry Thomas, an occupational therapist experienced in CBR, capacity building at national and community levels within a health and social context, and disaster context intervention.[91]

Thomas, during a few years as regional training adviser for Southeast Asia, described an integrated rural development project in Pakistan in which she was responsible for training the local trainers. The project included health care training, health education with school-aged children, agro-forestry, poultry rearing, vocational training, and marketing of local crafts such as carpets. The process of community development was slow because the villagers were mostly illiterate and they needed to see the results of activities of people who were participating before many of them became enthusiastic. Training and education were practical, and were assisted by role-plays, storytelling, and locally made pictures because of the low literacy skills.[92] Thomas, who has also worked with Aboriginal groups in Australia and in countries such as Ethiopia, Sudan, and Cambodia, promotes occupational therapy as "one of the best health-related bases" for entry into community development work, because its philosophy is compatible with "independence and self-reliance" and because of its "practical and functional approach," "broad-based training," and skills in "responsible problem-solving."[93] However, she believes specialized postgraduate experience or training is required to enhance knowledge of community development processes and particularly to assist in analysis and mediation of political, economic, and social factors and consequences of interventions.[93]

One good starting point for more occupational therapists to use an action-research approach to community development is CBR, which is defined as "strategy within community development for the rehabilitation, equalization of opportunity and social integration of all people with disabilities."[94] It is "implemented through the combined efforts of disabled people themselves, their families and communities, and the appropriate health, education, vocational, and social services."[94] The occupational perspective should be taken further, however, to include all people, not just those who are disabled. Opportunities for people differ from community to community. Exploration of the underlying reasons for these differences and how they impact on health and well-being needs to be undertaken using a community development, participatory approach that reflects the principles and practices of ecologically sustainable development. This is one of the most suitable approaches to increase awareness and promote action about the causes and effects of occupational and ecological alienation, deprivation, and imbalance, with the advantage of potential to also provide support and encouragement for the self-reliant, self-chosen occupation, which gives meaning, purpose, and social approval that, as earlier chapters demonstrated, are integral to health and well-being.

CBR has assisted remote and rural first nation communities in both the Tjalku Warra community and in the "Top End" of Australia to improve conditions and promote independence, healthier lifestyles, and improved quality of life.[95-97] An example was provided earlier of therapists using CBR working in various parts of Africa where, in grossly disadvantaged and poor countries, those who survive injuries caused by landmines, war, and accidents require rehabilitation but without the benefit of sophisticated and specialized centers.[79] Canadian occupational therapist Rachel Thibeault, who has a particular interest in psychosocial care, issues of meaning, and social justice in health services, also specializes in CBR with victims of war and landmines. She is a researcher with the UN World Rehabilitation Fund and has worked with disadvantaged Inuit peoples in their transition from hunter-gather lifestyles in Northern Canada, as well as in Sierra Leone, Cambodia, Lebanon, and Laos where she has centered on the reintegration of landmine victims as part of rebuilding civil society. Family and community violence, sexual abuse, and addictions are recurring problems to be addressed, while the principles of sustainable livelihoods and social inclusiveness are also central considerations of the rehabilitation program. Thibeault suggests that "to fully develop the potential of occupation in war-torn countries" requires 4 major steps.[98] These are:

1. The articulation of an intervention model based on the principles developed in the first edition of this text coupled with analysis of postconflict situations and growing evidence from occupational science.

2. The model should partner agencies with similar principles, values, vision, and commitment to social justice.

3. The model should be tested in postwar settings.

4. The model should have as its focus occupation/social justice and sustainable ecology. This should define political advocacy, representation, and action.

In their recent publication *Occupational Therapy Without Borders*, occupational therapists Kronenberg and Pollard reflect on a 1996 project undertaken with Mayan Indian families returning to Guatemala after 14 years as refugees in Mexico following the

1978–1983 "scorched earth" campaign in which thousands were murdered or displaced. An occupation-focused community development program over a 6-month period enabled children "to make contact with their Mayan inheritance through legends and stories."[43] Adolescents were engaged in carpentry that had potential economic and community benefits as well as training as community workers. Weaving as a basis for "trans-generational and cultural sharing" as well as for economic reasons was the basis of a program for the women, while elders were assisted to "recover their traditional role as guardians and transferrers of ancient wisdom" through the creation of a Council of Elders and regular meetings between them and adolescents.[43] Kronenberg and Pollard concluded that there is a need for occupational therapists to "develop transcultural, holistic, and community-centered interventions, and to work as social activists, fighting for occupational justice together with the populations we have the privilege to serve."[43]

While this type of program demonstrates the principles of sustainable community development in empowering local people in economically disadvantaged circumstances toward self-reliance,[99] occupational therapists have been using similar principles and theories on a smaller scale in economically advanced communities with people with physical, mental, or social difficulties. The following examples demonstrate a range of such programs:

* Planning and implementing a Community Integration Policy Project aimed at increasing access for disabled people to the Council's programs, employment opportunities, decision-making processes, and physical facilities. The project progressed through analysis of all the Council's functions, at all levels, and across all departments, staff development sessions, policy development, and implementation.[100]

* Participation in a Community Liaison Team at a general hospital "to assist raising the communities ideas about nursing homes, to support community groups, and to assist patients discharged from formal treatment to involve themselves in the community."[101]

* The design, development, and implementation of a quality-of-life project with older people. Four hundred twenty-two participants from 11 locations over a period of 6 weeks identified issues that affected the quality of their everyday lives. The process empowered them to establish a "Getting Out and About Club."[102,103]

* A group-learning project known as "Support" was conceived and designed by patients who completed a 24-hour occupational therapy stress management program offered at a community mental health day treatment center in New York. The patients had become a very close-knit group and as they moved to ex-patient status, they perceived a need to strengthen their community networks. They anticipated familial and community stressors and sought resources to provide knowledge and practice for themselves and their families in the management of those stressors.[104] Programs of this type extend occupational therapy into the sociopolitical arena.

Communal "doing" for the common and individual good has always been part of human activity. In modern societies, this has largely become superseded by governmental initiatives that lack a genuine community base. Occupational therapists and other public health practitioners who chose to take an OESCD approach need, initially, to enable people to recognize the impact of what they do, be, and become in communal and environmental health terms. Such education includes medico-socio-political leaders and organizations. By taking a holistic, enabling, participatory, and inclusive approach within a community, it is possible to enable attention to be given to the health and well-being needs of the environment, to those of others in the community and their own, and to take action about meeting those needs more effectively.

References

1. McMichael T. *Human Frontiers, Environments and Disease: Past Patterns, Uncertain Futures.* Cambridge, UK: Cambridge University Press; 2001:20, 21.
2. Lovelock J. *The Gaia Hypothesis.* Oxford: Oxford University Press; 1979.
3. The Gaia Hypothesis. Dr. C's remarkable ocean world. <www.oceansonline.com/gaiaho.htm> (last updated January 21 2005).Accessed February 2006.
4. Campbell B. *Human Ecology—The Story of Our Place in Nature from Prehistory to the Present.* New York: Aldine de Gruyter; 1983.
5. Suzuki D. *The Sacred Balance.* Vancouver/Toronto: Greystone Books; 2002.
6. Ecology. In: Norton AL, ed. *The Hutchinson Dictionary of Ideas.* Oxford, UK: Helicon Publishing Ltd; 1994:162.
7. The Asian NGO Coalition, IRED Asia, People Centred Development Forum. *Economy, Ecology and Spirituality: Toward a Theory and Practice of Sustainability.* 1993.
8. Schroyer T. Research programs from the Other Economic Summit (TOES). *Dialectic Anthropology.* 1992;17(4):355-390.
9. MacNeill J. Strategies for sustainable development. *Scientific American.* 1989;261(3):155-165.
10. Bello W. *Dark Victory: The United States, Structural Adjustment, and Global Poverty.* London, England: Pluto (in association with the Institute for Food and Development Policy and Transnational Institute); 1994.
11. Potter VR. Bioethics, the science of survival. *Perspectives in Biology and Medicine.* 1970;14:127-153.
12. Lander ES, Weinberg RA. Journey to the center of biology. *Science.* 2000;287:1777-1782.
13. World Health Organization, Health and Welfare Canada, Canadian Public Health Association. *Ottawa Charter for Health Promotion.* Ottawa, Canada; 1986:3.
14. Bush H, Zvelebil M, eds. *Health in Past Societies: Biocultural Interpretations of Human Skeletal Remains in Archeological Contexts.* Oxford: British Archaeological Reports International Series 567; 1991:6.
15. Wilcock AA. *Occupation for Health: A Journey from Self-Health to Prescription.* Vol 1. London, UK: COT; 2001.
16. Weiss J. *Conservatism in Europe 1770-1945: Traditionalism, Reaction and Counter-Revolution.* London: Thames and Hudson; 1977.
17. Fourier C. *Theory of the Four Movements, 1808* [1968, Oeuvres de Charles Fourier, vol 1 Paris: Editions Anthropos.; Le nouveau monde industriel et societaire; 1829.
18. Weiss J. *Conservatism in Europe 1770-1945: Traditionalism, Reaction and Counter-Revolution.* London: Thames and Hudson; 1977:60.
19. Ostergaard G. Proudhon, Pierre-Joseph. In: Bottomore T, ed. *A Dictionary of Marxist Thought.* 2nd ed. Oxford, UK: Blackwell Publishers; 1983:451-452.
20. Owen R. The address to the inhabitants of New Lanark. The Institute for the Formation of Character. January 1st 1816. In: Owen R. *Works of Robert Owen: Volume 1* (Pickering Masters Series). London: Pickering & Chatto (Publishers Ltd.); 1993:120-142.
21. Wilkinson KP. *The Community in Rural America.* Westport, Conn: Greenwood Press; 1991.
22. Bridger JC, Luloff AE. Sustainable community development: An Interactive Perspective; 1999. <www.cas.nercrd.psu.edu/ Community/Legacy/bridger_intro.htm>
23. Lorenz K. *Civilized Man's Eight Deadly Sins.* Latzke M, trans. London, England: Methuen and Co Ltd; 1974:12-13.
24. Stephenson W. *The Ecological Development of Man.* Sydney, Australia: Angus and Robertson; 1972:94.
25. King-Boyes MJE. *Patterns of Aboriginal Culture: Then and Now.* Sydney, Australia: McGraw-Hill Book Co; 1977:154-155.
26. Wilson EO. *The Diversity of Life.* Cambridge, Mass: Harvard University Press; 1992.
27. Livingston J. *One Cosmic Instant.* Toronto: McClelland Steward; 1973.
28. World Commission on Environment and Development. *Our Common Future.* New York: Oxford University Press; 1987:43.
29. Lele S. Sustainable development: a critical review. *World Development.* 1991;19(6):607-621.
30. Korten C. Sustainable development. *World Policy Journal.* 1992;9(1):157-190.
31. Van der Ryn S, Calthorpe P. *Sustainable Communities.* San Francisco, Calif: Sierra Club Books; 1986.
32. Kemmis D. *Community and the Politics of Place.* Norman, OK: University of Oklahoma Press; 1990.
33. Fowler EP. Land use in the ecologically sensible city. *Alternatives.* 1991;18(1):26-35.
34. Berry W. *Sex, Economy, Freedom and Community.* New York, NY: Pantheon Books; 1993.
35. Bray PM. The new urbanism: celebrating the city. *Places.* 1993;8(4):56-65.
36. Chamberland D. The social challenges of sustainable community planning. *Plan Canada.* 1994; July:137-143.
37. Gibbs D. Towards the sustainable city. *Town Planning Review.* 1994;65(1):99-109.

38. Sachs W. Global ecology and the shadow of development. In: Sessions G, ed. *Deep Ecology for the 21st Century.* Boston, Mass: Shambhala; 1995.

39. Wylie CM. The definition and measurement of health and disease. *Pub Health Rep.* 1970: 85: 100-104. (103).

40. Labonte R. Econology: integrating health and sustainable development. Part one: theory and background. *Health Promotion International.* 1991;6(1):49-64.

41. Labonte R. Econology: integrating health and sustainable development. Part two: guiding principles for decision making. *Health Promotion International.* 1991;6(2):147-156.

42. Werner D. Health and Equity: Need for a People's Perspective in the Quest for World Health. Conference: PHC21-Everybody's Business. Almaty, Kazakhstan: November 1998:2.

43. Simo Algado S Estuardo Cardona C. The Return of the corn men. Ch 25 In: Kronenberg F, Simo Algado S, Pollard N, eds. Occupational Therapy without Borders: Learning from the Spirit of Survivors. London: Elsevier Ltd, 2005; 336, 346.

44. Iwana M. Toward culturally relevant epistemologies in occupational therapy. *Am J Occup Ther* 2003; 57(5):582-587.

45. International Institute for Environment and Development. Whose Eden? Empowering local communities to manage their wildlife resources. *IIED Perspectives.* 1994;13:3-5.

46. Korten DC. *Sustainable Livelihoods: Redefining the Global Social Crisis.* New York, NY: People Centred Development Forum; 1994.

47. Korten DC. *Sustainable Development Strategies: The People Centered Consensus.* New York, NY: People Centred Development Forum; 1994.

48. Robertson J. *People Centered Development: Principles for a New Civilization.* New York, NY: People Centered Development Forum; 1994.

49. Vavrousek J. Human values for sustainable living. Edial. The Network. The Centre for our Common Future; 1993.

50. Atkinson A, Vorratnchaiphan CP. Urban environmental management in a changing development context: the case of Thailand. *Third World Planning Review.* 1994;16(2):147-169.

51. Marris P. Community development. In: Kuper A, Kuper J, eds. *The Social Science Encyclopedia.* London, England: Routledge; 1985:137-138.

52. Marris P. *Community Planning and Conception of Change.* London: Routledge; 1982.

53. Marris P, Rein M. *Dilemmas of Social Reform.* 2nd ed. Harmondsworth, England: Penguin; 1974.

54. Milio N. *Making Policy: A Mosaic of Australian Community Health Policy.* Canberra, Australia: Department of Community Services and Health; 1988.

55. McKeown T. *The Origins of Human Disease.* Oxford, UK: Basil Blackwell; 1988.

56. National Geographic Society. Archeology and Paleontology: Global Warming Preserved "Mass Kill" Fossils. <Nat.Geographic.com> Accessed December 2005.

57. Gugliotta G. Extinction tied to global warming: greenhouse effect cited in mass decline 250 million years ago. *Washington Post.* Friday, January 21, 2005;A03

58. Worldwatch Database. Worldwatch Institute; 1996.

59. Community Structure. Lecture 41: Carbon and Global Warming. Northern Arizona University. 1999. Available at: http://jan.ucc.nau.edu/doetqp/courses/env470/Lectures/lec41/Lec41.htm. Accessed December 2005.

60. Jones A. Fact Sheets: Ecological Sustainability. Australian Museum, 2003. Available at: http://www.amonline.net.au/factsheets/ecological_sustainability.htm. Accessed October 2005.

61. Egger G, Spark R, Lawson J. *Health Promotion Strategies and Methods.* Sydney, Australia: McGraw-Hill; 1990:107.

62. Corson WH. Changing course: an outline of strategies for a sustainable future. *Futures.* 1994;26(2):206-223.

63. Stead WE, Stead J. Can humankind change the ecological myth? Paradigm shifts necessary for ecologically sustainable business. *Journal of Organizational Change Management.* 1994;7(4):15-31.

64. The Greens/Green Party USA. Available at: http://www.greenparty.org. Accessed April 2006.

65. Pelton LH. *Doing Justice: Liberalism, Group Constructs, and Individual Realities.* Albany, NY: State University of New York Press; 1999:61, 93.

66. Ehrenfeld D. *The Arrogance of Humanism.* New York, NY: Oxford University Press; 1981:10.

67. Dubos R. *Only One Earth.* London, England: Doubleday; 1988.

68. Moore JC. 1975 Eleanor Clarke Slagle Lecture: behavior, bias, and the limbic system. *Am J Occup Ther.* 1976;30(1):11-19.

69. Vombrock J. Cardiovascular effect of human-pet interventions. *J Behav Med.* 1988;ii(5):509-517.

70. Hundley J. The use of pet facilitated therapy among the chronically mentally ill. *J Psychosoc Nurs.* 1991;29(6):23-26.

71. Harris M. Pet therapy for the homebound elderly. *Caring.* 1990;9(9):48-51.

72. Chinner T. An exploratory study on the viability and efficacy of a pet facilitated therapy project within a hospice. *Journal of Palliative Care.* 1991;7(4):13-20.

73. Fick KM. The influence of an animal in social interactions of nursing home residents in a group setting. *Am J Occup Ther.* 1993;47(6):529-533.

74. Southeast Asian contribution to the Earth Charter. In Our Hands. Southeast Asia Regional Consultation on a People's Agenda for Environmental Sustainable Development: Towards UNCED and Beyond. SEARCA. Philippines, 1991.

75. Bellamy DJ. Workaholics anonymous: putting people back into the equation of livelihood. *J Occup Sci: Australia.* 1997;4(3):119-125.

76. Trentham B, Cockburn L. Participatory action-research: creating new knowledge and opportunities for occupational engagement. In: Kronenberg F, Pollard N, eds. *Occupational Therapy Without Borders: Learning From the Spirit of Survivors.* London: Elsevier Ltd; 2005:440.

77. el Katsha S, Watts S. Environmental health interventions in Egyptian villages. *Community Development Journal.* 1994;29(3):232-238.

78. McDonough S. What's a practitioner to do? Challenging environments. In: Crepeau EB, Cohn ES, Boyd Schell BA, eds. *Willard & Spackman's Occupational Therapy.* 10th ed. Philadelphia: Lippincott, Williams & Wilkins; 2003:38.

79. Hobbs E, McDonough S, O'Callaghan A. *Life After Injury.* Penang: Third World Network; 2002.

80. Alary J, Beausoleil J, Guedon M-C, Lariviere C, Mayer R, eds. *Community Care and Participatory Research.* Montreal: Nuage Editions; 1992.

81. Coleman JS. Social Capital in the Creation of Human Capital. *American Journal of Sociology.* 1988; 94(Supplement):S95-S120.

82. Flora CB, Flora JL. Entrepreneurial social infrastructure: a necessary ingredient. *The Annals of the American Academy of Political and Social Science.* 1993;529(September):45-48.

83. Daly H. *For the Common Good: Redirecting the Economy Toward the Community, the Environment and a Sustainable Future.* Boston: Beacon Press. 1989.

84. Warren RI. *The Community in America.* 2nd ed. Chicago, Ill: Rand McNally and Company; 1972.

85. Meyrowitz J. *No Sense of Place: The Impact of the Electronic Media on Social Behavior.* New York: Oxford University Press; 1986.

86. Bender T. *Community and Social Change in America.* New Brunswick, NJ: Rutgers University Press; 1978.

87. Canadian Association of Occupational Therapists. *Enabling Occupation: An Occupational Therapy Perspective.* Ottawa: CAOT Publications ACE; 1997.

88. Wilcock AA. *Health Promotion Workshop.* Melbourne, Australia: World Federation of Occupational Therapists Congress; 1990.

89. do Rozario L. Keynote address. Purpose, place, pride and productivity: the unique personal and societal contribution of occupation and occupational therapy. Australian Association of Occupational Therapists 17th Conference Proceedings. Darwin; 1993.

90. Kronenberg F, Pollard N. Overcoming occupational apartheid: a preliminary exploration of the political nature of occupational therapy. In: Kronenberg F, Simo Algado S, Pollard N, eds. *Occupational Therapy Without Borders: Learning from the Spirit of Survivors.* London: Elsevier Ltd; 2005:61-62.

91. World Federation of Occupational Therapists. The Tsunami Disaster: A Situational Assessment to Inform WFOT's Response and Future Planning. World Federation of Occupational Therapists (WFOT) 2005.

92. Thomas K. A letter from Nepal. In: Wilcock AA, ed. *Health Promotion and Occupational Therapy.* Workbook: World Federation of Occupational Therapists Congress, Melbourne, Australia, 1990.

93. Thomas K. Comments on working in Sudan and Ethiopia. In: Wilcock AA, ed. *Health Promotion and Occupational Therapy.* Workbook: World Federation of Occupational Therapists Congress, Melbourne, Australia, 1990.

94. World Health Organization, ILO, UNESCO. *Definition of Community Based Rehabilitation.* Geneva, Switzerland: WHO; 1994.

95. Glynn R. Some perspectives on cross-cultural rehabilitation with remote area Aboriginal people. *Australian Occupational Therapy Journal.* 1993;40(4):159-162.

96. Pondaag B. Working with the Tjalku Warra community: a project report. The Australian Association of Occupational Therapists 15th Federal Conference. Sydney, Australia, 1988.

97. Walker V. An occupational therapist's contribution to Aboriginal health worker training. The Australian Association of Occupational Therapists 15th Federal Conference. Sydney, Australia, 1988.

98. Thibealt R. Occupation and the rebuilding of civic society: Notes from the war zone. *J Occup Sci.* 2002;9(1):38-47.

99. Burkley S. *People First: A Guide to Self Reliant Participatory Rural Development.* London, England: Zed Books; 1993.

100. Johnson V. The occupational therapist as a tertiary consultant in a local government agency. The Australian Association of Occupational Therapists 15th Federal Conference. Sydney, Australia, 1988.

101. Munro J. Community liaison team, Manly District Hospital. The Australian Association of Occupational Therapists 15th Federal Conference. Sydney, Australia, 1988.

102. Twible RL. Consumer participation in planning health promotion programmes: a case study using the Nominal Group technique. *Australian Occupational Therapy Journal.* 1992;39(2):13-18.

103. Twible RL. Journeying to a new land of hope: a promise for occupational therapy. The Australian Association of Occupational Therapists 18th Federal and Inaugural Pacific Rim Conference Proceedings. Hobart, Tasmania, 1995.

104. Hill L, Brittell TD, Kotwal J. A community mental health group designed by clients. In: Johnson JA, Jaffe E, eds. Health promotive and preventive programs: models of occupational therapy practice. *Occupational Therapy in Health Care.* 1989;6(1):57-66.

Suggested Reading

Bellamy DJ. Workaholics anonymous: Putting people back into the equation of livelihood. *J Occup Sci*: Australia. 1997;4(3):119-125.

Iwana M. Toward culturally relevant epistemologies in occupational therapy. *Am J Occup Ther* 2003;57(5):582-587.

Labonte R. Econology: integrating health and sustainable development. Part one: theory and background. *Health Promotion International.* 1991;6(1):49-64.

Labonte R. Econology: integrating health and sustainable development. Part two: guiding principles for decision making. *Health Promotion International.* 1991;6(2):147-156.

Lovelock J. *The Gaia Hypothesis.* Oxford: Oxford University Press; 1979.

Owen R. The address to the inhabitants of New Lanark. The Institute for the Formation of Character. January 1st 1816. In: Owen R. *Works of Robert Owen.* Vol 1 (Pickering Masters Series). London: Pickering & Chatto (Publishers Ltd.); 1993:120-142.

Simo Algado S, Simo Algado S Estuardo Cardona C. The return of the corn men. In: Kronenberg F, Pollard N, eds. *Occupational Therapy Without Borders: Learning From the Spirit of Survivors.* London: Elsevier Ltd; 2005,346.

Suzuki D. *The Sacred Balance.* Vancouver: Greystone Books; 2002.

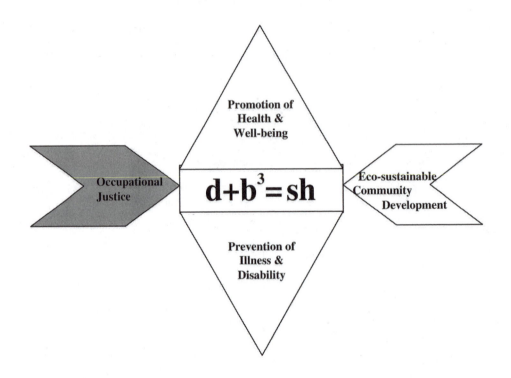

OCCUPATIONAL JUSTICE APPROACH

Theme 8:

"Health promotion action aims at reducing differences in current health status and ensuring equal opportunities and resources to enable all people to achieve their fullest health potential."
WHO, *The Ottawa Charter for Health Promotion,* 1986

The chapter addresses:
* The concept of occupational justice
* What is an occupational justice approach to health?
* Why an occupational justice approach is necessary
* An action-research approach to occupational justice

In the first edition of this book, I discussed a social justice approach to the promotion of health. Within it I talked about the concept of occupational justice and described my preliminary ideas about the direction this might take. Since then, Elizabeth Townsend and myself have taken a collaborative approach to explore and develop the concept further, Townsend having been exploring justice issues in relation to enabling people's occupations for some years previously. Apart from extensive debate, papers in journals, chapters in other texts, and formal presentations, this collaboration has been augmented by the input of attendees at workshops in many parts of the world where ideas were formed, discussed, and collected. Occupational justice has now become accepted as a useful concept and term within occupational therapy to the extent that it is appropriate to focus on this more relevant aspect of justice in this edition. The notion becomes clearer that occupational justice is an aspect of social justice that has been largely overlooked. Much of its substance, while not identified by this nomenclature, is addressed in several clauses of the UN *Declaration of Human Rights* that will be considered later in the chapter.

The Concept of Occupational Justice

Occupational justice concerns 2 complex sets of ideas:
1. The conceptual recognition of the occupational nature of people.
2. Respect for and equitable provision of resources to meet the differing occupational needs of individuals and populations as part of fair, enabling, and empowering societies.

Like social justice, the concept is based on beliefs about freedoms, rights, and responsibilities that determine cultural and political foundations and governance of societies and justice issues for both populations and for individuals.

Benjamin Disraeli, the 19th century British parliamentarian, described justice as "truth in action."[1] The action word links justice with doing and, perhaps, that is apt not only in the vernacular because it developed in the ancient world to adjudicate disputes over acceptable and unacceptable behavior among people, and how they shared resources and possessions.[2] It has been defined in many ways throughout time but is generally accepted as a societal ideal of ethical, moral, and civic principles,[2-5] mostly applied to legal systems within states but also concerned with equal distribution of resources and positive discrimination in terms of the underprivileged.[6] It is the latter aspect that is central to the branch of justice known as social justice, first named in 1840 by a Sicilian priest, Luigi Taparelli d'Azelglio, and given status by Utilitarian philosopher John Stuart Mill, who propounded belief in an "equitable and compassionate world where difference is understood and valued, and where human dignity, the Earth, our ancestors and future generations are respected."[7,8]

The recent rapid assimilation of social justice can be traced from the early 1970s when the American philosopher John Rawls identified individual rights, responsibilities, and liberties as moral principles of justice,[5] to over 2 decades later when Tara Smith explored respect and fair treatment of others in terms of justice as a personal virtue.[9] During that relatively short time, legislation began to appear in response to mass interest. The British Commission on Social Justice in 1994, for example, saw its application to the ethical distribution and sharing of resources, recognition of the equal worth of citizens, their equal right to meet basic needs, the diffusion of opportunities and life chances, and the reduction and elimination of unjustified inequalities. Social justice, now an accepted part of postmodern societies, is especially related to "the proper division of benefits and burdens within a society or other collective."[10]

Political dimensions of social justice have both public and private ramifications. Individuals and communities make decisions about what they need, want, or are obliged to do against a background of governmental or organizational regulations and business decisions. Public policy and funding and the associated regulation of justice, while largely invisible and unconscious in everyday life, are powerful determinants over what people can do despite individual motivation and energy. They set the stage for population, familial, and individual experiences of justice or injustice.[11] It is when people insist on fairness and equitable opportunity, respect, and shared responsibility in relationships that social justice is enacted through everyday life.[12]

To truly achieve social justice is difficult, as Iris Morton Young's critique of the distributive nature of social justice describes.[13] She argues that because distributive justice primarily addresses principles of allocation, it focuses on having and cannot sufficiently take into account biological or social differences that are based on unequal power relations. It, therefore, permits the continued exploitation, marginalization, disempowerment, and alienating experiences of particular groups such as women, people living in poverty, people with disability, or ethnic minorities.[13] Young talks instead about a justice of difference that is congruent with opportunity, empowerment, health, and quality of life that could create opportunities to enable people to live, work, and play without exploitation or violence.[13] Pelton, somewhat similarly, holds a view of justice that addresses "individual need, circumstances, merit, competence, and responsibility" even if they are members of a group the whole of which is discriminated against.[14]

"Justice is impersonal ... it ... must be applied equally to all.... Life is unfair. The 'starting gates' have never been equal for all individuals, and they never will be; they are different for each and every individual.

"Justice is an individual matter. It respects the individual and addresses individual need, circumstances, merit, competence, and responsibility. Group based discrimination ... is the differential treatment of individuals based on group identification ... or on the basis of inferences made from such a factor about other characteristics of the group's members."

"Current non-discriminatory laws typically specify group characteristics in regard to which discrimination is outlawed, such as race, gender, or religion.... What such laws sidestep is the positive right to be responded to on the basis of one's need, merit, ability, or what one does, rather than on the basis of group stereotypes ... people have the human right ... to be responded to as individuals, not as members of groups."

"In order to institute the principle of non-discrimination throughout our society, all public policies must be re-examined to ensure they meet fairness to individuals. This would mean that all individuals similarly situated in regard to need, merit, or deeds, must be treated similarly."

"It is time to recognize and respect group diversity and experiences as a pervasive fact of life, but as a poor and unjust basis for the formation of public policy. It is the far greater diversity of individuals that should be recognized and respected by policies that address the fundamental commonalities of all individuals: their human needs, their right to respect, and their potential to flourish when opportunity to do so is available."

LH Pelton. *Doing Justice: Liberalism, Group Constructs, and Individual Realities.* Albany, NY: State University of New York Press; 1999.

The concepts held by Young and Pelton sit well with that of occupational justice. Occupational justice and social justice are complementary ideas that overlap, sharing many common beliefs. Indeed, there are some that argue occupational justice is but a subset of the better-known concept: that occupational justice addresses what people need, want, or are obliged to do in their relationships and life as part of a broader social justice that addresses the social relations and conditions of living.

An occupational perspective of justice focuses on occupational equity; occupational fairness; occupational empowerment; occupational rights and responsibilities; occupational enablement, expression, and opportunity; occupational satisfaction; and occupational well-being. Equity, fairness, and empowerment do not call for all people to be able to do exactly the same things, rather they call for a justice of difference that enables the prerequisites of life to be obtained according to needs, matches meaning with competence, and value with capacity and opportunity. Occupational justice is challenged when people are not able to meet their basic requirements through what they do, not able to demonstrate their capacities and abilities, nor able to express themselves through opportunities for developing potential. It occurs when people are disempowered, deprived, alienated, or restricted so that they are unable to meet basic needs, find satisfaction, or experience well-being through their occupations in a society that appears not to value what they do. It also occurs when people feel unable to contribute to communal or societal endeavor.

Occupational injustice is not only a product of less developed nations, it is also common in overly governed systems of affluent nations afraid of litigation.

In the present day, it is rare to find the word *occupation* associated with those that address the ethics and principles of justice except, perhaps, in terms of opportunities and fair conditions of paid employment. This seems remarkable because apart from work everyday, life is characterized by the daily round of occupations, all or some of which can lead either to continued growth and well-being or eventual stunting of future potential and illness. While earlier chapters have demonstrated that people have a natural drive to engage in occupation to meet their biological natures and needs by circumstance and design, over millennia they have constructed unjust societies that fail to recognize the needs that created them. Unless the occupational nature and needs of people are recognized in occupationally just policies, the majority of the world's population will fail to flourish. This is already the case. While some people may find meaning and well-being through what they do, the majority are relegated to a life in which they are unable to meet even the occupational challenges of their environments to obtain the prerequisites of survival, quite apart from developing their becoming needs. Without occupational justice, people across the world experience inequities that touch the very essence of living.

What Is an Occupational Justice Approach to Health?

I define an occupational justice approach to health as the promotion of just socioeconomic and political conditions to increase individual, population, and political awareness, resources, and opportunity for people to participate in doing, being, and becoming healthy through engagement in occupations that meet the prerequisites of health and every person's different natures, capacities, and needs.

While occupational justice was recognized as a discrete entity and named during the last decade of the 20th century,[15] there have been much earlier initiatives linking health status with justice in regard to the things that people need, want, or have to do. A few examples of the varied nature of these earlier initiatives are worthy of mention at this point.

The first to be mentioned concerns the role of monasteries in feudal Europe that many consider to be a period of scientific decline because science and medicine became subordinate to the dogma of religious creeds. That may be so, but in other ways there was innovation. It was monastic establishments that initiated the first health and social welfare services for the masses based on an appreciation of human need.[16] While this was not explained in terms of justice at that time, Sigerist, the medical historian, suggested that Christianity applied "itself to the poor, the oppressed, the sinners, and the sick. It addressed itself to suffering humanity and promised healing and redemption" in a way that had not happened before.[17] The body though within this creed "was to be subordinated to the soul, and healing, like any other temporal activity had to be under ecclesiastical regulation."[18] Taking in the physically, mentally, and socially sick was considered by the monks not only a social duty but also a necessity because "morally good" occupations lead to good health while the opposite lead to illness, and labor was regarded as essential to spiritual health as its exercise components were to physical health.[16]

The second example is John Howard (1726–1790), a well-known Enlightenment philanthropist who, at his own expense and for his own interest, traveled widely inspecting prisons and hospitals throughout Europe. He published the facts of his visits, noting important aspects and injustices that were overlooked and in some places still are. For example, patients in hospitals then (and not infrequently now) did not have opportunity to maintain or upgrade occupations of daily life so that they were "often turned out very unfit to work, or the common mode of living."[19] Howard's ability to place the horrors, abuses, and injustices that were manifest in prisons before the public eye resulted in the British government taking responsibility for them and enacting some reforms. Included in his reports were details of the nature or the lack of occupation he saw, linking them to the state of health of inmates. He gave praise when he saw it, such as one penitentiary "...by providing airy apartments, free ventilation, plenty of water; and by promoting cleanliness, accompanied by wholesome food, and a proper degree of labour; the convicts may there enjoy better health...."[19] Howard's evaluation of most of the facilities in Europe must have led to his awareness of the possible ill-health effects of lack of occupation.[16]

As the Enlightenment movement declined, it left a lasting heritage in terms of a "literature of human freedom and (influenced well into the future) some institutions in which its values have been embodied."[20] Included in the latter, it can be argued, is the philosophy of occupational therapy that "embodies notions of self-realization, moral autonomy and independence, liberty and justice with regards to people's occupational health needs."[16] Turning that philosophy into action is required if this approach is to be followed by occupational therapists. It is also embodied in the spirit of public health that embraces an expanded mandate encompassing the social determinants of illness and the health and well-being needs of all people in whatever circumstance or environment. As that is inclusive of occupational determinants, action is also required of public health practitioners to ensure that this largely under-recognized aspect is considered.

Few would argue about the unjust lot of people with mental illness until fairly recent times. The impact of moral treatment has already been addressed in an earlier chapter, and the work of a 19th century psychiatrist W. A. F. Browne, who practiced in Scotland, was mentioned. Noteworthy with regard to occupational justice, in 1837, he based the treatment program at the Montrose Lunatic Asylum on justice, benevolence, and occupation, presenting his just approach to the asylum's managers in 5 lectures that were later published. He discussed some of the unjust conditions in asylums prior to 1815. These are presented below.

"Towards JUSTICE BENEVOLENCE AND OCCUPATION:

Lunatics in Gaols, in Cages, in Caves, in Dungeons—Associating of Lunatics with criminals - ... Modes of feeding Lunatics – "forcing"- Death from this process -... Lunatics exhibited for a sum of money; excited and induced to gorge themselves with food, or filth, for the amusement of visitors – Gangrene of extremities from cold – Insufficient supply of food, of clothing -... Terror as a remedy -... Deaths from the fury of keepers and patients. ..."

Browne went on to describe existing injustices in lunatic asylums at the time of his lectures despite moral treatment. Those injustices included:

"... Want of employment, want of bodily exercise ... Mental anxiety and disturbance produced by the oppressive, harsh, indelicate or derisive conduct of keepers - ... Solitary meals – Prejudices of public present obstacles to improvement - ..."

He asks "How are these to be removed?"

WAF Browne. What Asylums Were, Are, and Ought to Be. 1837:x,xi.

In his last lecture, Browne described a Utopian vision of asylums that called for physicians working within them to be conscientious, benevolent, and courageous. He envisioned within such communities there be no compulsion, chains, whips, or corporal chastisement. Instead, a graduation of employment would provide for individual occupational needs. There would be rooms for ladies to read, play the harp, or "flower muslin," for example, while others would be out walking, riding, or driving in the country or going to church or to the market. Working in the extensive and "swelling" grounds would be "the gardener, the common agriculturalist, the mower, the weeder, all intent on their several occupations, and loud in their merriment."[21] Work would be structured "so that it may be easy and well performed, and so apportioned that it may suit the tastes and powers of each labourer."[21] There would be handsome premises where gentlemen might follow intellectual pursuits or billiards and a news-room "for the politicians."[21] Everywhere would be a hive of industry with inmates "anxious to be engaged and toiling incessantly" at their own pleasure for the reward of lessening their pain and disagreeable thoughts, the approbation of others, self-applause, a sound sleep at night, and, perhaps, some small remuneration.[21] Such was Browne's vision of just and effective treatment by occupation for those with mental illness.

Those 3 scenarios depict how in different ways occupational justice approaches to health can be participatory, community models that enable change. The change is directed to meeting the occupational needs and natures of people and to recognizing those as health issues and a matter of justice. Change will often require equitable but different resources and opportunities to enable occupational participation sufficient for both individual and population well-being. Concentrating on justice for an individual without considering the justice of social policies for the total community or environment is unlikely to succeed in the longer term and injustices will be enacted later with others.

Over the last 25 years particularly, public health practitioners have concentrated their efforts on issues of social justice usually prompted by or in line with WHO directives. Indeed, it is they who lead much of the action toward those directives. They have not, however, addressed sufficiently the injustices caused by lack of recognition of the holistic occupational nature and needs of people and the relationship of those to health. Occupational therapists, too, have an implicit concern with social justice as well as occupational justice as part of their philosophical base but have failed to recognize or to act sufficiently upon injustices of all kinds. Issues of justice have not been central in their documented approach to health promotion even though, from my own experience, more clients from socially disadvantaged groups than from affluent groups receive occupational therapy services. Townsend has suggested that occupational therapists need to become conscious of how "the social vision which forms the foundation of occupational therapy" is "narrowed to comply with dominant community, managerial, and medical approaches..."[22] She advances the idea that "enabling people to participate as valued members of society despite diverse or limited potential" is central within the vision.[22] In *Good Intentions Overruled,* she explains that justice usually depends on processes that recognize, approve, celebrate, and provide meaningful experiences as well as, apart from, or instead of money. The governance of injustice, she writes, is through laws, rules and regulations, policies, procedures, penalties, disincentives, disempowerment, mistreatment, exclusion, and domination.[23] Conveying messages about social expectations, justice, and injustice to populations, however, is mainly achieved through informal rather than formal ways, such as via cultural materials, telecommunications, films, and Websites.[24,25]

The basis for the approach is that, currently, there are inequities in the experience of health and of ill-health in all populations around the globe because of a lack of awareness or policies to enable people to participate in the occupations they want, need, or are obliged to do in order to provide the necessities of life; find meaning, purpose, satisfaction, and belonging; and reach toward their potential as human beings as part of communities and populations. The lack of awareness, the policies, and the inequities all need to be recognized and addressed. Although, in the main, the approach is based on social, political, and occupational sciences, it requires a holistic attitude that enables the gathering of data from every possible source and discipline and is proactive in increasing understanding, raising awareness, and promoting change. It fits well with WHO directives in that it is person-centered; enabling and empowering; and encourages participatory diverse, inclusive, and shared advantage.

In the WHO *Declaration of Alma Ata*,[26] OCHP,[27] and *Jakarta Declaration*,[28] social justice surfaces as one of the fundamental prerequisites of health. The earlier documents claimed that to achieve "health for all by the year 2000," it would be essential to "close the gap between the 'haves' and 'have nots'" and to achieve "more equitable distribution of health resources within and among countries, including preferential allocation to those in greatest social need so that the health system adequately covers all the population."[29] This distributive justice view of equal access for everyone to the same health services is well recognized.[30-37] More than that, at the core of health equity is the "right to the highest attainable standard of health as indicated by the health status of the most socially advantaged group."[38] It is those who are already socially disadvantaged by poverty, gender, ethnicity, or disability, for example, who are further disadvantaged by inequities in health.

Occupational justice, like social justice, accepts that ill health can be an outcome of the inequitable distribution of power and resources, resulting from factors such as the type of economy, national priorities and policies, and cultural values.[13,37,39,40] Those underlying determinants, as shown in earlier chapters, can result in people experiencing occupational deprivation, imbalance, and alienation; fatigue; hunger and thirst; boredom; and stress that can lead to ill-health or premature death. Alternatively, the underlying determinants may lead to health and well-being if they enable people to:

* Engage in doing that meets the prerequisites of health.
* Find meaning, purpose, satisfaction, and belonging that promotes physical, mental, and social well-being, including spiritual meaning.
* Aim toward becoming what they have the potential to become.

This occupational justice approach to health aims both at enabling the latter and at changing the underlying determinants that lead to ill-health.

In the interests of understanding the relationship between issues of justice and of health, there have been calls for change in institutional processes in national and civic arenas, that set forth ethical and moral expectations of citizens as well as toward more equal distribution of resources to reduce gaps between the "haves and have-nots." There have also been calls for a critical analysis of the cultural processes that shape both the medical care system and the broad social concern with medical care. This is because standard rehearsals of equity, in the liberal tradition, ignore the underlying determinants and processes of health experiences and the extent to which they arise from factors beyond individual control.[41-43] Many analyses have pointed to discrimination or unjust conditions that disadvantage some groups over others. Doyal and Gough, for example, identified civil and political rights, the right of access to "need satisfiers," and political participation as preconditions for the satisfaction of basic needs.[44] Those are central to this occupational justice approach to health. In occupational terms, underlying factors such as the type of economy, national priorities and policies, and societal values as determinants of health status have been identified earlier in this text. The personal and population consequences of occupational injustice are not discrete. They are the foundations of illness or health and well-being for individuals and communities. At stake is not only the reduction of illness or disability, which may be outcomes for people participating in occupation to obtain the prerequisites of health, but also the promotion of physical, mental, and social well-being. That is dependent on the ability, opportunity, and meaningfulness of living, working, and playing in safe, supportive communities in accord with the WHO 1986 mandate[27] and its follow-up *Health for All in the 21st Century*.[28] This mandate touches on one of the difficulties of health systems and approaches controlled by medical science. Medical science places social health largely outside its boundaries, thus separating it from physical and mental health. Yet people are social and occupational beings whose doings are embedded in the social values, rules, and constraints of different cultures and populations and in the nature of their physical environment.[44]

The basis of this occupational justice approach to health can therefore be described as holistic because it encompasses the interactive nature and complexity of people within natural and human-made environments. Another requirement is for the institutions and services that result from the underlying conditions and policies to create means and opportunities in tune with people's occupational, as well as social, natures. Sociopolitical planners have to envision whether or not such services will motivate people to engage in the occupations emanating from them and whether or not they might lead to stress-related illness or to the experience of well-being. The latter calls for appreciation of human need in ways described in earlier chapters—that all individuals are different in nature, capacity, need, and deed, needing to express that difference with and for others, supporting, supported, and appreciated by them. Most people in the world need to draw on those differing capacities to provide the prerequisites of health such as food and shelter for the sustenance and safety of families and communities. Others, more fortunate in many ways, without such a fundamental cause still need purpose in their lives and can be bereft without the obvious goals of survival. Without occupation of an apparent essential nature, they fail to experience quality of life, health, or well-being because they cannot find adequate substitutes. The removal of the fundamental requirement to do to obtain the prerequisites of health has not reduced the biological need for health-giving engagement in occupation. Many people appear to be lost without that motivation. This is a challenge in affluent societies that have started along the social justice path and provide funds and other resources to those without means of providing for themselves. The total removal of providing for self and family may be a health risk in itself. This brings into play the concept of enablement put forward by the WHO as one of the 3 means of promoting health.[27] This same notion underpins this occupational justice approach that aims to draw out individual occupational needs, strengths, and potential.[11]

The major underlying determinants of occupational justice control what occupations are valuable, acceptable, or even of interest to a population. For example, in the present day, some societies and the institutions and services they have developed embrace peace while in others, war-making occupations are considered essential to a population's beliefs and needs. Hence, the particular structure and ideologies of these determinants sets out the possibilities and limits of occupational justice or occupational injustice and governs socially-determined occupational forms. Depending on the ways they are organized, socially-determined occupational forms could prevent or increase occupational injustices.

Within many populations, there appears to be a conflict between a valuing of the new and different, named by Watson as neophilia,[45] and a valuing of conformity and standardization, described by Stein as a "cult of efficiency."[46] There is a danger that distributive justice without the moderating effects of a justice of difference and in the interests of efficiency may result in standardization that restricts the diversity of people's natures, needs, and capacities. This is already happening in many arenas of education, paid employment, and provision of health services. Diversity throughout the world is reducing as populations succumb to the lure of fast food chains, designer clothes, electronic doing, and preoccupation with following the trends set by the West, whether or not they are healthy in the long term. This occupational justice approach deplores the reduction of diversity because it recognizes the health-promoting aspects of participation in doing, being, and becoming according to different natures and needs. It is based on an inclusive rather than a hierarchical classification of occupations in which status given to the things that people do is reduced and where "no one would be denied participation in occupation that he or she needed or wanted to do to build their individual lives or communities."[11]

The beliefs that underlie this approach have mainly arisen from 2 sources: the wide-ranging exploration of health from an occupational perspective recorded in this text and the collaboration between Townsend and myself to consider the notion of occupational justice and bring it to the attention of interested others. The beliefs are that humans are occupational beings, that satisfying and meaningful participation in occupation is a determinant of health and well-being as well as quality of life, and that people participate in occupations as autonomous beings in diverse sociocultural and economic systems. Such participation is interdependent and contextual. To harness the health-promoting properties of occupation depends on coordinated action across different sectors of communities. Such coordinated action will lead to health and social policies aimed at fostering just, safe, satisfying, stimulating, and enjoyable occupational conditions as a global responsibility.

The principles of this approach are founded on opportunities for participation in occupation as a human right and on empowerment through occupation. The *Universal Declaration of Human Rights* recognizes as the "foundation of freedom, justice and peace in the world" the "equal and inalienable rights of all members of the human family" in the determination "to promote social progress and better standards of life in larger freedom."[47] It calls for "every individual and every organ of society" to "strive by teaching and education to promote respect for these rights and freedoms and by progressive measures, national and international, to secure their universal and effective recognition and observance."[47] Everyone without distinction "such as race, color, sex, language, religion, political or other opinion, national or social origin, property, birth or other status" is entitled to the rights and freedoms named in the *Declaration*.[47] In terms of occupation, specifically, the document mentions everyone's rights to:

* "Take part in the government of his country, directly or through freely chosen representatives."

* "Social security... in accordance with the organization and resources of each State, of the economic, social and cultural rights indispensable for his dignity and the free development of his personality."

* "Work, to free choice of employment, to just and favorable conditions of work and to protection against unemployment" and to "equal pay for equal work."

* "Just and favorable remuneration ensuring for himself and his family an existence worthy of human dignity, and supplemented, if necessary, by other means of social protection."

* "Rest and leisure, including reasonable limitation of working hours and periodic holidays with pay."

* "A standard of living adequate for the health and well-being of himself and of his family, including food, clothing, housing and medical care and necessary social services, and the right to security in the event of unemployment, sickness, disability, widowhood, old age or other lack of livelihood in circumstances beyond his control."

* "Education… directed to the full development of the human personality and to the strengthening of respect for human rights and fundamental freedoms."
* "Participate in the cultural life of the community, to enjoy the arts and to share in scientific advancement and its benefits."
* "Duties to the community in which alone the free and full development of his personality is possible."

These rights are inclusive of the notions about doing, being, and becoming addressed in earlier chapters and are complementary to the concept of health held by the WHO.

These rights are reflected in WHO initiatives that are guidelines to workers in the field of public health who could look more widely, inclusively, and extensively at the relationship between health and all the things that people need, want, or are obliged to do. They are also reflected in Occupational Therapy Associations *Codes of Ethics*, but they, too, could be more widely applied. In those of the American Occupational Therapy Association (AOTA), for example, is a public statement of commitment to promote inclusion, diversity, independence, safety, and empowerment for all recipients of occupational therapy, including the community and society at large. This is to be done in various stages of life, health, and illness "in a variety of contexts to support engagement in everyday life activities that affect health, well being and quality of life."[48] Ethical action is seen to transcend application of the AOTA's principles being a commitment "to beneficence for the sake of others… to genuinely good behaviors, and to noble acts of courage."[48] To implement occupationally just programs to meet physical, mental, and social health and wellbeing as that *Code of Ethics* requires, will take "noble acts of courage" to challenge existing ways of delivering services and extending them to the people in most need.

Other principles about the nature of occupation are central to this occupational justice approach to health, such as the requirement of a greater understanding of occupation as a holistic concept and a more inclusive classification of occupations. The nature of the action required to use this approach effectively as well as understanding the basic ideology relating to the connection between occupation and health is called for, and for many this could be difficult. This is because health, over the last century, has been largely the domain of experts with a narrower view of what it is about: namely the discrete physiological workings of the body and mind and the pharmaceutical remedies to right any abnormalities. The ideology of that domain is powerful because of the great success it has achieved in terms of surgery and medicinal remedies. This much more holistic view demands a closer look at every level of the population but without asking for a denial of the benefits of medicine per se. If these difficulties can be overcome, accepting the notion of enablement of occupational potential as paramount for healthy populations and individuals is a first principle. Following acceptance of that is the requirement to also accept the principle of diversity, and that a more socially inclusive acceptance of the value of participation in many types of doing is needed. Inequities in opportunities for participation in diverse occupations for health and well-being can be reduced, but both a justice of distribution and a justice of difference will be required to achieve that (Table 8-1).[11]

Why an Occupational Justice Approach Is Necessary

The relationship between occupational justice and health is seldom considered because the concept is in its infancy and largely unknown. However, social justice continues to be the subject of numerous investigations in terms of health and because the 2 types of justice cannot be separated, those are useful to examine. In one of the most notable investiga-

Table 8-1

Foundations of an Occupational Justice Approach to Health

Basis of Approach	Underlying Beliefs	Underlying Principles
Applicable to populations, communities, and individuals	Humans are occupational beings	Occupational opportunities as a human right
Aimed at reducing inequities in the experience of health/ ill health	Participation is a determinant of health and well-being	Inequities in opportunities for participation can be reduced
Based on social, political, and occupational science	People need to participate in occupations as autonomous beings in diverse socioeconomic systems	Both justice of distribution and justice of difference required
Holistic concept of people within natural and human-made environments	Participation is interdependent and contextual	Enablement of occupational potential for populations and individuals
Is person centered, enabling and empowering	Coordinated action leads to health and social policies that foster justice	Empowerment through occupation
Is participatory-diverse and inclusive	Safe, satisfying, stimulating, and enjoyable occupational conditions are a global responsibility	Diversity and inclusivity of occupational participation

tions related to Western societies, Hart reported in 1971 that in the United Kingdom the availability of good medical care tended to vary inversely with the need of the population served, and in areas where there was the greatest proportion of illness and death, both general practitioners and hospitals had the largest caseloads and the fewest resources.[49] A little later, *The Black Report* on "Inequalities in Health" in Britain gave an account of the inverse relation between health status and social location and called for a radical overhaul of health service activities and resources.[50] Similarly, in Australia, Broadhead found in an investigation in which occupation (paid employment), education, and affluence were used as variables of social status that the 4 indicators of morbidity—recent illnesses, chronic conditions, days of reduced activity, and mental health—showed significant relationships to affluence for both sexes after standardization for age.[51] According to Opit in 1983, approximately 15% of the Australian population suffered from poverty and from lack of autonomy or power, with subsequent anxiety, depression, risk taking, injudicious alcohol consumption, and premature death all exacerbated by the inability to take advantage of the limited resources committed to their welfare.[52] Those suffering most were Aboriginals, single parents, the unemployed, large families with a single wage earner, the elderly, and many recent migrants, and the degree of deprivation and the numbers were increasing.[52] By the late 1980s, Gallagher and Ferrante claimed there was no indication that "any Western democracy has the political will to make the massive redistribution involved in recommendations such as those of *The Black Report.*"[41] This remains the case. In the United States, for example, which unlike other developed countries does not have national health insurance, poorer health and less access to medical care are similarly associated with race, ethnicity, and poverty.[53-56] Despite what Sussenberger describes as an idealized version of the social system and views of equality, "inequalities are socially and materially enacted through the dynamic and changing interrelationships of such variables as class, gender, race, ethnicity, age, and disability."[57]

The polarization of wealth lies, to a large extent, in the hands of giant multinational corporations and speculative investors whose financial support of governments provides them with overwhelming influence that results in trade agreements counterproductive to health giving and humane societies.[58,59] To change the polarization of wealth today in America, for example, the "Green Party" claims, would require attention to the tremendous and unfair gap between the rich and the poor, or even between the very rich and the average person.[60] One-fifth of the population receives about one-half of all national income, while the bottom one-fifth receives less than 4%, and that behind this unjust distribution are a few giant corporations who own or control nearly all sources of information and communication.[60] In terms of the global distribution of wealth, Kronenberg, Simo Algado, and Pollard provide figures based on reducing proportionally the Earth's populations to 100 people.[61] This eases the difficulties of coming to grips with the magnitude of many of the global problems. Six people, all from the United States, own 59% of the whole world's wealth, "80 live in substandard housing, 70 are illiterate, 50 are undernourished, 10 are disabled, 1 is dying, 2 are newborns, 1 has a computer," and only 1 "has higher education."[62]

Werner recognizes that the cruelly inequitable and lopsided global economy poses the biggest obstacle to health, particularly in the developing world.[59] The regulation or transformation of the prevailing market system is required to put need before greed:

> In such a transition, the World Health Organization and UNICEF need to reclaim their mandate as world coordinators of well-being of the disadvantaged. They need to gain strong enough popular support to stand up to the transnational corporations—the pushers of weapons, cigarettes and infant-formula—without fear of funding cuts by the US Government. Likewise, financial institutions such as the World Bank must be structurally adjusted to place basic human needs before unregulated corporate profits.[59]

The rhetorical commitment to social justice and egalitarianism in most liberal economies cannot be achieved without structural change or political will. Yet, even in conventional international health education, it has been noted that worldwide there is shrinking from acknowledgment of "the social roots of grotesque inequalities"[63] and that:

> Regardless of their origins, social and economic inequalities are reflected epidemiologically: disparities of outcome in and between countries are now major challenges in medicine and public health. If health is ever to be construed as a human right, such disparities must be seen as the chief challenge for medical education.[63]

Similar challenges are evident in conventional international education of other health workers, such as public health, occupational health and safety, and occupational therapy. That is not always because they are not addressed within curriculum. I have spent close to 2 decades trying to instill such values, only to watch practitioners carry on with those of earlier times when such inequities were disregarded, except perhaps rhetorically. I have also observed such contributions to curriculum being axed in favor of other requirements deemed more relevant. Maybe this is a result of occupational therapy appearing to be perceived by its practitioners as apolitical, as the authors of the 2005 *Occupational Therapy Without Borders* observe.[61] In relation to occupational injustice, they introduce the notion of occupational apartheid to raise critical awareness and understanding about the political nature of occupation.[61] They provide the following working definition:

The segregation of groups of people through the restriction or denial of access to digni-
fied and meaningful participation in occupations of daily life on the basis of race, color,
disability, national origin, age, gender, sexual preference, religion, political beliefs, sta-
tus in society, or other characteristics. Occasioned by political forces, its systematic and
pervasive social, cultural, and economic consequences jeopardize health and well-being
as experienced by individuals, communities, and societies.[64]

Lack of attention to or action taken about issues of justice often appears to be because of
sociopolitical, economically driven, work-place directives. While the evidence of health
inequities is growing, structural change to put thought into action is lagging behind.
Farmer, Furin, and Katz suggest in terms of medicine and public health that "goods are
still parochial, limited to few beneficiaries" because "medicine is developing evidence, but
has no equity plan: we lack a rights-based approach to its distribution."[63]

It is more than 2 decades since the call for health for all by the year 2000 made its
debut at the break-through conference held at Alma Ata in Kazakhstan. It was there that
it became widely recognized that through comprehensive multisectoral primary health
care, the underlying political and socioeconomic causes of health problems could, and
should, be confronted. David Werner some 20 years ago, again in Kazakhstan, regret-
ted the failure of attaining a "New Social Order" based on equity and social justice. He
points to "Structural Adjustments and World Trade Agreements" as political initiatives
that have placed "the cost of health and foods beyond the reach of millions" and made it
difficult for equity-minded nations to sustain basic-needs oriented policies.[59] The irony
is that today in affluent postindustrial nations, the problems of obesity from overeating
and lack of physical occupations is a major thrust of public health. This bipolar unhealthy
outcome is rooted in unequal power relations with large population groups being culturally subordinated, exploited, marginalized, and disempowered.[13] Concerns of justice and
injustice can be linked without much effort to the politics of economic growth that show
insufficient regard to empowerment or to the overall human health and environmental
health costs:

The well-being of the poorer half of humanity is compromised by landlessness, job-
lessness, insupportably low wages, cut-backs in health and welfare services, and the
resultant pandemic of anger, crime, violence, despair, unrest, with consequent harsh
measures in social control—all of which arise from the growing disparity of wealth
and power.[59]

At the opposite spectrum are others who may appear empowered to direct their lives, but
flounder in policies that create situations in which people, unable to realize their talents
or achieve their aspirations, seek to satisfy their unanswered needs in risky or unhealthy
behaviors such as overeating or substance abuse. Empowerment, not just access to services, is closely linked with health.[11]

An age-old issue that has been commented on by philosophers throughout time concerns the distribution of work according to its apparent pleasant or unpleasant characteristics. John Ruskin (1819–1900), for example, in *Sesame and Lilies*, asks "Which of us... is
to do the hard and dirty work for the rest—and for what pay? Who is to do the pleasant
and clean work, and for what pay?"[65] Along similar lines, Ramazzini in an earlier time
raised very practical health concerns that pointed to gross disorders and early death that
were the lot of workers in many types of basic but necessary-to-societies employment
and that was out of proportion with the well-to-do occupation and health experiences of
the more affluent.[66] The division is less obvious in the 21st century within post-industrial
nations, although still a major concern. However, the division is great between countries. The affluent postindustrial nations have passed the more dangerous, repetitive,
and unhealthy forms of employment associated with industry to newly industrialized

nations, and another group of nations remain reliant on subsistence agriculture or a mixture of that and hunter-gathering lifestyles. That, too, is compromised by action in the West. Their populations grow, their lands reduce in size and fertility at the same time as the ecology is degraded and the climate changes, resulting in widespread famine and long-term population illness. Effectively, the same divide as in earlier times within countries is now enacted across the globe.

In the developing world, economic decline leads to an increase in infectious diseases and a decrease in the provision of health care and education.[67] There is also growth in the tobacco and fast-food industries. This coupled with routine preventive programs being unavailable or unaffordable except to a small minority, and the fact that chronic diseases start at earlier ages, results in people arriving at old age "in poorer shape with fewer reserves."[68-70] The compression of morbidity apparent in the West is far from the case in the developing world.[71] As disease and illness are perpetuated and resources are expended on more and more needing cure, less is available for programs aimed at prevention, well-being, community development, and so on. This medicalization of health has led to overwhelming concentration on repair after something goes wrong. The idea that health can be improved for all people, including those without resources to access such medical expertise, is poorly understood. Yet, the WHO clearly outlines as a prerequisite for health those basic amenities and needs that are obtained through what people do despite injustices apparent to all, such as the number of homeless children throughout the world being seen as outside the "medicalized" health systems until they become ill.

The UN believes it is impossible to state the number of homeless and street children. They are to be found in every country in the world, including those thought to have well-organized and kindly social welfare systems. In Australia, for example, there are an estimated 26,000 young people homeless each night of the year, and the number is increasing. They leave home because of issues such as family conflict, violence, physical and sexual abuse, or sometimes, because of dissatisfaction or boredom, peer pressure, and substance abuse. The lot of this growing population of alienated, deprived, desperate, and disenfranchised group is of particular concern to large numbers of the more advantaged, to politicians, to social welfare, and to the WHO and UN.

The UN General Assembly adopted *The Convention on the Rights of the Child* in November 1989. It became international law in 1990, having been ratified by all but 2 countries in the world (the United States and Somalia).[72] Its roots can be traced from the work of Eglantyne Jebb, who founded Save the Children in 1923, through the *Universal Declaration of Human Rights*, and an earlier *Declaration of the Rights of the Child* in 1959 that provided a statement of general principles but was not legally binding. These special rights were created because of the physical and mental immaturity of children that makes them particularly vulnerable and in need of special care, safeguards, assistance, and appropriate legal protection. Unfortunately, this has not prevented children from suffering because of decisions and actions taken by adults and being viewed collectively rather than as individuals with personal needs and rights.[73] The basic principles of the convention bring together civil, political, social, economic, and cultural rights of the child in a holistic way. Claiming that society has an obligation to satisfy the fundamental needs of children and to provide assistance for the harmonious development of their personalities, talents, and abilities, it calls for their right to[73]:

∗ Survival, "including nutrition, shelter, an adequate standard of living and access to healthcare."

∗ Development, so that children "reach their full potential" including education, play, leisure, and cultural activities.

✳ Protection from all forms of abuse, neglect, and exploitation, including "rehabilitation for children who have suffered any form of abuse or exploitation."

✳ Participation including enablement of active roles in "decisions affecting their own lives, in their communities and societies in preparation for responsible adulthood."

The number of children living on the streets is aggravated by war, and increasing numbers live in war-torn countries. They have often experienced family separations or disintegrations, destruction of their homes and communities, and lack of trust among people. Many suffer physical injury and psychosocial distress or experience gender-based violence. Some have witnessed their parents' murder, torture, or rape or have been threatened with death personally. In Rwanda, for example, more than one-third of 3030 children surveyed by UNICEF in 1995 had witnessed family murders, and nearly 80% had lost immediate family members.[74] Additionally, disruption to agriculture or food supplies; displacement of populations; and destruction of basic hygiene, education, and health services all impact on children's development—physically, mentally, and emotionally, accumulating and interacting with each other. Even without personal exposure to armed conflict, a child in a country at war will experience some of the many causes of injustice because of the transfer of resources from investment in development to investment in armaments.[75] The UN claims:

> *If countries continue to employ four times as many soldiers as teachers, education and social systems will remain fragile and inadequate, and Governments will continue to fail children and break the promises made to them through ratification of the Convention on the Rights of the Child.*[76]

Braveman points to "the massive aftershocks resulting from destruction of infrastructure (for example, clean water) critical for survival and health; many more deaths occurred for this reason in the wake of the first Gulf War than as a direct result of the military action itself."[77] In Iraq, he maintains the war will exacerbate inequities, taking "its heaviest toll on the poor and especially poor children."[77]

The list of inequities and the illness resulting from them in poorer countries of the world are horrendous so that it becomes possible to forget that they are also apparent in the postindustrial affluent world. These, too, require attention. In a socially and occupationally just community, respect and fairness would be evident in everyone's dealings with each other. As well, understanding would be explicit of how policies, economics, industry, education, social welfare, and health systems empower what and how people do, be, and become. At present, many decisions of these powerful agencies are invisible. Similarly, people are unable to be fully aware of how market force or cultural bias affects possibilities for participating or not in various occupations. In that case, it is possible to experience injustice as a result of taken-for-granted beliefs, values, and assumptions or power conflicts and tensions between competing interests. Power is a central feature in defining justice. Political dimensions of justice have interpersonal, private ramifications, although the ruling apparatus of an organized society is largely unconscious in everyday experience.[11]

Individual motivation and energy make a difference. As I write this text, an example of that is unfolding. Tasmanian vegetable growers in recent weeks took to their tractors and journeyed in them to the mainland of Australia, for thousands of kilometers, in a very roundabout route to the nation's capital. This incredible caterpillar-like expedition was a result of a multinational decision to replace their high quality produce with that from overseas. The vegetable growers recognized serious long-term ramifications of this decision, as well as the short-term financial difficulties, and decided they needed to make their plight widely known. They sought "source of origin" labeling on their products, and public awareness of what such multinational decisions could mean in terms of everyone's future. State and national leaders became involved because communities demonstrated their support as the convoy passed through their streets, and at least one noticeable immediate effect has been that a large supermarket chain is now identifying source of origin of the vegetables they sell.

While that example appears to be mainly concerned with national economic policy, it is also about health and well-being from an occupational and social justice point of view. It is worth teasing out further so that the relationship becomes more obvious. Tasmania is an island state with a small population; predominantly rural, its economy is mainly dependent on tourism, forestry, and agriculture. Its climate is conducive to rural occupations and the growing of vegetables and fruit that thrive in temperate zones. If these were to be reduced to any extent, unemployment and its subsequent ill effects would inevitably take their toll. The already high dependence on social welfare in the rural zones of this rural state would climb higher with the subsequent burdens associated with social and later mental and physical disease. Because of distance and separation from the mainland, the island state is not attractive to large business enterprises and much of its land is protected from development, so it makes sense to base its economy on the growing of high-quality foods that require small but dense areas for crop cultivation. The farmers are proud of their products and aware of the benefits of their way of life. They are also aware of the benefits to the nation's population in terms of the quality of the food they grow. In terms of social and economic justice and its understood relationship to health, and in terms of occupational justice of achieving health and well-being through what these growers do, be, and become, the probable loss of this means of livelihood because of the greed of a multinational company is a matter of health.

Weaving these ideas together, this approach to health requires its practitioners to develop interventions aimed at, and leading to, equitable opportunity and resources that enable all people across the globe to survive and develop through what they do. It is a very necessary approach because its substance is largely overlooked. If appreciated at all, the occupational needs and natures of people as a health issue are given lip service and, despite the efforts of health professions aimed at people's doings, there is scant acknowledgment of their contribution, occupational therapy, for example, having been described as a neglected or invisible profession.[78,79] Survival is dependent on occupation, and meaning and potential are embedded in what people do as both expressions of personal capabilities and spirituality and as connectedness with communities. Ensuring ways for people to engage in survival and meaningful occupations is more than icing on the health cake; rather, it is a practical means through which health, personal, and community transformation becomes possible. Such transformation requires action for it to be recognized politically and organizationally, and practitioners taking this approach would need to direct their efforts to that end as well as toward survival, health, well-being, and happiness for populations and individuals.

An Action-Research Approach to Occupational Justice

An action-research approach would primarily explore and focus debate on and action toward underlying occupational policies, economics, attitudes, institutions, and activities. It would call attention to those that reduce the meeting of occupational needs and occupational choice, belonging, satisfaction, balance, and meaning. It would take action to

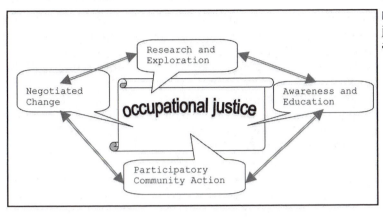

Figure 8-1. Occupational justice—action-research approach.

overturn those injustices that prevent people from satisfying the prerequisites of health; from reaching their potential; or that lead to the experience of occupational imbalance, alienation, deprivation, or apartheid, early preclinical health disorders, disease, and disability. It would do so in consultation, exploration, and participation with population groups and focus on enabling action for change. Action would include mediation, advocacy, and negotiation. Outcomes would suggest further exploration, awareness raising, and action. The process could continue in a spiraling pattern, monitoring and effecting change toward occupationally just solutions in accord with the needs of the population (Figure 8-1).

An example of how increasing community awareness can lead to social action comes from Kinnell's account of how rising levels of literacy, which resulted from the increased emphasis on education in England during the late 18th and early 19th centuries, fostered the growth of trade in children's books. Because the books dealt increasingly with themes such as the right to exercise individual moral judgment and social justice, this development was instrumental in disseminating radical ideas and raising the level of people's political consciousness and dissent.[80] This example suggests that information about occupational justice and health, packaged in an attractive and consumer-oriented manner, perhaps using the Internet or popular magazines, might be one way to approach the raising of consciousness on a population scale. Werner agrees with that view when he suggests:

> *Perhaps, most important of all, we need to become popular educators, helping ordinary people to see through the disinformation of the mass media, to analyze local and world events, to understand the roots of their hardships, and then to mobilize a massive demand for more responsible, democratic, and humane global leadership.*[59]

Interventions designed to approach occupational justice issues might involve developing community awareness about inequities in occupational opportunities through action involving community groups and the media, along with providing individual and community laboratories to practice relevant skills that lead to political lobbying for structural change. As with all action-research, it would be an ongoing spiraling of exploration, awareness raising, and action toward change, moving forward in small or large steps according to responses or to the critical nature of the action required. The timing of various stages of the approach could vary considerably. It may, for example, be necessary to raise community or political awareness about the concept of occupational justice prior to researching or exploring issues in more depth because so little and so few know about it. Alternatively, a researcher or a group of researchers may become aware of particular issues, suspect the occupation for health outcomes, and carry out appropriate research before raising community awareness toward action. A combination of those 2 approaches has been taken with regard to the establishment of the first Australasian Occupational Science Centre (AOSC) as an education and research center at the University of Wollongong. This aims to provide community education about the relationship between what people do and their health through occupation-based community projects and research and to make recommendations for public health policy. Based on those aims, AOSC is undertaking its first major project called, appropriately, "To do or die" (Wicks A, oral communication, August 2005).

The project focuses on fostering health for older people by educating retirees, community agencies, businesses, and local governments about the occupational nature and needs of local retirees. Adopting a population approach to health, the project is based on 4 of the OCHP directives: to develop personal skills, to create supportive environments, to strengthen community action, and to build healthy public policy,[113] and on 3 key beliefs that people need and have a right to participate in occupations:

1. For their health and well being.

2. Relevant to their community.

3. That promotes healthy individuals, communities, and populations.

In seeking funding for the project, AOSC is using the opportunity to increase awareness of occupational science and the relationship between occupation and health generally. For this project specifically, it will increase awareness of justice issues in terms of older people in the community needing to maintain and enhance their health through participation in occupation and community life. In order to do that, it will gather information about barriers that are limiting participation. Advertising in local media, radio, television, and press and reporting of events associated with the project will contribute to increasing awareness and educating a wide range of people about the connections, as will the strategic seeking of resources from the university sector; local business and peak bodies; and local, state, and national governments (Wicks A, personal communication, August 2005).

That project is an important one in terms of future occupational justice for a fast growing sector of communities. Government and health bodies are both concerned about the resource implications of an aging population and an anticipated "blow out" of medical costs. The WHO's *Ageing and Life Course Programme Policy Framework*, and subsequent publications about aging, are useful guides to inform discussion and to form action plans that promote healthy and active aging.[81,82] Practitioners working with older people should be delivering programs, raising awareness, and enabling older people to maintain and increase their health through what they do. Action-research is a great "way to go" with both well and "not so well" older people.

Despite apparent lip service to the notion of active aging, there remains much more media coverage about governmental concerns regarding estimates of the likely soaring health and pension costs. That has not led to better provision of occupation-based services to reduce illness, either in the community or in residential care. The UN report of the "International Year of Older Persons" stressed the importance of meeting, recognizing, involving, and consulting older people as potential societal resources and keeping in mind that stereotyping can lead to discrimination and violations of human rights.[83] It is, therefore, occupationally unjust to not engage in strategies such as action-research when such violations are obvious, as in the case of many aged-care facilities. There, it is not uncommon for older people like Joe, aged 83, and Marianne, who is 90, to sit alone in the midst of others day after day, often unable to talk or share similar interests. Unqualified personnel who have little understanding of the need for choice, interest, difference, and participation run the programs they are expected to join. Ironically, organization was Joe's forte. A sing-song 1 day a week, and seated exercise classes or social events often with colored balls or balloons on another 2 days, do not satisfy his needs. They are taken on outings, in which neither Marianne nor Joe have interest, and are expected to sit in front of a television that shows program after program that they did not choose. Marianne finds it hard not being attended too when she talks about what she has done in her life as a teacher or being ignored when she asks questions or offers advice to younger relatives who visit infrequently. Joe squirms when told by caring staff not to do something for his own good, and being given no chance to help others in a way that he has done with considerable skill throughout his adult life. Although both have been seen by an occupational therapist, her activities on the 1 day each week she is employed were confined by the agency-to-risk management, safe mobility, independent hygiene, and dressing assessments. This scenario is enacted across the developed world, contributing considerably to the health costs incurred in such facilities. For those who work in the sector, an action-research approach approved by local, state, or national governments would not only raise their awareness of the plight of many, it would, in the long term, reduce expenditure, and most importantly, involve the participants in establishing their own criteria for a healthy and just lifestyle.

In the United States, a research and educational arm of Partners in Health known as the Institute for Health and Social Justice was established in 1994 to link critical scholarly analysis with community-based experience. Following ratification of The Millennium Declaration of the UN General Assembly 2000, the Institute became involved in a 5-year effort to formulate pragmatic solutions to many global health injustices on individuals, communities, and nations. There are 10 specialized task forces addressing different aspects of global inequality, such as hunger, poverty, gender and education, maternal and child health, infectious disease and access to essential medicines, and access to technology. It is probably safe to say that the relationship between occupation, health, and justice will not be recognized as central in these efforts, although aspects of that relationship will be obvious even if not spelled out in the terms addressed here. This is one important reason for strategies to be developed to bring this aspect to the attention of international health organizations. It is necessary to raise awareness continuously and repetitively as a 1985 study funded by the Rockefeller Foundation and reported by Werener demonstrates.[59] That study showed a number of poor countries—China, Sri Lanka, Costa Rica, and Kerala State of India—at that time had achieved basic health care at a low cost, universal primary education, outreach to rural and vulnerable communities, and that every person had enough to eat. This was achieved through sociopolitical efforts aimed at meeting all people's basic needs equitably rather than prioritizing economic growth. The resultant rates of child survival and longevity were comparable to those of richer nations. By the 1990s, it was becoming increasingly difficult for these equity-oriented nations to sustain this basic needs approach. All experienced some reversals in their quality of life indicators as a result of changed political commitment to equity. The latter can be laid at the feet of free market globalization policies, structural adjustment programs, and "mandates for lop sided economic growth."[59]

Werner, in his address to delegates at Kazakhstan, points to the necessity for all people involved in health promotion needing to become more cognizant of economic issues and the strategies of global organizations[84] and demonstrate a willingness to become involved in serious dialogue at that level. This is so that it becomes possible to "work toward more humane and sustainable alternatives to our current top down policies."[59] It is also imperative that all health workers educate for peace. Action-research aimed at different sectors of society building "ethical frameworks," integrating traditional values with international legal standards "promote peace, social justice, respect for human rights and the acceptance of responsibility."[59]

Increasing awareness might be through community workshops. Occupational therapy participants in early workshops about occupational justice, for example, experienced a sense of the need for major change in sociopolitical, population, and individual thinking to fully address issues of occupational injustice. They identified as important "redefining the way resources are shared and moneys distributed" in ways that "nourish development of the mind, body, and spirit of individuals and communities" through "choice," "empowerment," and "participation," and "personal, environmental, societal, cultural and communal opportunity."[85] The concept of "sharing in and contributing to the community" was associated with the political enabling of "equal opportunity for meaningful and diverse occupations" that might mean the "reduction of disadvantage" through "changing cultural values" toward "equity in living."[86] Participants discussed contradictions, tensions, and dilemmas between the rights of individuals for personal responsibilities as the notion of "acceptable or unacceptable occupations," such as drug dealing or gun recreation, was debated when discussion turned to the "social and ethical standards of a community."[87] Because of such contradictions or tensions, it is useful to have and to use documents such as *The Declaration of Human Rights*[88] or *The Convention on the Rights of the Child*[73] to steer awareness exercises and to use as back-up in presenting new directions to "powers-that-be." The greater the awareness of rights, the more chance there is of securing them.

With that in mind, we can consider what form occupational justice action-research approaches for children might take as an example. The Convention's 2 conceptions of the child—as a recipient of adult and State concern and protection and as a contributing participant to decisions affecting his or her own life and to his or her communities and societies—suggest it is a matter of justice that children should be enabled to actively prepare for responsible adulthood as young citizens.[73] Additionally, the UN provides recommendations for action toward the enabling process. For them to experience the least physical, mental, and emotional trauma from the results of war, it is recommended that[73]:

* Exploration includes the related effects on women, families, and the community support systems because "children's well-being is best ensured through family and community-based solutions that draw on local culture and an understanding of child development."

* Families and communities are empowered to take part in the healing process. "Helping war-affected children to build on their own strengths and resilience, in collaboration with trusted caregivers, is an important strategy in the process of healing."

* There should be knowledge of the way child development is understood locally, "a deep understanding of and respect for the societies," and local culture and practices, such as the rites and ceremonies related to growing up, adulthood, death, burial, and mourning.

* Attention to children's primary health, chronic, or acute conditions, and rehabilitative requirements should facilitate "the fullest possible social integration."

* "Child-focused health needs assessments" should be expedited while taking into account "food, health and care factors and the coping strategies likely to be used by the affected population."

* Approaches must be holistic, addressing psychological recovery and social reintegration as well as physical vulnerability.

* Training and raising awareness of caregivers, such as parents, teachers, and community health workers, will assist development of diverse programs. Preferably, these should focus on supporting healing processes and re-establishing a sense of normalcy.

* Education should continue despite difficult circumstances even in situations of armed conflict. Such was the case in the former Yugoslavia when "classes were held in the cellars of people's homes, often by candlelight" during the height of the fighting. In situations such as that, use might be made of a teacher's emergency pack (TEP), developed by UNESCO and UNICEF. Described as "school-in-a-box," this contains basic teaching materials (eg, brushes and paints, chalk, paper, pens, pencils, and exercise books). Other creative ways to maintain education might include use of pre-packaged teaching materials for distance learning. "In Sierra Leone, non-traditional teachers, including mothers and adolescents, were trained and deployed."[127]

In the particular case of an occupational justice approach to health, it is worth noting the UN claim that:

A number of activities have been identified as supporting healing by fostering in children a sense of purpose, self-esteem and identity. These include establishing daily routines such as going to school, preparing food, washing clothes and working in the fields; providing children with the intellectual and emotional stimulation through structured group activities such as play, sports, drawing, drama and story-telling; and providing the opportunity for expression, attachment and trust that comes from a stable, caring and nurturing relationship with adults.[73]

Occupational therapists are intimately concerned with occupations of that type and for such reasons. They use similar programs, adjusted case by case, for people of all ages. Incorporating such programs into action-research approaches for situations in which occupational injustice is apparent or rife is a necessary step to be taken in:

* War torn countries: Inspiration might be drawn from work such as that of Rachel Thibeault with the Inuit of Northern Canada or in Lebanon or postwar Sierra Leone.[89-92] It might also be found in readings from *Occupational Therapy Without Borders*. Within this recent text are many examples of approaching the more daunting and, to most, the unfamiliar problems of working in areas of troubled and unjust physical, mental, and social health. Readers are provided with rich anecdotes and stories from the field to inspire. These include interventions in war-torn countries and with street kids.[61]

* Needy communities or populations: Street kids present an occupational justice problem across many communities, populations, and countries. Kronenberg tells of street children in Mexico for whom "occupational and social participation is denied or restricted to survival at the margins of society, where the predominant occupations are derived from crime, drugs, prostitution, and affiliation with gang culture."[64] He, rightly, critiqued the occupational therapy profession for not having addressed the phenomenon or needs of street children and provides some insights for future action.[64] It is a daunting but common problem, but there are national and international organizations and local agencies that can assist with programs or at least need to be contacted prior to beginning a new action-research project. "Street Kids International" is one such organization. They use a "Street Business Toolkit" in conjunction with youth outreach programs and health training. In Zambia, over 300 youth have been trained, some now have businesses, and others plan to start a business cooperative.[93] Work with street kids can provide a useful fieldwork experience for occupational therapy students and practice in using an action-research approach.

Such an experience was very successful in Adelaide a few years ago when students worked with street kids who produced a video depicting their lives that resulted in them receiving an award.[94]

* Daily practice with people within established health care systems: In many places, both rehabilitative and health promotion opportunities have reduced with tighter time lines and program resourcing policies since the 1980s when Hodges identified that action toward social justice for, and with, the disabled did not occur.[95] Those concerns remain a challenge for occupational therapists in their regular employment fields. The challenge is to promote change to environments as well as for people and to influence the development of person-centered policies and laws toward occupationally just situations in health care settings.[22] Being responsive to "conditions within the patients' primary systems" is a starting place "to bring about changes in conditions that are detrimental to health." Johnson proposed the setting up of laboratories in which "patients acquire skills they need to influence change in their environments."[96] Such a laboratory could be envisaged as part of critical action and is in line with the action-research approach.

* Daily life of total population: Many people are straitjacketed into roles set by their communities. For example, there is enormous pressure for older people to stop, or substantially reduce, their activities at a given age, or for adolescents and even young children to excel in a restricted range of subjects at school to be fitted for particular jobs or to go to college. In many instances, a child's particular talents are set aside in the interests of potential material reward or educational and societal expectations. Those scenarios are not surprising within basic national frameworks characterized by "economic division of labor organized for private profit rather than human need," a gender-based division of occupation "that separates privatized child rearing from recognized and remunerated work," "paid labor markets that generate a marginalized underclass," and a globalized international political economy that increasingly subjugates its poorest workers and must then "engage in crisis management in the form of segmented social welfare concessions."[97,98] In addition, legislative changes that reduce risks, individuality, and experimentation can also reduce occupational opportunity, meaning, belonging, and satisfaction and lead to occupational alienation, deprivation, and imbalance. It is timely to consider social and political mechanisms that influence people's access to necessary, meaningful, and health-promoting occupation. Even social justice and equity models are, on the whole, biased toward current social, economic, educational, and health opportunities, which can lead to reduced occupational choice because they do not sufficiently encompass egalitarian ideas about individual and community uniqueness. Occupational therapists could take up this particular aspect of justice. With regard to occupational justice per se, Kronenberg and Pollard suggest it is "not only an issue of professional responsibility: for us it is a issue of ethical responsibility and global citizenship in which there is not really a choice."[64]

For those who embrace the notion of occupational justice, the way ahead will be a struggle, but as Werner argues:

> *The Struggle for Health is essentially a Struggle for Equity and Compassion, not just in the Provision of Health Services, but in all sectors and aspects of life. Therefore we health planners need to reach far beyond conventional medical and health services. We need to join with social activists, alternative economists, grassroots organizers, progressive educators, and other agents of change, to advance a multi sectoral strategy that puts the basic needs of all people—especially the disadvantaged—before the myopic power plays of the global rulers.*[64]

Pelton sees "the ultimate test of any policies and programs must be demonstration of improved outcomes [such as] ... reduced violence, drug abuse, mortality rates, child placement rates, child abuse, and homelessness."[14] It is very important that work to those ends is reported widely so that outcomes, whether negative or positive, are transparent for occupational justice action-research teams that follow.

Weaving these ideas together, occupational justice can be described as equitable opportunity and resources to enable people's engagement in meaningful occupations. Meaning is embedded in occupation as an expression of personal capabilities and spirituality, and as connectedness with communities that create and reflect the meanings that humans, as occupational beings, give to their occupations. Engagement in meaningful occupation then appears to be a practical means through which personal and community transformation becomes possible. Furthermore, such transformation could be politically and organizationally directed toward health, well-being, happiness, and even the survival of humans.

References

1. Disraeli B. *Speech in the House of Commons.* London, UK: 11th February, 1851. Available at: http://www.crystalclouds.co.uk. Accessed April 25, 2006.
2. Irani KD, Silver M, eds. *Social Justice in the Ancient World.* Westport, CT: Greenwood Press; 1995.
3. Habermas J. *The Philosophical Discourse of Modernity: Twelve Lectures.* Cambridge, Mass: MIT Press; 1995.
4. Pitkin HF. Justice: on relating public and private. *Political Theory.* 1981;9:327-352.
5. Rawls J. *A Theory of Justice.* Cambridge, Mass: Belknap Press of Harvard University Press; 1971.
6. Justice. In: Norton AL, ed. *The Hutchinson Dictionary of Ideas.* Oxford, UK: Helicon Publishing Ltd; 1994.
7. Definitions of social justice on the web. Available at: http://www.aworldconnected.org/. Accessed August 2005.
8. Mill JS. *Utilitarianism.* London; 1863.
9. Smith T. Justice as a personal virtue. *Social Theory and Practice.* 1999;25:361-384.
10. Geras N. Justice. In: Bottomore T, ed. *A Dictionary of Marxist Thought.* 2nd ed. Oxford, UK: Blackwell; 1991:275.
11. Townsend EA, Wilcock AA. Occupational justice. In: Christiansen CH, Townsend EA, eds. *Introduction to Occupation: The Art and Science of Living.* Upper Saddle River, NJ: Pearson Education Inc; 2004.
12. Marshall G, Swift A, Roberts S. Social justice. In: Marshall G, Swift A, Roberts S, eds. *Against the Odds? Social Class and Social Justice in Industrial Societies.* Oxford: Clarendon Press; 1997.
13. Young IM. *Justice and the Politics of Difference.* Princeton, NJ: Princeton University Press; 1990.
14. Pelton LH. *Doing Justice: Liberalism, Group Constructs, and Individual Realities.* Albany: State University of New York Press; 1999:13,32.
15. Wilcock A, Townsend E. Occupational justice: occupational terminology interactive dialogue. *Journal of Occupational Science.* 2000;7(2):84-86.
16. Wilcock AA. *Occupation for Health: A Journey from Self-Health to Prescription.* Vol 1. London, UK: COT; 2001.
17. Marti-Ibañez F, ed. *Henry E. Sigerist on the History of Medicine.* New York: MD Publications, Inc.; 1960:7-8.
18. Porter R. *The Greatest Benefit to Mankind: A Medical History of Humanity from Antiquity to the Present.* New York: Harper Collins; 1999:110.
19. Howard J. *An Account of the Principle Lazarettos in Europe; with Various Papers Relative to the Plague: Together with Further Observations on some Foreign Prisons and Hospitals; and Additional Remarks on the Present State of those in Great Britain and Ireland.* Warrington: William Eyres; 1789:140-142.
20. Emerson RL. *Enlightenment. Grolier Multimedia Encyclopedia 1995.* Danbury, Conn: Grolier Electronic Publishing, Inc; 1995.
21. Browne WAF. *What Asylums Were, Are, and Ought to Be.* Edinburgh: Adam and Charles Black; 1837:229-230.

22. Townsend E. Muriel Driver Memorial Lecture: occupational therapy's social vision. *Can J Occup Ther.* 1993;60(4):174-184.
23. Townsend E. *Good Intentions Overruled.* Toronto: University of Toronto Press; 1998.
24. Giddens A. *Modernity and Self Identity: Self and Society in the Late Modern Age.* Stanford, Calif: Stanford University Press; 1991.
25. Smith DE. *Texts, Facts and Femininity: Exploring the Relations of Ruling.* New York: Routlege; 1990.
26. World Health Organization. *The Declaration of Alma Ata.* International Conference on Primary Health Care, Alma Ata, USSR; 1998.
27. World Health Organization, Health and Welfare Canada, Canadian Public Health Association. *Ottawa Charter for Health Promotion.* Ottawa, Canada; 1986.
28. World Health Organization. *Jakarta Declaration on Leading Health Promotion into the 21st Century.* 4th International Conference on Health Promotion, Jakarta, Indonesia, 21-25th July, 1997.
29. World Health Organization. *Formulating Strategies for Health for All by the Year 2000.* Geneva: WHO; 1979.
30. Cookson R, Dolan P. Principles of justice in health care rationing. *Journal of Medical Ethics.* 2000;6(5):323-329.
31. Daniels NB, Kennedy P, Kawachi I. Why justice is good for our health: the social determinants of health inequalities. *Daedalus.* 1999;128(4):215-251.
32. Emanuel EJ. Justice and managed care: four principles for the just allocation of health care resources. *Hastings Center Report.* 2000;30(3):8-16.
33. Jennings B. Democracy and justice in health policy. *Hastings Center Report.* 1990;September/October:22-23.
34. Maynard A. Inequalities in health: an introductory editorial. *Health Econ.* 1999;8:281-282.
35. McGary H. Distrust, social justice, and health care. *Mt Sinai J Med.* 1999;66(4):236-240.
36. Moskop JC. Rawlsian justice and a human right to health care. *J Med Philos.* 1983;8:329-338.
37. Veatch RM. Justice in health care: the contribution of Edmund Pellegrino. *J Med Philos.* 1990;15:269-287.
38. Braveman P, Gruskin S. Defining equity in health. *J Epidemiol Community Health.* 2003;57:254-258.
39. Moscovitch A, Drover G. *Inequality: Essays on the Political Economy of Social Welfare.* Toronto, Canada: University of Toronto Press; 1981.
40. Bunton R, Macdonald G, eds. *Health Promotion: Disciplines and Diversity.* London, England: Routledge; 1992:171.
41. Gallagher EB, Ferrante J. Medicalisation and social justice. *Social Justice Research.* 1987;1(3):377-392.
42. Le Grand J. Equity, health and health care. *Social Justice Research.* 1987;1(3):257-274.
43. Sen A. *Commodities and Capabilities.* Amsterdam: Elsevier; 1985.
44. Doyal L, Gough I. *A Theory of Human Need.* Houndmills, Hampshire: Macmillan; 1991.
45. Watson L. *Neophilia: The Tradition of the New.* Seven Oaks, Kent, UK: Sceptre Books; 1989.
46. Stein JG. *The Cult of Efficiency.* Toronto, ON: House of Anansi; 2001.
47. Office of the High Commission of Human Rights. Universal Declaration of Human Rights. United Nations Department of Public Information.
48. American Occupational Therapy Association. Definition of Occupational Therapy Practice for the AOTA Model Practice Act; 2004.
49. Hart JT. The inverse care law. *Lancet.* 1971;Feb 27:405-412.
50. Report of a 1977 working party, chaired by Sir Douglas Black, Hart JT. The Black report: a challenge to politicians. *Lancet.* 1982;Jan 2:35-36.
51. Broadhead P. Social status and morbidity in Australia. *Community Health Studies.* 1985;IX(2):87-98.
52. Opit LJ. Economic policy and health care: the inverse care law in Australia. *New Doctor.* 1983;41-42:9-12.
53. Bee HL. *The Journey of Adulthood.* 4th ed. Upper Saddle River, NJ: Prentice Hall; 2000.
54. Shi L, Singh D. *Delivering Health Care in America: A Systems Approach.* Gaithersburg, Md: Aspen; 1998.
55. Marmot M, Smith G, Stansfield S, et al. Health inequalities and social class. In: Lee P, Este C, eds. *The Nations Health.* 4th ed. Boston: Jones & Bartlett; 1994.
56. Berger K. *The Developing Person Through the Lifespan.* New York: Worth; 1994.
57. Sussenberger B. Socioeconomic factors and their influence on occupational performance. In: Crepeau EB, Cohn ES, Schell BA, eds. *Willard & Spackman's Occupational Therapy.* 10th ed. Philadelphia: Lippincott, Williams & Wilkins; 2003:99.
58. Korten D. *When Corporations Rule the World.* West Hartford, Conn: Kumerian Press; 1955.
59. Werner D. *Health and Equity: Need for a People's Perspective in the Quest for World Health.* Conference: PHC21-Everybody's Business. Almaty, Kazakhstan: November 1998:2.
60. The Greens/Green Party USA. Home Page. Available at: http://www.greenparty.org. Accessed April 20, 2006.

61. Kronenberg F, Simo Algado S, Pollard N. *Occupational Therapy Without Borders: Learning From the Spirit of Survivors*. London: Elsevier Ltd; 2005:xv.

62. Smith DJ. *If the World Were a Village*. Toronto: Kits Can Press; 2002.

63. Farmer PE, Furin JJ, Katz JT. Global health equity. *Lancet*. 2004;May 29 (363):1832.

64. Kronenberg F, Pollard N. Overcoming occupational apartheid: a preliminary exploration of the political nature of occupational therapy. In: Kronenberg F, Simo Algado S, Pollard N, eds. *Occupational Therapy Without Borders: Learning From the Spirit of Survivors*. London: Elsevier Ltd; 2005:67.

65. Ruskin J. *Sesame and Lilies*. 13th ed. Orpington and London: George Allen; 1892:107.

66. Ramazzini B. *A Treatise of the Diseases of Tradesmen, Shewing the Various Influence of Particular Trades upon the State of Health; with the Best Methods to avoid or Correct It, and Useful Hints Proper to Be Minded in Regulating the Cure of all Diseases Incident to Tradesmen*. London: Andrew Bell et al; 1705.

67. Kalache A, Aboderin I, Hoskins I. Compression of morbidity and active aging: key priorities for public health policy in the 21st century. *Bulletin of the World Health Organization*; 2002;80(3):Genebra.

68. Kalache A, Keller I. The greying world. A challenge for the twenty-first century. *Science Progress*. 2000;83(Pt 1):33-54.

69. King H, Aubert RE, Herman WH. Global burden of diabetes, 1995-2025. *Diabetes Care*. 1998;21:1414-1430.

70. Kalache A. Future prospects for geriatric medicine in the developing countries. In: Yallis RC, Fillit HM, Brocklehurst JC, eds. *Textbook of Geriatric Medicine and Gerontology*. London: Churchill Livingstone; 1998:1513-1520.

71. Fries JF. The compression of morbidity. *N Eng J Med*. 1980:303(3);130-135.

72. Children's Rights Alliance. *UN Convention on the Rights of the Child*. Available at: http://www.childrensrights.ie/convention.php - 29k. Accessed January 2006.

73. United Nations. *The Convention on the Rights of the Child*. 1990. Available at: http://www.unicef.org/crc/. Accessed January 2006.

74. UNICEF. Rwanda Emergency Programme. Progress Report No. 1—May 1994-March 1995. Kigali, Rwanda: UNICEF; March 1995.

75. United Nations. State of the World's Children. United Nations Children's Fund (UNICEF), 1996.

76. United Nations. Impact of Armed Conflict on Children. United Nations, 1996.

77. Braveman PA. Health, equity, human rights, and the invasion of Iraq. *J Epidemiol Community Health*. 2003; 57:593.

78. Blom Cooper L. *An Emerging Profession in Health Care. Report of a Commission of Inquiry 1989*. London, UK: Duckworth; 1990.

79. Bockhoven JS. *Moral Treatment in Community Health Care*. New York: Springer Publishing Co, Inc; 1972.

80. Kinnell M. Sceptreless, free, uncircumscribed? Radicalism, dissent and early children's books. *British Journal of Educational Studies*. 1988;36(1):49-71.

81. World Health Organization. Ageing and Life Course Programme Policy Framework. Madrid, Spain: WHO Second UN World Assembly on Ageing; April 2002.

82. World Health Organization. International Association of Gerontology (IAG). Active Ageing: From Evidence to Action. Available at: http://www.who.int/hpr/aging. Accessed April 25, 2006.

83. United Nations. *International Year of Older People. Towards a Society for all Ages*. 1999. Available at: http://www.un.org/ecosocdev/geninfo/aging/aging-e.htm. Accessed January 2006.

84. International Forum on Globalization, 950 Lombard Street, San Francisco, CA 94133, USA.

85. Starbuck RA, Whitehead BJ, Holdsworth CR, et al. Occupational Justice Workshop. Australian Association of Occupational Therapists Conference. Canberra, Australia, April 1999.

86. Crombie S, French G, Wright-St Claire V. Occupational Justice Workshop. Australian Association of Occupational Therapists Conference. Canberra, Australia, April 1999.

87. Howard L, Gamble J, Bye R, Arblaster K, Dean P, Casley L. Occupational Justice Workshop. Australian Association of Occupational Therapists Conference. Canberra, Australia, April 1999.

88. United Nations. Declaration of Human Rights. Available at: http://www.hrweb.org/legal/udhr.html. Accessed April 20, 2006.

89. Thibeault, R. Fostering healing through occupation: the case of the Canadian Inuit. *Journal of Occupational Science*. 2002;9:153-158.

90. Thibeault R, Forget A. From snow to sand: CBR perspectives from the Arctic and Africa. *Canadian Journal of Rehabilitation*. 1997;10(2):134-140.

91. Thibeault R. Connecting health and social justice: a Lebanese experience. In: Kronenberg F, Simo Algado S, Pollard N, eds. *Occupational Therapy Without Borders: Learning From the Spirit of Survivors*. London: Elsevier Ltd; 2005.

92. Thibeault R. Occupation and the rebuilding of civic society: notes from the war zone. *Journal of Occupational Science*. 2002;9(1):38-47.

93. Meredith. Postcards from the Field. Summer 2004. Zambia, Africa: street kids international. Available at: http://www.streetkids.org. Accessed April 25, 2006.

94. School of Occupational Therapy. University of South Australia; 1998.

95. Hodges A. Health promotion and disease prevention for the disabled. *Journal of Allied Health*. 1986;Nov.

96. Johnson J. Wellness and occupational therapy. *Am J Occup Ther*. 1986;40(11):753-758.

97. Denzin NK. *Symbolic Interactionism and Cultural Studies*. Oxford, UK: Blackwell; 1992:145.

98. Fraser N. *Unruly Practices*. Minneapolis, Minn: University of Minnesota Press; 1989:107.

Suggested Reading

Bockhoven JS. Occupational therapy: a neglected source of community rehumanization. In: *Moral Treatment in Community Health Care*. New York: Springer Publishing Co, Inc; 1972.

Daniels NB, Kennedy P, et al. Why justice is good for our health: the social determinants of health inequalities. *Daedalus*. 1999;128(4):215-251.

Office of the High Commission of Human Rights. *Universal Declaration of Human Rights*. United Nations Department of Public Information.

Ramazzini B. *A Treatise of the Diseases of Tradesmen, Shewing the Various Influence of Particular Trades Upon the State of Health; with the Best Methods to Avoid or Correct It, and Useful Hints Proper to Be Minded in Regulating the Cure of All Diseases Incident to Tradesmen*. London: printed for Andrew Bell et al; 1705.

Thibeault, R. Fostering healing through occupation: the case of the Canadian Inuit. *Journal of Occupational Science*. 2002;9:153-158

Thibeault R. Occupation and the rebuilding of civic society: Notes from the war zone. *Journal of Occupational Science*. 2002;9(1):38-47.

Townsend E. Muriel Driver Memorial Lecture: occupational therapy's social vision. *Can J Occup Ther*. 1993; 60(4):174-184.

Townsend EA, Wilcock AA. Occupational Justice. In: Christiansen CH, Townsend EA, eds. *Introduction to Occupation: The Art and Science of Living*. Upper Saddle River, NJ: Pearson Education Inc; 2004.

Werner D. Health and Equity: Need for a People's Perspective in the Quest for World Health. Conference: PHC21- Everybody's Business. Almaty, Kazakhstan: November 1998.

Young IM. *Justice and the Politics of Difference*. Princeton, NJ: Princeton University Press; 1990.

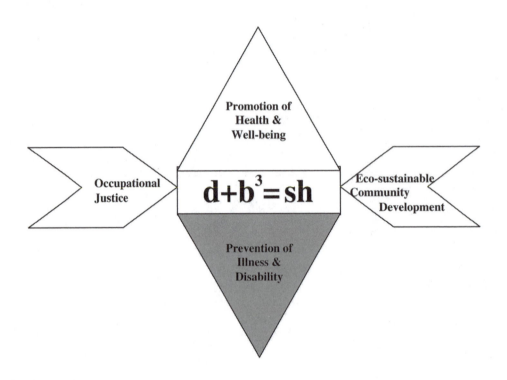

9

OCCUPATION-FOCUSED PREVENTIVE APPROACH TO ILLNESS AND DISABILITY

Theme 9:

"A few largely preventable risk factors account for most of the world's disease burden. This reflects a significant change in diet habits and physical activity levels worldwide as a result of industrialization, urbanization, economic development and increasing food market globalization."
WHO, *Global Strategy on Diet, Physical Activity and Health*, 2004

"It is often less costly to prevent disease than to treat it. For example, it has been estimated that a one-dollar investment in measures to encourage moderate physical activity leads to a cost saving of $3.2 in medical costs (US Centers for Disease Control, 1999)."
WHO, *Active Aging: A Policy Framework*, 2002

The chapter addresses:
* The concept of occupation-focused prevention of illness and disability
* What is an occupation-focused preventive approach to illness and disability?
* Why an occupation-focused preventive approach to illness and disability is necessary
  * "Poverty is the greatest threat"
  * Urbanization
  * Increased drug abuse and civil and domestic violence
  * Decrease of physical activity
* An action-research approach to occupation-focused prevention of illness and disability

The third of the 4 approaches to be considered in the final chapters is concerned with occupation-focused prevention of illness and disability (OPID). Its title suggests that illness and disability could be reduced and in some cases prevented by what people do or do not do. This points to the need to become clearer about the negative, as well as the positive, health consequences of occupation. That there are negative consequences has been identified throughout the text, as well as some aspects having been recognized as particular problems within public health. This is so with regard to paid employment specifically and to some of the effects of lack of physical exercise. The latter is reflected in the first of this chapter's themes that could apply to all occupation, not just physical activity. However, few studies have addressed preventing illness and disability in the holistic terms of all the things that people want, need, or have to do; what it means to them; or the physical, mental, and social outcomes. In this sphere, as in others, prevention of social problems is usually considered separately. Perhaps because of the enormity of the task, health studies have not yet managed to concertedly research the effects of national policies about a range of social issues from this holistic occupation and health perspective. The concept is very complex but unless it is addressed more thoroughly, occupation-specific preventive approaches would be incomplete, even though beneficial, in some respects.

To illustrate the complexity in a small way, the public health concerns about cigarette smoking can be considered briefly. Approaches to stop the habit have concentrated, in the main, on shocking people about the hazards of smoking itself rather than on why they might find it so necessary or comforting to take up the habit in the first place and what other forms of doing it replaces, supplements, or enhances. Peer pressure, the greed of multinational tobacco companies, and advertising are often blamed and rightly so, but to take a more holistic stance, from an occupational perspective for example, requires consideration of what basic needs are fulfilled by taking it up, what occupational needs are not met to make it necessary or possible to ignore the many and various warnings, a teasing out of what cigarette smoking replaces in terms of millennia past, and whether or not there could be changes in lifestyle and occupation across the board that would reduce the incidence. It reminds me of Lorenz's very useful question about behavior in general, but applied to smoking: what has smoking to do with survival? Restated: can the origins of behavior that have similar traits, benefits, or challenges to smoking be traced and what purpose did they serve? Alternatively, are there occupations that reduce the incidence of smoking or that are so appealing that they replace the habit? Armed with such knowledge, strategies to reduce the incidence of smoking might be more wide ranging.

To illustrate the complexity in another way that is true to the notion of physical, mental, and social health is to consider the range of "prevention organizations"—that is, those organizations that are committed to preventing some aspect of present existence that is deemed counterproductive to personal, community, or world health. Types of prevention such organizations address often include prevention of poverty; prevention of illness such as cancer, HIV/AIDS, STDs, TB, obesity-related disorders, noncommunicable disorders, and mental illness; prevention of work-related illness or accidents; prevention of behaviors such as suicide, drug, alcohol, or other substance abuse; school drop outs; bullying; cruelty to or abuse of children; teen pregnancies; family, sexual, and youth violence; juvenile delinquency; gang behavior; and terrorism; as well as pollution and ecological degradation.

A holistic occupation-focused approach could be useful for any of those issues and would be new to public health practitioners but complementary to or extending other forms of prevention that they commonly use. To them, uncovering the causes of medical diagnosed illness and disease has been, and remains, the lynch pin of practice. It is also the focus of epidemiological research notwithstanding the holistic philosophy of the OCHP[1] and *Jakarta Declaration*,[2] which have been adopted as the basis of the "new public health" movement.[3] Preventive approaches generally take for granted a medical science explanation of the cause of disease and the mechanisms for prevention. On the whole, these approaches have been remarkably successful, especially as primary prevention of illness and disability is important to people in all parts of the world. However, perhaps because of that focus, little attention has been paid to OPID, except to a limited degree in control of obesity, cardiovascular disease, and work-related occupational disorders.

OPID is, perhaps, 1 of the 4 approaches nearest to occupational therapy practices of the past few decades because it addresses illness and disability as defined by conventional medicine. However, to be true to the potential range of issues it could address that would only provide the starting place for a much more holistic stance. Another difference for occupational therapists would be that it seeks to prevent the occurrence of illness and disability, as well as providing services to assist people to reduce the ongoing impact of them. It is both preventive approaches to medically defined physical and mental illness and disability at primary, secondary, and tertiary levels as well as social and occupational illness that will be considered in this chapter. Consideration will focus on occupational causation or intervention strategies with particular reference to current and anticipated disorders or issues of concern because of their actual or expected prevalence.

The first section considers the concept of this approach. This will tell some of the tale of the battles that initiated the development of public health and preventive medicine. The story is fascinating but readers can do more than be interested; they can also learn about how changing the status quo can be achieved with determination and belief in the justice and truth of the potential outcome and the action required, whatever the odds. Additional to that story is another of the long-held belief that occupational therapists have a valuable contribution to make to the prevention of illness for all people, not just those who are sick or disabled. Now, with the WHO call for partnerships to make better health for all a reality, might be the time to reawaken occupational therapy's "preventive" potential.

The Concept of Occupation-Focused Prevention of Illness and Disability

A simple definition of prevention is "fending off problems before they emerge."[4] Disease prevention is the name given to action usually emanating from the health sector about risk factors and risk behaviors.[5] It is commonly referred to as preventive medicine. In affluent countries, preventive medicine is often implemented by general medical practitioners who use population-based studies as a foundation for advice or prescriptions to protect individuals against disease agents. In developing countries, it is best known for methods such as immunization, vaccination, and screening, as well as for social initiatives like encouragement of breast feeding, particularly where nutrition is poor, and environmental engineering pertaining to matters like quarantine and sanitation. The OPID approach could come under the umbrella of preventive medicine that is closely linked to public health, both historically and at present, but adding to it innovative thought and direction and a broader approach to social illness and disability that reflects some of the ideas raised in previous chapters.

Preventive medicine emphasizes early diagnosis with consequent retardation of disability and illness and it is viewed erroneously by many as what is meant by the term *health promotion*. This misconception has a historical foundation when the 2 ideas were frequently discussed together and became entwined in thought. Leaders of public health such as Last, an author of some note in the field, provide an example of such entwining when writing of the need for "... more effective health promotion programs aimed at smoking cessation, reduced alcohol use, nutrition, exercise, stress reduction, and control of violent behavior...."[6] that are largely preventive initiatives. Such issues are heavily represented in the research topics that are most frequently addressed within preventive medicine with the addition of prevalent diseases across the world and the hazards of paid employment.[6,7] Last believes that all public health practitioners "share a common reliance on one scientific discipline, epidemiology"[6] despite the different strategies of health educators, industrial hygienists, and sanitary engineers. The most fundamental purpose of epidemiology, he says, is to "supply information, and ways to interpret it, for the diagnosis and measurement of the health problems of the population."[6]

Prevention of illness through epidemiological research aimed at "early preclinical factors" is the most influential aspect of public health in affluent societies and attracts the most resources. This has been the case for at least 2 decades despite a stated commitment to social health, as evident in the Australian Commonwealth Department of Community Services and Health's brief summary of WHO's appeal for "Health for All by the Year 2000":

> *In addition to the availability of suitable health services at a cost the country can afford, it also means a personal state of well-being and a state of health that enables each person to lead a socially and economically productive life. Therefore, member states will continue to consider obstacles to health such as ignorance, malnutrition, poor housing, unemployment, and contaminated drinking water just as important as other considerations such as the lack of nurses and doctors, drugs, vaccines, or hospital beds.*[8]

The medical view of prevention is so pervasive that the pursuit of a medically defined disease-free state is the idea that prevails, although in recent years, public health has recovered the notions of social medicine, which studies the "social behavior of human beings and their external environment."[9] Occasionally, this extends to how people "work and play" in many different cultures. Epidemiologists' concentration though is on specific, known social habits and their effects on physical and mental states of health, and it does not, to any extent, extend preventive approaches into the realm of social or occupational (in the broader sense) illness. That still, largely, remains the domain of social planners and economic policy.

While epidemiological research embraces some, but not all, notions about occupation and health, at least since the mid 1970s it has been accepted that there are "associations between much of this human behavior and human health and disease."[9] Douglas Gordon, who was a medically trained pioneer of social medicine in Australia, suggests that the practice of social medicine includes coming to understand the motives, values, social organizations, and structures of different cultures, as well as the "philosophies and essential mysteries of human behaviors insofar as these affect health."[9] At about the same time, Reilly was arguing for occupational therapists to recognize better the power of occupation and the basic links between it and health.[10-13] Additionally, a group of leaders in the field with a preventive and wellness perspective to health care was encouraging them to aim, through occupation, at "maintaining optimum health rather than ... intermittent treatment of acute disease and disability."[14] Some occupational therapists have speculated on reasons for this, with Brown advancing that it erupted from the illness-oriented medical model for several reasons, such as advances in technology, concurrent escalation of health care costs, a general increase of health care knowledge leading to the dominant role of physicians being challenged, and a societal reaction against the complexities of modern medicine toward simpler, more natural remedies.[15] Johnson suggested that the interest was part of the human potential and countercultural movements, in which many groups, particularly women and minorities, reacted to social forces that seemed to ignore their individual, perceived needs.[16] Like Brown, she cited growing dissatisfaction with medicine and perceived dehumanization in the medical care system as important factors, along with increasing recognition of ways in which the world was being polluted.[16] In that vein, West (Figure 9-1) envisaged that health and medical care in the future would "emphasize human development by programs designed to promote better adaptation, rather than technologically oriented programs offering specific solutions to specific disabilities."[17] She held that the occupational therapist should function as "health agent [rather than therapist] with responsibility to help ensure normal growth and development,"

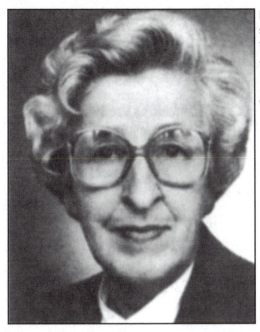

Figure 9-1. Wilma West. (Republished with permission of American Occupational Therapy Association, from American Occupational Therapy Association. *A Professional Legacy: The Eleanor Clarke Slagle Lectures.* Rockville, Md: Author; 1985:309. Permission conveyed through Copyright Clearance Center, Inc.)

considering more fully the "socio-economic and cultural as well as biological causes of disease and dysfunction," but all in a "new mold" rather than a recast of an earlier prototype.[14,17,18] Shortly afterward, she proposed a health model for occupational therapy practice based on the assumption that health care in the decade ahead would be as concerned with prevention as with rehabilitation. Therefore, she advocated more effective methods to enhance and enrich development of physical, mental, emotional, social, and vocational abilities and suggested a "timely translation" of occupational therapists' "long time focus on activities of daily living for the disabled to advocacy of the balanced regimen of age appropriate, work play activities for man in the pre-disease/disability phase."[19] Her view that such a role required only a "broader application of existing knowledge about the effects of activity—or its absence—on health"[19] was an invitation to occupational therapists to revisit and use their underlying philosophy in a way advocated in this text.

Along similar lines, Cromwell advocated for occupational therapists to become specialists in human behavior in ordinary environments where patients live, work, and play. She stated a need to think about the global trend toward preventive rather than curative programs, about world health care, and about searching for more universal systems of care by considering, for example, how different nations combat the problems facing them.[20] These views were compatible with emerging conceptualizations about the nature of health held by other leaders in the field at that time such as Mosey and Fidler. Mosey defined health needs as "inherent human requirements that must be met for an individual to experience a sense of physical, psychological and social well-being,"[21] and Fidler held that health is the ability to carry out activities that are essential for developmentally appropriate self-maintenance and meeting of intrinsic needs according to the social context.[22]

Some therapists, such as Wiemer, Finn, Grossman, and Laukaran, promoted preventive approaches as potentially important aspects of occupational therapist's work in community health.[23-27] Finn observed that for the majority of therapists who practiced in the community at that time, there was a trend to select programs and services at the levels of secondary and tertiary prevention, an observation that still holds some truth. To encourage involvement in primary prevention, in line with Reilly, she proposed the development of a model of practice addressing the issue of the significance of occupation to human life. She argued that because primary prevention is directed toward an understanding of both the relationship between the basic structural elements of society and health and of what keeps people in a state of health, occupational therapists should make their contribution with a greater understanding of the effects of occupation on health.[25]

Occupational therapists have a surprisingly long history of interest in prevention, although many will be unaware that as early as 1934 in Canada it was being recognized that occupational therapists had a potential role in the community in preventing ill health. At that time, Le Vesconte suggested that, in combination with social workers, occupational therapists should be involved in social and economic reorganization to that end.[28,29] Unfortunately, this direction got lost in medicalization of professional offerings and did not re-emerge until the work already discussed in the 1960s and 1970s drew attention to it once more. The concerted push from those far-sighted leaders was optimistic at that time; few real changes to practice eventuated, perhaps because of economic constraints that curbed the development of trends toward prevention that were not yet a priority in health planning. The work itself may have appeared less defined, less sophisticated, less measurable, more isolating, and daunting in the face of the massive social, economic, and political conditions that interfere with health.[26] Other reasons could have been limited opportunities or lack of professional incentives for service in positions not specifically designated for occupational therapists, competition with other professionals, and inability to cross boundaries.[27] The lack of action at that time may have been compounded by occupational therapy's long-term association with clinically based medicine concerned with ill, rather than all, people. People in need of "occupation-focused preventive approaches" may not be "referred through medical channels, since they are not diseased but are disengaged from daily life."[30]

The concept of OPID extends into the concept of social and occupational illnesses, as mentioned earlier. These are not necessarily manifest in medically defined mind or body ailments, although they may be. Such illnesses are evident in maladaptive behaviors, stress, frustration, boredom, aggression, and so forth and in some cases, can be early identifying factors in later manifest medical diagnosis or lead to death though suicide. Epidemiological methods could be used to assist with discovering sequelae or connections; however, exploration of OPID must also depend on other quantitative and qualitative tools to capture the holistic, interactive, and complex nature of human doings and their relationships to illness and disability. Some of the complexity is obvious in a pre-public health summation by Robert Owen (mentioned earlier and obviously a man of great vision) who recommended in the 19th century "the discovery of the means, and the adoption of the practice, to prevent disease of body and mind are necessary."[31] The scroll on the next page provides some insights into Owen's views on a preventive approach to illness.

> ... members of the medical profession know that the health of society is not to be obtained or maintained by medicines; that it is far better, far more easy, and far wiser, to adopt substantive measures to prevent disease of the body or mind, than to allow substantive measures to remain continually to generate causes to produce physical and mental disorders.
>
> *Owen R. Works of Robert Owen: Volume 3: Book of the New Moral World. (Pickering Masters Series). London: Pickering & Chatto (Publishers Ltd.);1993:156.*
>
> ...the prevention of disease will be obtained only when arrangements shall be formed, to well educate, physiologically, every man, woman, and child, so as to enable them to understand their own physical and mental nature; in order that they may learn to exercise, at the proper period of life, all their natural faculties, propensities and powers, up to the point of temperance; neither falling short, nor exceeding in any of them, or discontent and disease must necessarily follow.
>
> *Owen R.* Paper: Dedicated to the Governments of Great Britain, Austria, Russia, France, Prussia and the United States of America. *London: New Lanark Conservation; 1841.*

Owen's early 19th century occupation-focused preventive doctrine was founded on his belief that "disease is not the natural state of man"[31] and that what people do, be, and become is integral to their health or illness. Pre-empting the ideas about occupational alienation, imbalance, deprivation, and boredom set out in this book, he suggested that in a "perfect" world, "the physical sciences will have rendered unnecessary all severe, unhealthy or even unpleasant labour" and "idleness and uselessness will be unknown."[31,32] A well-read social reformer with great insight, Owen might well have been aware of the work of Lettsom, a late 18th century British medical reformer who had warned that the filthy, overcrowded slums that housed workers in the emerging industrial economy, combined with ignorance, had created ideal conditions for epidemics to occur. As a result of his warning, parishes were empowered by an act of Parliament to levy a rate for civic maintenance such as street cleaning and refuse-disposal.[33]

The act was insufficient to counter the illness resulting from the occupational change from agriculture to industry and subsequent escalating populations in town and cities. Additionally, pollution, slum housing, and lack of amenities such as water, sanitation, and waste disposal led to regular outbreaks of cholera in plague proportions. As mentioned in Chapter 1, it was a lawyer, Sir Edwin Chadwick (1800–1890), who led the social reform that resulted in the emergence of public health. His 1842 *Report on the Sanitary Condition of the Labouring Population of Great Britain* warned the public of the unhealthiness of urban areas.[34] Chadwick was an "anti-contagionist" and, with like-minded sanitarians, believed that disease resulted from atmospheric contamination caused by sewage, polluted water, and industrial waste. It was clear to them that sanitary engineering such as plentiful supplies of clean drinking water and underground drainage was necessary in urban environments. In 1848 a public health act was passed, and Chadwick was appointed a member of a general board of health empowered to act or prosecute on such issues as water, drainage, disposal of rubbish, slaughterhouses, poisonous fumes, and suspect food establishments. Those were the understood concerns of public health for over a century, and it was these that are deemed to have resulted in a decrease in morbidity and mortality statistics that overshadows significantly those attributable to modern medicine.[33,35]

Chadwick's interests in public health encompassed planning healthy home environments, the provision of public recreation grounds, and the conditions in which children worked.[36] Prior to the industrial revolution, children's work was an integral aspect of family life and economy, where they learned adult skills, roles, and traditions from their parents. In the world of industry, their work was radically transformed. Children often had to endure a harsh regime and long working hours that were deemed to be acceptable even by spokespeople for the medical profession. Physician Edward Holme, for example, denied the harmful effects of long hours of labor, while surgeon Thomas Wilson saw no necessity to permit recreation.[37] Not all members of the medical profession held those views. Indeed, it was physician and social reformer Thomas Southwood-Smith's *Report on the Physical Causes of Sickness and Mortality to Which the Poor Are Particularly Exposed* that was influential in developing Chadwick's ideas. Southwood-Smith early in his career argued for the alleviation of suffering and an increase of human happiness no matter what social change was required. With that in mind, he tackled social reform head on, and played a significant role in overturning occupational health and safety hazards in industry and the mines.[37] In 1832, when he was appointed by a parliamentary commission to look into the issues of concern, he, with Chadwick and economist, Thomas Tooke, ensured that a questionnaire on the health of employed children was sent to medical practitioners in the heartland of industrial development. The Factory Act of 1833 incorporated the work of the commission, including clauses that spelled out that children under 13 could not work for more than 8 hours a day and not at night, and those less than 9 were not permitted to work in textile mills at all. Additionally, children were subject to medical inspection and were to receive a minimum of 2 hours schooling each working day.[32] In a supplementary report, the incidence and nature of industrial disease and injury was identified. These included respiratory problems, fatigue, and monotony as dangers, as well as accidents from unprotected machinery.[37] It was 7 years later that a Royal Commission of Inquiry was established to look into conditions in mines. Tooke and Southwood-Smith were 2 of the commissioners. The report addressed the conditions of employment such as hours, wages, meal-breaks, clothing, holidays, the incidence and type of accidents, and health issues. It found that women and children as young as 6 were employed underground in certain pits. Ten or 12 hours a day was usual, many in conditions that were socially, mentally, and physically brutal with the result that many suffered rheumatism caused by continuous damp and appeared old and worn beyond their years (Figure 9-2). Southwood-Smith's medical evidence graphically illustrated, in a unique addition to a parliamentary report, how the work produced fatigue, extraordinary muscular development, stunted growth, crippled gait, and skin disorders providing an unequivocal link between occupation and ill health. This report shocked the nation and despite clamorous opposition of mine-owners, public outrage led to the 1842 Act to Prohibit the Employment of Women and Girls in Mines and Collieries, and to Regulate the Employment of Boys.[34,37]

Sir William Osler (1849–1919) claimed there is no doubt:

> … that it was in the field of prevention of disease that modern medicine attained its greatest achievements. Our life is no longer shortened by diseases such as leprosy, plague, smallpox, and rabies. Our life expectation is about twice as long as it was half a century ago.[38]

Despite this accolade, medicine was not the dominant force in early public or preventive health even though it is regarded as one of its branches.[32] American medical historian Sigerist hypothesized that what he described as the new hygienic movement started in

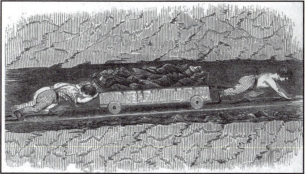

Figure 9-2. Drawing by Margaret Gillies in the 1840 "Blue Book" recording the Royal Commission of Inquiry into Conditions in Mines shows 3 young children pulling and pushing a loaded wagon of coals. The child in front is harnessed by chain and belt. (Reprinted with permission of The Wellcome Library.)

England in a practical way because the industrial revolution began there and dominated life in the 19th century. He claimed that medicine could not successfully fight disease alone largely because "hygiene and public health, like medicine at large, are but an aspect of the general civilization of the time, and are largely determined by the cultural conditions of that time."[38]

Preventive approaches based on social and environmental engineering grew and continued in affluent societies as departments of public health largely outside medicine but, perhaps, with a medical officer in charge. As epidemiological research advanced, that began to change, more medically trained health workers became interested, and the nature of prevention focused more on internal physiology and the detection of factors that might lead to epidemics of both infectious and other diseases. The new public health revitalized by the WHO "health for all" rhetoric of Alma Ata and OCHP expanded to embrace a new social consciousness of ecological, cultural, and behavioral factors that urgently required attention. The promise has still to be realized because resources are limited, the public of affluent societies remains captivated by the promise of cure, and it is only from time to time that their conscience is stirred to address illness, disease, and death in massive proportions outside their experience and nations.

One of the major tasks of the WHO is preventing and combating disease through both medical and social engineering, especially in developing countries such as in Africa, South America, and an expanded Europe. Perhaps, surprisingly, the latter has almost as many social health problems as Africa (Ziglio E, oral communication, June 10, 2005). In the field of prevention, WHO coordinates international efforts to monitor outbreaks of infectious disease, delivers programs to combat and eradicate diseases by developing and distributing vaccines, conducts research, carries out worldwide campaigns to boost or discourage consumption of products according to their health effects, and issues binding scientific and medical assessments of drugs and recommendations as to their use.[39] By its publications, declarations, and charters, the WHO most importantly leads debate about ways forward and challenges those involved in public health and prevention of illness to think and act outside the "medical square."

The concept of occupation-focused prevention presented here is one way to do that. It is appropriate to consider whether occupational risk factors can be prevented even though they are very complex. It is certainly possible to identify "occupational" risk factors to health and well-being by considering already completed research undertaken for other reasons. With a focus on occupational imbalance, deprivation, and alienation as risks to health, studies from education and sociopolitical fields are relevant as well as what is reported in health, medical, and preventive medicine literature. More research is needed, but even so, there is sufficient knowledge to claim that the concept is in line with public health conventions as well as WHO directives aimed at the "absence of illness" through preventive approaches based on known risks.

What Is an Occupation-Focused Preventive Approach to Illness and Disability?

I define an occupation-focused approach to the prevention of illness and disability as the application of medical, behavioral, social, and occupational science to prevent physiological, psychological, social, and occupational illness; accidents; and disability; and to prolong quality of life for all people through advocacy and mediation and through occupation-focused programs aimed at enabling people to do, be, and become according to their natural health needs.

In the first edition of this book, I addressed a preventive approach in a way that was closely compatible with and based on a wide variety of preventive medicine literature. I defined it then as "the application of Western medical and social science to prevent disease, prolong life, and promote health in the community through intercepting disease processes." I have chosen in this edition to extend the approach to emphasize the direction that an occupational perspective might provide. Like conventional medicine, the original version was a reductionist, illness model aimed at populations and individuals, often underpinned by population-based epidemiological studies. It was aimed at protection against disease agents by methods such as immunization, vaccination, screening, and some social and environmental engineering, emphasizing early diagnosis with consequent retardation of disability and focused on preventing illness that was deemed complementary to or the same as promoting well-being.

This new approach is occupation-focused; is also applicable to populations, communities, and individuals; and is aimed at reducing not only the experience of physical and mental illness, but also social and occupational illness that may or may not manifest in medically related conditions. Based on medical, epidemiological, behavioral, social, and/or occupational science, it accepts that people influence the state of their health through what they do. That is, they can improve their experience of health or reduce illness as well as disability as a direct or indirect result of what they do, feeling satisfied or good about what they do, and meeting their needs and biological potentials. These mechanisms have been explored within the text as natural means to maintain and improve health and to ensure long-term survival. In this chapter, it is maintained that doing, being, and becoming advisedly and wisely can assist with overcoming illness and disability. This is the central tenet of OPID.

The approach is one that supplies information for the other approaches, as well as being a platform of intervention in its own right. It is here that research is undertaken to test the truth or strength of associations that can then be applied to advice or intervention strategies. The information can be reductionist or holistic in nature dependent on the best type of research to elicit particular forms of knowledge. All types are needed if this and the other approaches are to be holistic. Large scale empirical studies are usually undertaken by full time researchers over a long period of time so it is unlikely, but not impossible, that action-research groups from within a community will choose this type of approach, but they could use the data from other large studies in combination with their own to inform what they do or to assist with advocacy or mediation processes. Qualitative and critical forms of research will generally form the substance of the action-research because, for example, it is difficult to find out how people feel about what they do by reductionist methodologies that seek at all costs to reduce bias. It is also difficult to find out about people's aspirations and potential through those means. The chosen ways of gaining such information are often small-scale studies in comparison to those deemed acceptable by epidemiologists, research granting, or national funding bodies who have been influenced by the rhetoric and effectiveness of that type of research. This means that, often, epidemiologists, the medical research fraternity, the media, or the general public may not take some valuable research seriously. Much that is useful and good lays molding in archives. That is probably truer for qualitative rather than quantitative studies. On the other side of the coin, much that is useful and good may be overlooked in striving to be holistic; for example, it might be easy to overlook the significance of information about chronobiology or biological rhythms when grappling with preventive issues such as bullying, binge drinking, or accidents.[40]

Research concentrating on why people succumb to unhealthy lifestyles and habits is necessary but is rare. Public health maintains a long tradition of epidemiological research that could be useful for some aspects of discovery but does not embrace the most suitable research methods to explore the more complex interactive occupation-based determinants of illness. This necessitates both critical and qualitative, phenomenological methodologies being recognized as valid research tools to use in conjunction with conventional quantitative epidemiology. Qualitative methodologies are well suited to exploring the occupational aspects from this wider view of public health, as well as the more restricted perspective of the relationship between illness and occupational hazards. Using qualitative methodologies, along with critical research approaches, it is possible to extend both the direction and the range of exploration to include underlying determinants based on long-held occupational beliefs and structures.

Occupational science is a new discipline and its research is particularly vulnerable to neglect. Closely allied time-use researchers have a longer history, and the results of studies in that field could be particularly useful as foundation material for OPID action-research. All types add to the knowledge base, and important to the OPID approach is an understanding of how to promulgate valuable findings of either a positive or negative nature widely so that effort is not wasted and new ways forward are found. The new ways might be based on combining apparently vastly different findings and types of research into a new synthesis in the same way that histories of ideas unify and correlate things that often appear unconnected. Table 9-1 outlines contrasting research paradigms.

That people are occupational beings is the foundation belief of this approach as it is of the other three. The approach also holds that natural health is attained and maintained and illness prevented through engagement in occupation in line with the results of the exploration that provides the basis of the text. Such engagement has got to meet the physiological requirements for physical, mental, and social exercise that results in the well-working of the organism as a whole and, as well, provides socioculturally valued and individual meaning and purpose, and the opportunity to grow and develop according to biological capacity. If such engagement is also inclusive of meeting the basic prerequisites for survival and health for all members of the world's population, then physical, mental, social, and occupational illness will be reduced.

The WHO in the *Jakarta Declaration* points out the current challenges to the prerequisites for health. All are related in some way to people's occupations, but among them are some that are very closely associated. "Poverty is the greatest threat" and "demographic trends such as urbanization," "increased sedentary behavior," "increased drug abuse, and civil and domestic violence threaten the health and well-being of hundreds of millions of people."[2] Other factors with a significant impact on what people do or do not do and that could be damaging or beneficial to health, include transnational factors relating to:

Table 9-1

Contrasting Research Paradigms That Could Inform Occupation-Focused Approaches to Prevention of Illness and Disability

Research Paradigms

	Quantitative	Qualitative	Critical
Nature	Reductionist Positivist Predetermined structure	Holistic Interpretive Flexible as ideas emerge	Embedded in society Interactive, participa-tory Flexible and dynamic
Purpose	Test hypotheses Test empirical observation Measure Discover laws Generalize	Explore Understand subjective realities Discover meanings	Uncover inequity Facilitate social action
Values	Value free Objective	Value bound Subjective	Value laden Cannot be value free
Examples of research methods for OPID	Cohort, case-control, and cross sectional studies Vital, health, and popula-tion statistics Measurement of bio-rhy-thms, biomechanics, etc Surveys and questionnaires Time-use diaries Experience sampling	Questionnaires Time-use diaries Experience sampling In-depth interview Focus groups Field observation	Quantitative data Questionnaires Time-use diaries Experience sampling In-depth interview Focus groups Field observation Critical praxis Self-reflection History of ideas

Adapted from Wilcock A. Biological and sociocultural perspectives on time use studies. In: Pentland WE, Harvey AS, Powell Lawton M, McColl MA, eds. *Time Use Research in the Social Sciences.* New York: Kluwer Academic; 1999:195.

> ... the global economy, financial markets and trade, wide access to media and com-munications technology, and environmental degradation as a result of the irresponsible use of resources. These changes shape people's values, their lifestyles throughout the lifespan, and living conditions across the world.[2]

People need information about how what they do results in or changes the experience of physical, mental, and social illness because they need information about other causes of or factors in illness. Indeed, it is perhaps even more important because it is informa-tion that people can work with day by day to improve health for themselves. It is here, particularly, that the modern world could learn from the approaches used to promulgate the *Regimen Sanitatis*. This implies that the information given out about physical, mental, social, and occupational illness should be inclusive of every aspect possible, however basic or apparently insignificant. What is required is not only the great medical break-throughs of contemporary science that are the meat of current media releases. To begin to understand the diverse complexity of occupational impacts on illness, quantitative, qualitative, and critical research needs to be diverse, inclusive, and integrated prior to dissemination. Integration of research findings from various fields has the potential to both assist policy development and personal and community action to reduce illness. Broad-minded watchdogs are probably required to make this happen.

Because of such diverse and complex issues, limited attention to or selectivity with regard to types of research that are attended to slows down the process of understanding and ignores people's interactive physiology and sociopolitical environmental dependence. Information about the social and occupational nature of illness is as important as the physical and mental factors but infinitely more complex. Prevention of physical, mental, social, and occupational illness is a global responsibility, not the responsibility of medical science alone.

The underlying principles of this OPID are based on the notion that occupation should be a factor in the repair of illness as well as a source of health. In many cases, when people seek medical help or communities call for change in order to meet very real needs, the type and structure of what they can do day by day is seldom addressed except perhaps, sometimes, for minor adjustments. Instead, for individuals, medication is prescribed, x-rays ordered, food intake advised on, or exercise suggested. In terms of communities, peripheral adjustments are made such as changes of personnel, or investigative bodies are set up that carry out enquiries over months or years. The whole picture is seldom recognized, investigated, or attended to even though physical, mental, social, and occupational illness results from many interactive causes. The picture is too large and the societal structure of occupation to complex to grapple with. Yet, finding out how structural factors impact on what people do to meet basic requirements, the meaning they find, and the opportunity to meet biological potential for the majority rather than a few high achieving go-getters are important. Consider for a moment the accuracy of the oft-quoted saying that anyone could be president of the United States. It is far from accurate, even if true in theory. The same is true of all communal structures, for in none are everyone's different capacities recognized equally or even as positive factors; occupational chances are not given equally; potential is not recognized equally; and so it is only those who thrive in existing and particular societal structures who are advantaged in an ongoing way. That implies that some people are more likely than others to experience illness because of their occupations. Getting the balance as right as possible with as many as is practicable experiencing good health, or of engaging in occupations that improve their health if they become ill or disabled, would be a desirable outcome of OPID.

The *Jakarta Declaration* recognizes a clear need for new forms of action to prevent illness by addressing emerging threats to health. The boundaries that exist between public and private sectors and organizations throughout the world require breaching because cooperation is essential. The call for "the creation of new partnerships for health" provides the opportunity to those who recognize the connection between occupation and health to come together "on an equal footing" to help everyone address the prevention of illness through their daily doings. This may be achieved through research, through promoting social responsibility to reduce illness and disability, through protecting environments, and through helping to increase awareness of unhealthy aspects of occupation in all facets of life in an equitable and just way.[2]

In short, this approach looks to implement WHO objectives for preventing disease and reducing disability with a view to eventual integration of the understanding that occupation and health can impact on illness and disability in a negative or a positive way.

Table 9-2

Foundations of an Occupation-Focused Approach to Prevention of Illness and Disability

Basis of Approach	Underlying Beliefs	Underlying Principles
Applicable to populations, communities, and individuals	Humans are occupational beings, natural health is attained and maintained, and illness prevented through doing	Occupation should be both a source of health and a factor in the repair of illness
Aimed at reducing the experience of physical, mental, social, and occupational illness	Physical, mental, social, and occupational illness can be reduced	Physical, mental, social, and occupational illness result from many interactive causes
Based on medical, epidemiological, behavioral, social, and occupational science	Research and information given out about physical, mental, social, and occupational illness should be inclusive; holistic, as well as reductionist	Limited attention to or selectivity with regards to particular types of research slows down the process of understanding and ignores people's interactive physiology
People influence the state of their health through what they do	People need information about how what they do affects physical, mental, and social illness	Information about the social and occupational nature of illness is as important as the physical and mental factors
Is informative, can be reductionist and/or holistic	Integration of research findings from various fields will assist policies and action to reduce illness	Quantitative, qualitative, and critical research needs to be integrating and disseminated
Is diverse, addressing many different and interactive causes of illness	Prevention of physical, mental, social, and occupational illness is a global responsibility	Diversity and inclusiveness of preventive research

Increasing awareness within the population at large would be a valuable starting place. Encouraging sociopolitical processes and policies to consider occupational health effects of legislation in a much broader way than currently is essential in the longer term and will not be achieved without a gradual increase of understanding (Table 9-2).

Why an Occupation-Focused Preventive Approach to Illness and Disability Is Necessary

The *Declaration of Alma Ata* proclaimed that "primary health care includes at least: education about the prevailing health problems and the methods of preventing and controlling them...."[41] The WHO claims that:

Chronic diseases are now the major cause of death and disability worldwide. Noncommunicable conditions, including cardiovascular diseases (CVD), diabetes, obesity, cancer and respiratory diseases, now account for 59% of the 57 million deaths annually and 46% of the global burden of disease.[42]

The WHO and others in the public health fraternity have also recognized that policies to improve a population's social experience and environment could be more important than improving individual health using medicine.[43] As previously shown, this was certainly the case in the 19th century. While the societal and environmental changes are different in the present time, they are similarly injurious to health. It has been said that the greatest effects could be achieved by "investing in policies that promote sustainable development, protect the environment, promote equity and tackle the social gradient of health."[43] These can be as varied as reducing inequalities in child development and education, improving the quality of life of older people,[44-46] improving parenting, improving recreational opportunities, reducing consumption of fossil fuel by encouraging walking or cycling,[47-52] or persuading politicians to adopt innovative population-based policies, all of which can be tackled from an occupational perspective.[43]

Also requiring urgent preventive measures are new and re-emerging infectious diseases, mental health problems, and a high prevalence of chronic NCDs, as the number of older people increases in all parts of the world.[2] McKeown has pointed to NCDs being a response to "conditions that have arisen in the last few centuries"[53] acting on a genetic constitution suited to the lifestyles of at least 100,000 years ago, some of which have occurred on a large scale only from the last century:

Living conditions have changed profoundly since industrialization, in ways that might be expected to prejudice both physical and mental health: increased size and density of populations; transfer from rural to urban life; reduction of fibre and increase of fat, sugar and salt in the diet; increased use of tobacco, alcohol and illicit drugs; reduction of physical exercise; changes in patterns of reproduction, with fewer and later pregnancies.[53]

While that account indicates several occupational initiatives, the perspective taken here makes it possible to add to the list. Changes required in respect of the impact of illness or premature death also include those associated with paid employment, occupational imbalance, deprivation, or alienation. They are also needed as a result of many sociopolitical initiatives that indicate a lack of awareness of occupational determinants that lead to illness.

It has already been noted that national priorities and policies, the type of economy, and cultural values determine occupational risk factors and behaviors such as overcrowding, loneliness, substance abuse, lack of opportunity to develop potential, imbalance between diet and activity, and ecological breakdown. They can also result in ongoing unresolved stress from occupational imbalance, deprivation, or alienation, which are risk factors in themselves; may result from other risk factors; or lead to the development of health risk behaviors. These risk factors can lead to early, preclinical health disorders such as boredom; burnout; depression; decreased fitness, brain, or liver function; increased blood pressure; and changes in sleep patterns, body weight, and emotional state, and ultimately to disease, disability, or death. It is timely to consider some particular examples of occupation-based disorders with comment relating to "doing, being, and becoming" to make the occupation connection clear. Four examples will be discussed according to priorities identified by the WHO and others of the public health fraternity.

"POVERTY IS THE GREATEST THREAT"

"Poverty is the greatest threat"[2] was a major topic in the last chapter on occupational justice, but at this point it is important to reiterate that engagement in occupation has, historically, been the method to obtain the basic needs of health. If opportunities "to do" this diminish, a combination of survival requirements are affected. Poverty through lack of means of doing is often accompanied, for example, by hunger, disease, illiteracy, and child labor, or, as is the case for many Arctic Inuit communities, with addiction, violence, depression, and unemployment.[54] Poverty is more than income. The poor have described it as "ill-being." This includes "doing" experiences such as living and working in risky, unhealthy, or polluted environments, and "being" and "becoming" experiences such as bad feelings about self, perceptions of powerlessness, voicelessness, anxiety, and fear for the future, as well as more obvious experiences of poverty such as lack of food, work, money, shelter, and clothing.[55] People with disability often experience poverty particularly in developing countries where prejudicial attitudes are common and access to education and employment limited. They are, for example, often excluded from opportunities to develop farming skills—a basic means of livelihood for many.[56]

The last decades have been marked by global poverty and debt crises around the world, including the newly industrialized countries of Southeast Asia and the Far East, those of the former Soviet block, and in Western Europe and North America. There have been famines in sub-Saharan Africa, South Asia, and parts of Latin America. In developing countries, Eastern Europe, and the Balkans, a resurgence of infectious diseases has been rife. Health services and schools have closed.[57] While natural disasters can account for some of the present experience of poverty, much more can be laid at the doors of political and multicorporate initiatives, will, and greed. It is, as the *Jakarta Declaration* argues, "the global economy, financial markets and trade" that shape "living conditions across the world" and both the values and what people do throughout their lives.[2] It is not only people but all other living things and the ecology that have been degraded by what a very few humans with money and power have done, and continue to do, in its pursuit.

URBANIZATION

In many countries, but in postindustrial societies particularly, the centralizing of paid employment and big business leads to a massing of people all living together often without any sense of community and sometimes with increasing experience of isolation. While for people with more outgoing natures the chance to meet others who share like interests and do things together appears to be increased by urban living, for many others it leads to being lonely, bored, and alienated. It is easier to be unknown and remain so in a crowded city than in a smaller community where people are recognized for their ability to contribute in special ways according to their capacities and interests. There are fewer places to walk in safety and fresh air, the pace of life is faster, and demands on attention are more frequent. While cities obviously appear to be less healthy places to live in than rural environments, doing things, becoming fulfilled, and being with others is so important that the effects are felt in the "left-behind" rural sector.

There are less and less opportunities for people to live out their lives in rural communities with the diverse advantages of modern amenities and services. Services are centered in large urban settings or, increasingly, moved "off-shore." The demands on local government escalate in line with the legislative requirements in urban centers where there are more residents to pay for the services. The bureaucracy of necessity increases, while essential services and occupational opportunities decrease. When the local government can no longer exist financially, centralization follows. Support facilities continue to decline, yet more occupational deprivation occurs and illness follows. Child care, education, recreation, sporting, communal, commercial, and employment opportunities dwindle, and older people are left with decreasing support from diminishing family, social, health, or public service facilities or activities in which they can participate. For many, active aging is reduced to domestic and garden chores. For people living outside urban centers, long and tiring travel is an ongoing and increasing necessity as rural services are closed down. Road accidents are a major concern. These and suicide are becoming common for rural youth because often the most obvious forms of local recreation are alcohol and "going to town." Earlier and simpler ways to spend free time in the country such as walking, swimming, fishing, and other "naturally" based occupations are frequently discouraged in childhood as unsafe, are not deemed "cool" for an electronically focused youth culture, and are dependent on a type of personal occupational enterprise that is reducing as rules and regulations increase across the board to an unhealthy point. Depression, not surprisingly, is on the rise for all ages and in some countries exceeds the incidence in urban centers.[58] The need for rural community redevelopment is a growing and critical need in terms of those populations preventing illness through what they do, be, or strive to become.

INCREASED DRUG ABUSE AND CIVIL AND DOMESTIC VIOLENCE

With urbanization and the grouping together of large groups of people has come an increasing facility to engage in the use of legal or illicit drugs and of civil and domestic violence. These unhealthy methods of doing, being, and becoming have multiple causes, but can be blamed not least on decreasing opportunities for people to learn about looking after themselves in practical ways and their responsibilities to the community and to others. Engagement in pleasurable doings is becoming more expensive and elitist as it becomes tied to material artifacts like the right shoes, clothes, and tools; specialty venues; and making money. Such exclusion can lead some people to seek other forms of self-expression through, for example, fundamentalism. Others experience boredom, self-depreciation, envy, ennui, and more, which can be magnified if social welfare support becomes preferable to unwanted types of paid employment. Getting back at "the system," at "the establishment," at those closest, or at those who are different is a maladaptive form of doing, being, and becoming that increases as socioeconomic policies fail to recognize doing, being, and becoming as basic health needs.

Substance abuse is unhealthy occupational behavior that is learned from families, friends, and from community and media sources. The young seem particularly at risk, and the age at which some start "becoming" a user is early. Exposure, particularly to other young people "doing their own thing" apparently having fun and growing up through what appears to be risky and adventurous, can appear exciting. With other risk-taking behaviors, such as driving recklessly or becoming part of antisocial or aggressive "gangs," substance abuse almost appears to have taken over earlier puberty rights of passage. For some young people, perhaps of an adventurous or rebellious nature or those who are more easily led, and particularly for those whom education systems and processes fail, it provides a means of forgetting failure or getting back at established norms.

Sometimes changes in sociocultural, community, and family occupations lead to boredom and loss of direction for the young. In communities where there are increasing numbers of both parents working, problems with child care, boredom, and teenage freedoms may be a factor. Alternatively, modern adult occupational behavior can result in overprotection of the young from the realities of living. Health problems such as substance abuse can occur when there appears to be not enough "to do" that holds meaning or purpose for them or there may be an imbalance of too much or too little responsibility in what they are expected to do or to become. Overprotection might also be a factor in disguising the need for young people to develop responsible doing to meet life's needs, dangers, and potentials. In the present day, this appears to have resulted in decreased attention being given to learning of adult self-care behavior, future "survival" activity, and personal responsibility. Coupled with frequent media coverage of substance abuse and of incidents of aggression, this amounts to glorification of "ill-doing." Those examples, of course, oversimplify the complex matter of the search for self-worth, meaning, and purpose that are essential elements of doing, being, becoming, and belonging healthily.

DECREASE OF PHYSICAL ACTIVITY

Physical doing has altered throughout time as a result of accelerating changes in societies across the world. On the whole, people in postmodern cultures are no longer required to undertake either sustained or substantial physical exercise. They undertake it at will rather than for necessity. This contrasts markedly with the situation that existed until fairly recent times:

> *Vigorous physical activity was part of everyday life for most people, at home, at work, and in transit between them. Even as recently as 1850, human muscles provided up to one third of the energy used by workshops, factories, and farms. Today the figure is less than 1%; the human body is becoming redundant as a source of energy in the workplace [with physical activity having become] largely a recreational option rather than a survival necessity.*[7]

Very few people in the postmodern world would run or walk for several hours every day, as early humans did, and as some in hunter-gathering or agricultural economies still do. This lack of physical activity is despite considerable media exposure to the claims that exercise of sufficient vigor and regularity is protective of cardiovascular disease and conducive to general well-being. Commonly accepted standards about what a protective level of fitness entails vary from a mixture of regular daily physical activity[42] to vigorous, repetitive, rhythmical activity such as walking, running, swimming, or cycling, for at least 20 minutes, 3 to 4 times a week.[59] In Britain, the United States, and Australia in the 1990s, less than half the adult population met that standard, with women less likely at that time to engage in physical activity than men.[7,60-62] This continues to be the case today.[42] Physical inactivity remains a major concern as it declines with age from as early as adolescence, and many studies have found differences between groups not only according to age and gender but also according to ethnicity, sociocultural status, education, and employment.[42,63-66] Despite growing interest, "the study of physical activity as it relates to health is in its infancy," and it is difficult to estimate and measure because most investigations use different criteria to define physical activity or describe and quantify its many variations.[67] The WHO reports that "the most data was available for leisure time activity, with less direct data available on occupational (paid employment) activity, and little direct data available for activity related to transport and domestic tasks."[42]

In many respects, the use of the phrase *physical activity* is a misnomer, although its usage in that way is probably related to concerns about the growing incidence of obesity and the interrelationship between physical energy expenditure and food intakes that are important to stress. However, its current use maintains the myth that physical, mental, and social health can be separated. The constituents of the WHO argument, though, substantiate the interaction between them and, I believe, would be strengthened if the word *occupation* was used instead of *physical activity*. This view is offered because the suggested preventive benefits include those from work, domestic chores, and leisure pursuits, all of which are occupations with social and mental attributes as well as physical attributes.

Physical inactivity (or sedentary occupation) is a significant contributor to the global burden of chronic disease "estimated to cause 2 million deaths worldwide annually."[42] Throughout the world, "about 10-16% of cases each of breast cancer, colon cancers, and diabetes, and about 22% of ischemic heart disease" result from sedentariness.[42] It is as strong a risk factor as increased blood pressure, smoking, and high levels of cholesterol, and adults who are inactive are twice as likely to die from cardiovascular disease than those who are very active.[68]

The protective effect of vigorous activity is part of the occupation/survival-based health mechanism of biological evolution. The protective effects have been found to include strengthening of heart muscle,[69,70] increased production of protective HDL cholesterol,[71,72] reduction in triglycerides,[67] reduced blood pressure,[42,73,74] improved glucose metabolism,[42,75] increased resting metabolic rate, maintenance of weight loss,[42,76] and reduction of fibrin stickiness (and therefore the formation of blood clots).[77] Apart from cardiovascular disease, several studies have shown the protective effect of physical activity against osteoporosis, some cancers,[78] anxiety, and depression.[42,79] Additional benefits result from the way it discourages substance abuse, "helps reduce violence, enhances functional capacity and promotes social interaction and integration," and "interacts positively with strategies to improve diet."[42]

The WHO *Global Strategy on Diet, Physical Activity and Health* provides the following facts:

*   Appropriate regular physical activity is a major component in preventing the growing global burden of chronic disease.

*   At least 60% of the global population fails to achieve the minimum recommendation of 30 minutes moderate intensity physical activity daily.

*   The risk of getting a cardiovascular disease increases by 1.5 times in people who do not follow minimum physical activity recommendations.

*   Inactivity greatly contributes to medical costs—by an estimated $75 billion in the United States in 2000 alone.

*   Increasing physical activity is a societal, not just an individual problem, and demands a population-based, multisectoral, multidisciplinary, and culturally relevant approach.[42]

Those 4 examples provide some indication of where to begin tackling the enormous task of preventing physical, mental, social, and occupational illness through strategies based on notions about doing, being, and becoming.

An Action-Research Approach to Occupation-Focused Prevention of Illness and Disability

As described in Chapter 1, the terms *primary*, *secondary*, and *tertiary prevention* are used to differentiate different stages of the preventive process:

*   Primary prevention is about preventing the occurrence of illness or injury.

*   Secondary prevention is about early detection or arrest.

*   Tertiary prevention is about the reduction of chronicity or possible relapse.

In line with public health preferences, the thrust of this chapter has been concerned with the primary prevention of illness, disability, and premature death. It is aimed both at well populations or those at risk because of what they do or do not do. It demands an

Figure 9-3. Action-research approach.

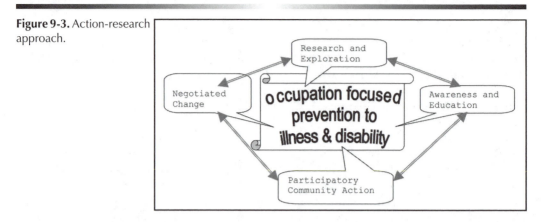

appreciation that what people do, how they feel about it, and whether they are able to use their innate capacities in ways that allow them to grow toward potential. They are central within the experience of health. It has been clearly shown throughout the text that this fact is understood and promoted by the WHO. However, because those facts are fragmented according to other ways of considering them, they are less obvious, easy to overlook, and cannot be seen as a whole phenomenon. Their fragmentation is according to sociocultural patterns that emerged with industrialization, such as paid employment away from the home, leisure apart from work, self-care that is taken for granted for all but the very young and the very old, education that is separate from families and community life, health behaviors that are provided for by trained personnel, and political action that is remote from real life and has to be accepted as the way things are. Another way they are considered, especially by health practitioners, is in terms of a division between what is considered physical, mental, or social. This also makes it difficult to appreciate or take into account the interactive nature of physiology, health, and occupation. Occupation that crosses the physical, mental, and social domain is more difficult to research but is more functional and very necessary so that people are better able to equate what they do in their everyday lives to their health.

The major difference of the approach taken here is to explicate the occupational determinants of health and illness from other aspects of population health and to consider them as a whole so that the interaction between them is made clear. So the action-research approach to the prevention of illness through what people do or do not do would primarily explore particular aspects of occupation within a community or population that appear to lead toward physical, mental, and social illness and are of concern to its members. It would go on to focus debate and raise awareness and action toward preventing members of the community or population from being ill, experiencing disability or premature death, using occupation as the medium of intervention. It would do so in consultation and participation within the population to enable action for change. Action would again include mediation, advocacy, and negotiation. Outcomes would suggest further exploration, awareness raising, and action. The process could continue in a spiraling pattern monitoring and effecting change toward preventing illness, caused or worsened by occupation in accord with the needs of the population (Figure 9-3).

Preventing illness and disability through advice about doing or not doing and active programs aimed at the same ends were lynch pins of medical practice for about 2000 years as part of the ancient rules of health, although such practice was aimed at individuals rather than populations. Such intervention needs to be reactivated from a population point of view but based on close scrutiny of the occupational nature and needs of people according to modern explanations of health and illness. Such scrutiny has many of the same requirements as inquiry into the social nature of illness. Clearly, not all risk factors have been established. Other possibilities, and the underlying determinants of risk factors, need to be studied with the rigor applied to the study of risks already known. So too do the methods of implementing change require ongoing scrutiny in the same way as other aspects of population health initiatives.

The public health preoccupation with risk factors of illness (medically defined) suggests that it may be necessary to demonstrate the linkages between engagement in occupation and illness if research pertaining to prevention through "doing" initiatives are to be valued and resourced by public health authorities. Much of occupational therapist's or other social scientist's studies of occupation are effectively ignored or studied only within their own disciplines. They appear to be seldom brought to the attention of public health authorities. Even major Harvard studies, such as that by Glass and colleagues[80] about the positive effects of social and productive occupation on mortality rates in older Americans, do not seem to have effected changes in policy or emphasis. To try to address both the linkages and the apparent lack of interest, this text is addressed to both public health practitioners and occupational therapists. To that end, it has provided a broad, contextual picture of the interaction between occupation and illness based on the changing occupational behaviors of humans. In retrospect, occupational behavior can be seen as central to changes in morbidity and mortality. This has been recognized (although not described in the same way) by the WHO and noted public health researchers such as Dubos,[81] McKeown,[53] and McMichael.[82] Even those authorities do not draw together the occupational inferences in a holistic way that provides the different and potentially useful way of looking at the evidence provided here. Public health practitioners or occupational therapists could both gather relevant evidence from this holistic point of view. Any particular action-research could and should draw on a range of existing generic to reductionist studies to provide validity and to convince funding sources of the worth, usefulness, and potential benefits that could result.

To raise awareness of preventing illness through what people do in their everyday lives, the various promulgation strategies of the *Regimen Sanitatis* could be revisited, adopted, and adapted, such as using state of the art technology and popular media. An example, is the excellent Australian "Life: Be In It" campaign that is being revisited on television at the present time after a 10-year lapse. Additionally, reminder strategies could be used, for example, by prominently displaying posters of an "Occupation for Public Health Pyramid" aimed at prevention. The poster could center on an occupation-focused approach to prevention such as in Figure 9-4.

Preventing occupation-generated illness and disability by using occupation-focused action programs can be based on WHO findings that a "few, largely preventable, risk factors account for most of the world's disease burden."[42] This is increasingly so in developing countries as well as in postindustrial nations. The risk factors reflect the changes that the history in this text has made clear. As people changed their predominant occupations from hunting and gathering to agriculture, to industry, and to highly technical computerized lifestyles, significant changes to activity, diet, and substance use also occurred. At the same time, mental and social demands altered with those of the new occupations, and sociopolitical structures encroached more and more, altering what people did naturally to maintain their health and feelings of well-being.

Reducing the rates of the known "largely preventable risk factors" can be implemented in occupation-focused, community-based programs to effect a change in physical activity, dietary habits, and substance use such as cigarette smoking. The WHO claims the scien-

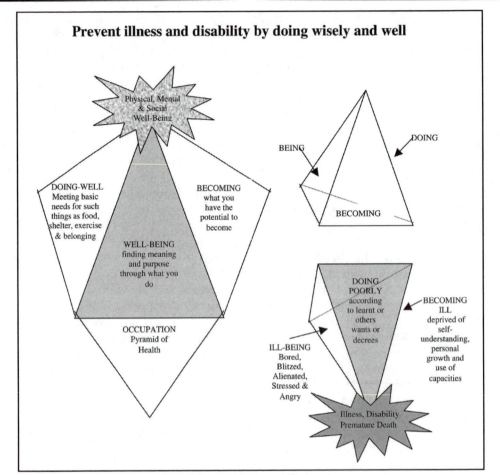

Figure 9-4. An "Occupation for Public Health Pyramid" aimed at prevention.

tific evidence is strong that such changes can have a major impact on chronic diseases in a relatively short time. It has been found that occupations of a physical nature lower the risk of breast cancer (possibly through hormonal metabolism), help to lower blood pressure, reduce body fat, improve glucose metabolism, benefit musculoskeletal conditions such as low back pain, and reduce osteoporosis and falls among older people. It has been suggested that playing sports is relaxing because "one is using the mind and body the way they were intended to be used in fighting or running away" in response to the fight or flight reaction.[42]

Physical activity also reduces symptoms of depression, anxiety, and stress just as other types of occupation.[42] The WHO recognizes that social health and economic benefits also accrue from policy changes toward increasing physical occupation. Not only do they have a beneficial effect on social interaction throughout life, they can also provide enjoyment, reduce violence, increase productivity, create healthier environments, and reduce health care costs. Sustained behavioral interventions have been shown to be effective in reducing global risk factors to the extent that WHO has adopted the broad-ranging *Global Strategy on Diet, Physical Activity and Health* that has informed this chapter.[42] Linking in with this strategy by informing or seeking advice from WHO would be strategic and useful in that it would begin to air a holistic rather than a fragmented view of occupation as an important aspect of prevention to a wider and potentially influential audience. For the 60% of the world's population who do not engage in sufficient physical activity,[42] more could be achieved if such activity were attuned to mental and social needs for meaning, purpose, belonging, and self-actualization; to the doing, being, and becoming occupation-focused natures of people for whom exercise alone does not appear to be motivating.

Occupation-focused programs reflecting the WHO strategy "Move for Health" could work with communities to increase regular physical activity for all people, not only during leisure or sporting activities but also at work, whatever the physical demands, during domestic duties, and in regular travel from place to place.[42] Additionally, the provision of education and advice in the way that commonly occurs at present, supporting exercise programs in schools and communities, being vigilant about what is sold in cafeterias, for example, suggesting daily walks or "gym" attendance, and taking every available opportunity to provide information about the dangers of poor eating habits, not exercising, and the impact of smoking or alcohol abuse. However, while sensible exercise programs are clearly beneficial, the occupational perspective that has emerged suggests that problems can best be addressed if moving for health is associated with occupations that meet people's doing, being, and becoming natures and needs.

Present global initiatives and national occupational structures in developing and affluent countries alike differ significantly from the occupational freedoms of earlier ages. Rules and regulations, even if originally intended to reduce the incidence of illness or to improve safety or equitable lifestyles, have altered the freedom of people to follow their built-in health needs in natural ways that provide for different natures and capacities. Modern expectations as well as regulations segregate people according to what they do and judge or reward those who succeed in very particular ways. When there are such parental, societal, or cultural pressures or political directions, it is very easy for people not to become aware of particular talents or capacities outside those parameters or, if they are aware, to be unable to use them in ways that are satisfactory in the longer term. This means that regularly many feel alienated or deprived, become stressed or inactive, become food and substance users and abusers, and fall victim to NCDs. This view is also in line with the WHO perspective that recognizes, for example, that increasing the level of "physical activity is not merely about individual behavior. Multi-sectoral policies and initiatives are needed to create environments that help people to be physically active."[42] It recommends such policies and initiatives be population-based and involve both public and private stakeholders, including health, sport, education, transport, and culture and recreation policy makers; urban planners; and local government about relevant "physical activity in all life settings."[42]

Partly because of word usage (physical activity equates in many minds to exercise regimes), virtue is accorded to those who do well in terms of walking or jogging regularly or attending the gym. It is hardly surprising that people do not equate the physical activities of daily living with their health. In a retrospective study conducted on 100 people older than 60, it was found that the majority of the sample did not associate their life's occupations with their health.[83] The justice of condemning those for whom gym attendance or such like fails to meet their basic needs, capacities, or learned behaviors is largely unfair and certainly counterproductive. Patterns of doing acquired early in life are often maintained unconsciously, establishing the foundation for health or illness patterns, and are difficult to overturn. A more just way of assisting populations as a whole is to advocate for the development of structures and ways of life that enable a greater number of people to become active and involved in occupations from childhood that:

* Fulfil occupational natures and needs rather than being "add-on" requirements.

* Provide for basic requirements.

✳ Provide meaning, purpose, and a sense of belonging.

✳ Provide opportunities to develop and grow.

Health is more likely to be maintained if individuals have the skills and resources to cope effectively with the diversity of life's challenges.[84]

Healthy diets have been at the forefront of health education campaigns for many years and appear to be heeded by those who are health conscious. They are heard but not accessed efficiently by many others who are diet conscious for the sake of fashion rather than health; those with poor skills in terms of acquiring or preparing food; those whose lifestyles are unbalanced; or those who are alienated, deprived, depressed, or unhappy in other ways. It is important to address the underlying problems as well as those primarily concerned with eating. This should be with varied approaches, not least the learning of practical food skills and strategies, to assist understanding of calorie intake and occupation demands in very down-to-earth and practical ways.

In terms of reducing substance use and abuse, attempts to "change existing environments and conditions" include "the creation or strengthening of regulations and normal population behaviors."[85] These are strategies that the U.S. Department of Health (Behavioral Health Services Division) employs. They advise that the prevention of alcohol, tobacco, and other drug use needs to be "an active process that promotes the personal, physical and social well-being of individuals and families not in need of treatment services,"[85] as well as those deemed to be at greatest risk in the future. By taking primary, secondary, and tertiary prevention approaches, the prevention process needs to integrate various strategies to target the general population, those at average to high risk, and those already using to prevent chronic use.[85] Because adolescents are particularly vulnerable and health problems developing at that time are likely to carry through into later life, some experts propose action approaches be developed specifically targeted to their needs.[86]

Particularly in postindustrial nations, recognizing and providing programs to enable people to become more active, diet conscious, and satisfied without excessive or destructive use of tobacco, alcohol, or other drugs requires sociopolitical activism to change the system. It also requires grass roots programs in which people with similar natures and occupational needs have a chance to meet and develop with the support of like-minded others. That occurs naturally for those who recognize their interests and capacities and live in a place where such connection is feasible, but it is not available everywhere or possible for everyone. Bringing potentially like-minded people together might be useful in some cases. Providing advice about lifestyle development that enables the following of capacities whether or not they involve physical activity so that emotional needs are met is another way. Managed risk-taking activities might also meet unconscious needs that if not met might result in dangerous and unhealthy risk taking. A better time to assist people to incorporate physical activity of a more appealing kind is when life is satisfying and with the support of or in the company of like-minded others.

We could learn from how the ancient health rules provided the foundation for several experts of different periods and places to advocate daily health maintenance regimes for people of different trades and callings. For example, for scholars it was suggested when and what to eat, when to work at scholarly activity, when to take physical exercise each day, and when to rest:

> *The Professors of Learning ought therefore to pursue the Study of Wisdom with Moderation and Conduct, and not be so eager upon the Improvement of their Mind, as to neglect the Body: they ought to keep an even balance, so that the Soul, and the Body may like Landlord and Guest observe the dure Measures of Hospitality, and do Mutual Offices, and not trample one another under Foot.*[87]

Different regimes were advised for those with other occupations, interests, duties, or skills.

In affluent societies, the 8- to 10-hour day in a working week is a common expectation whether people are involved in physically demanding, mentally demanding, or socially demanding work. No recent research has considered whether there are different requirements for different occupations, and what happens outside designated work time is largely forgotten except for the new mandates to exercise regularly. Neither is there a general understanding of the day-night occupation continuum in health terms, although some experts might hold very specific views. The research addressing the perils of shift-work points to numerous health concerns that are seldom addressed fully or applied to potential problems across the board. In a similar vein, the WHO recommends "a 'Life Course' approach to eating and physical activity that begins with prepregnancy, includes breast feeding, and extends to old age"[42] and argues for multifaceted, multi-institutional approaches because:

> The evidence (of behavioral interventions in reducing the rates of CVD, cancers and diabetes in populations have been well-proven in countries such as Finland, Japan and Singapore) is overwhelming that prevention is possible when sustained actions are directed both at individuals and families, as well as the broader social, economic and cultural determinants of NCDs.[42]

In countries where poverty is rife, occupation-based programs might need to center on skills to increase access to food, shelter, peace, equity, and other prerequisites of health. Practical programs to help people with food production or preparation on a small, personal, as well as a community or population scale could be useful in some situations, shelter building, clothing manufacture, first-aid, or ways to maintain rudimentary education when disaster occurs might be other useful occupational programs that could snowball into community-based action should needs arise. This can be important, too, for people with disability who may have been excluded from learning such skills. If poverty is a result of war or conflict, action-research to prevent further social illness and to reduce the possibilities of physical and mental illness might include communal occupations that meet the people's needs for belonging and building trust. Thibeault tells how home building in war-torn Sierra Leone assisted community members to gradually come together again after having been on different sides in the conflict.[88]

Rewarding occupation,[89] relaxation techniques,[90] and learning to cope with stress through regular or occasional participation in life's mundane or relaxing activities can provide resistance to stress-related disorders that appear to lead to other forms of illness. Fear of stress-related illness and of litigation has prompted many programs aimed at risk reduction. Antonovsky, following Selye's lead, asked the important question of not whether stress is bad for health, but for whom and under what conditions is it good or bad. Successful coping with stressors requires some experience of stress, and, indeed, moderate stress that augments the functional capacities of all systems is necessary for maintaining positive health and vitality as well as providing a reserve against extreme stress. "Heart attacks are not the result of shoveling snow or running for a train, ... they are the product of a lifetime of not doing things like shoveling snow or running for a train."[91]

Other types of occupation-focused prevention could assist population groups to work at political structural change to well-established occupational institutions such as the division of labor, the effects of the rampant growth of technology in daily living, and legislation that potentially leads to risk factors impinging on the individual, such as lack of opportunity to develop potential, occupational imbalance, deprivation, and alienation as well as early, preclinical health disorders such as boredom, burnout, or sleep disturbance.

This may well include identification of occupational factors that lead to:

*   Stress-related and mental illness, lack of learning to cope with stress.

*   Ineffective parenting, child exploitation; deprivation, food abuse.

*   Child cruelty/abuse, family/sexual violence, juvenile delinquency, teen pregnancies.

*   Bullying and people abuse (women, children, elders, disabled, ethnic, or religious groups).

*   School drop-outs, street-living, suicide, aggression, substance abuse.

*   Work-related alienation, dissatisfaction, illness, or accidents; welfare fraud.

*   Exclusion of older people from work or chosen occupations that ensure active aging.

*   Terrorism, gang behavior.

*   Pollution, ecological degradation.

   Some occupational therapists have worked in the preventive sphere for many years, although their contributions to public health appear to have been largely overlooked. Within paid employment, the mining industry in Australia was the venue for programs in health and safety education for back injury prevention and management,[92] and for all levels of the workforce in ergonomics, assessing and monitoring work methods, and advising on the adaptation of heavy vehicles and mining equipment being used in geographically hostile environments.[93] Workers at a major Texas grocery distribution center were the recipients of an industrial accident/injury primary prevention program combining educational psychology principles with back care education, body mechanics, environmental modification, and work simplification at work stations. The program expanded into a comprehensive accident/injury prevention project within the company.[94] Strategies for children have enabled the safe transportation of those with physical handicaps[95] and community outreach programs using play and group process for preschool children at risk of developing psychiatric disorders.[96] Home safety programs for older adults are becoming fairly common. These include education about ways to modify the environment and activities of daily living to lessen the risk of accidental injury, the prevention of falls, improvements for individual homes, and community education.[97-99]

   The probability of more radical changes in occupation as the century progresses holds potentially serious health consequences. Dubos' warning that people's biological inheritance only enables adaptation up to a point and that chronic disease states develop over time[100] is a precursor of Maslow's concerns that the rapidity of the changing world calls for "a different kind of human being ... who is comfortable with change" because the huge acceleration in technology could lead to death for those unable to adapt.[101] The WHO expresses similar concerns associated with socioecological change, calling for a "systematic assessment of the health impact of a rapidly changing environment, particularly in areas of technology, work, energy production, and urbanization."[1] Unfortunately, the concerns are real and are made more so by the culturally constructed global community. It appears that the 21st century is beginning to uncover some of the connections between people's doings and illness, and an occupation-focused preventive approach is needed to help people to understand the connections and to overcome them.

References

1. World Health Organization, Health and Welfare Canada, Canadian Public Health Association. *Ottawa Charter for Health Promotion.* Ottawa, Canada; 1986.

2. World Health Organization. *Jakarta Declaration on Leading Health Promotion into the 21st Century.* Geneva; 1998.

3. Ashton J, Seymour H. *The New Public Health: The Liverpool Experience.* Milton Keynes: Open University Press; 1988.

4. Prevention. Available at: http://www.finnevo.fi/eng/contents/iso9000_terms.htm> Accessed January 2006.

5. Nutbeam D. Health promotion glossary. *Health Promotion International.* 1998;13(4):349-364.

6. Last JM. *Public Health and Preventive Medicine.* Stamford, Conn: Appleton and Lange; 1987.

7. Hetzel BS, McMichael T. L S Factor: Lifestyle and Health. Ringwood, Victoria: Penguin; 1987:186-187.

8. Commonwealth Department of Community Services and Health. *World Health Organization: A Brief Summary of Its Work.* (Clause 24). Canberra: Australian Government Publishing Service; 1988:10.

9. Gordon D. *Health, Sickness and Society: Theoretical Concepts in Social and Preventive Medicine.* St. Lucia, Queensland: University of Queensland Press; 1976:5.

10. Reilly M. 1961 Eleanor Clarke Slagle Lecture. Occupational therapy can be one of the great ideas of 20th century medicine. *Am J Occup Ther.* 1962;16:1-9.

11. Reilly M. The challenge of the future to an occupational therapist. *Am J Occup Ther.* 1966;20:221-225.

12. Reilly M. The modernisation of occupational therapy. *Am J Occup Ther.* 1971;25:243-246.

13. Reilly M. A response to: defining occupational therapy: the meaning of therapy and the virtues of occupation. *Am J Occup Ther.* 1977;31(10):673.

14. West W. The occupational therapists changing responsibilities to the community. *Am J Occup Ther.* 1967;21:312.

15. Brown KM. Wellness: past visions, future roles. In: Cromwell FS, ed. *Sociocultural Implications in Treatment Planning in Occupational Therapy.* New York: Haworth Press; 1987.

16. Johnson JA. *Wellness: A Context for Living.* Thorofare, NJ: SLACK Inc; 1986.

17. West W. The 1967 Eleanor Clarke Slagle Lecture. Professional responsibility in times of change. *Am J Occup Ther.* 1968;22(1):9-15.

18. West W. The growing importance of prevention. *Am J Occup Ther.* 1969;23:223-231.

19. West W. The emerging health model of occupational therapy practice. Proceedings of the 5th International Congress of the WFOT, Zurich, 1970.

20. Cromwell FS. Our challenges in the seventies. Occupational therapy today—tomorrow. Proceedings of the 5th International Congress. Zurich, 1970:232-238.

21. Mosey AC. Meeting health needs. *Am J Occup Ther.* 1973;27:14-17.

22. Fidler GS, Fidler JW. Doing and becoming: purposeful action and self actualization. *Am J Occup Ther.* 1978;32:305-310.

23. Wiemer RB. Some concepts of prevention as an aspect of community health: a foundation for development of the occupational therapists role. *Am J Occup Ther.* 1972;26(1):1-9.

24. Finn GL. The 1971 Eleanor Clarke Slagle Lecture. The occupational therapist in prevention programs. *Am J Occup Ther.* 1972;26(2):59-66.

25. Finn GL. Update of Eleanor Clarke Slagle Lecture: the occupational therapist in prevention programs. *Am J Occup Ther.* 1977;31(10):658-659.

26. Grossman J. Preventive health care and community programming. *Am J Occup Ther.* 1977;31(6):351-354.

27. Laukaran VH. Toward a model of occupational therapy for community health. *Am J Occup Ther.* 1977;31:71.

28. Le Vesconte HP. The place of occupational therapy in social work planning. *Can J Occup Ther.* 1934;2:13-16.

29. Le Vesconte HP. Expanding fields of occupational therapy. *Can J Occup Ther.* 1935;3:4-12.

30. Johnson J, Kielhofner G. Occupational therapy in the health care system of the future. In: Kielhofner G, ed. *Health Through Occupation: Theory and Practice in Occupational Therapy.* Philadelphia: FA Davis Co; 1983:191.

31. Owen R. *Paper: Dedicated to the Governments of Great Britain, Austria, Russia, France, Prussia and the United States of America.* London; 1841. (New Lanark Conservation)

32. Wilcock AA. *Occupation for Health.* Vol 1. A Journey from Self Health to Prescription. London: British College of Occupational Therapists; 2001.

33. Porter R. *Disease, Medicine and Society in England 1550-1860.* London: MacMillan Education; 1987.

34. Chadwick E. *Report on the Sanitary Condition of the Labouring Population of Great Britain.* London: British Parliamentary Report; 1842.

35. Girling DA, ed. *New Age Encyclopedia.* Vol. 6. London: Bay Books; 1983:150.
36. MacDonald EM. *World-wide Conquests of Disabilities: The History, Development and Present Functions of the Remedial Services.* London: Bailliere Tindall; 1981:88-89.
37. Guy Rev Dr. JR. *Compassion and the Art of the Possible: Dr. Southwood Smith as Social Reformer and Public Health Pioneer. Octavia Hill Memorial Lecture.* December 1993. Cambridgeshire: Octavia Hill Society & The Birthplace Museum Trust; 1996:5.
38. Sigerist HE. *On the History of Medicine,* ed. Marti-Ibañez F. New York: MD Publications, Inc; 1960:16.
39. Wikipedia. World Health Organization. Available at: http://www.en.wikipedia.org/wiki/World_Health_ Organization. Accessed October 2, 2005.
40. Parmeggiani L, ed. *ILO Encyclopedia of Occupational Health and Safety.* 2 Vols. 3rd rev ed. Geneva, Switzerland: International Labour Organisation; 1983.
41. World Health Organization. *The Declaration of Alma Ata.* International Conference on Primary Health Care, Alma Ata, USSR; 1998.
42. World Health Organization. *Global Strategy on Diet, Physical Activity and Health. Chronic Disease Information Sheets.* World Health Organization Documents and Publications: 2004. Available at: http://www. who.int/dietphysicalactivity/publications/facts/chronic/en/. Accessed December 2005.
43. Richards T. News extra: Social Policy more important for health than medicines, conference told. *BMJ.* (18th December)1999;319:1592.
44. Bassuk SS, Glass TA, Berkman LF. Social disengagement and incident cognitive decline in community dwelling elderly persons. *Ann Intern Med.* 1999;131(3):165-173.
45. Iwarsson S, Isacsson A, Persson D, Scherston B. Occupation and survival: a 25-year follow-up study of an aging population. *Am J Occup Ther.* 1998;52:65-70.
46. Rudman D, Cook J, Polatakjo H. Understanding the potential of occupation: a qualitative exploration of senior's perspectives on activity. *Am J Occup Ther.* 1997;51:640-650.
47. Evans R. Doctors—get on your bikes. *BMJ.* bmj.com, 31Mar 2000 (full text).
48. Mason B. Prescribed cycling. *BMJ.* bmj.com, 2 Apr 2000 (full text).
49. Xavier G. Bicycle use is even more important to poor countries. *BMJ.* bmj.com, 2 Apr 2000 (full text)
50. Wardlaw M. Of steel and skulls. *BMJ.* bmj.com, 17 Apr 2000 (full text)
51. Chiheb Z. Why do school children cycle on the continent, but not in the UK? *BMJ.* bmj.com, 14 May 2000 (full text)
52. Wardlaw M. Segregating cyclists is not the answer. *BMJ.* bmj.com, 19 May 2000 (full text)
53. McKeown T. *The Origins of Human Disease.* Oxford, UK: Basil Blackwell; 1988:154.
54. Thibeault, R. Fostering healing through occupation: the case of the Canadian Inuit. *Journal of Occupational Science.* 2002:9;153-158.
55. Listen to the Voices. Available at: http://www.worldbank.org/poverty/voices/listen-findings.htm> Accessed 2005.
56. Yeoman S. Occupation and disability: a role for occupational therapists in developing countries. *Brit J Occup Ther.* 1998:61;523-527.
57. Chossudovsky M. Global poverty in the late 20th century [Electronic version]. *Journal of International Affairs.* 1998;52:293-311.
58. Probst JC, Laditka S, Moore CG, Harun N, Paige Powell M. *Depression in Rural Populations: Prevalence, Effects on Life Quality, and Treatment Seeking Behavior.* Rockville, Md: Office of Rural Health Policy, US Government of Health and Rural Services; 2005.
59. American College of Sports Medicine. *Guidelines for Exercise Testing and Prescription.* 4th ed. Philadelphia: Lea and Febiger; 1991.
60. Caspersen CJ, Christensen GM, Pollard RA. Status of the 1990 physical fitness and exercise objectives—evidence from NHIS 1985. *Public Health Reports.* 1986;101:587-592.
61 Blaxter M. *Health and Lifestyles.* London: Tavistock/Routledge; 1990.
62. Clee J. Unpublished study. University of South Australia; 1991.
63. Gilliam TB, Freedson PS, Geenen DL, Shahraray B. Physical activity patterns determined by heart rate monitoring in 6-7 year olf children. *Med Sci Sports Exer.* 1981;13:65-67.
64. Stephens T, Jacob DR, White CC. A descriptive epidemiology of leisure time physical activity. *Public Health Reports.* 1985;100:147-158.
65. Shea S, Basche CE, Lantigua R, Weschler H. The Washington Heights-Inwood healthy heart program: a third generation community-based cardiovascular disease prevention program in a disadvantaged urban setting. *Preventive Medicine.* 1991;21:201-217.
66. King AC, Blair SN, Bild DE, et al. Determinants of physical activity and interventions in adults. *Med Sci Sports Exer.* 1992;24:S221-S237.
67. Kaplan RM, Sallis JF, Patterson TL. *Health and Human Behavior.* New York: McGraw-Hill Inc; 1993:350.

68. Powell KE, Thompson PD, Caspersen CJ, Kendrick JS. Physical activity and the incidence of coronary heart disease. *Ann Rev Public Health.* 1987;8:253-287.
69. Blair SN, Kohl HW, Paffenbarger RS, Clark DG, Cooper KH, Gibbons LW. Physical fitness and all-cause mortality: a prospective study of healthy men and women. *JAMA.* 1989;262:2395-2401.
70. Ekelund LG, Haskell WL, Johnson JL, Whaley FS, Criqui MH, Sheps DS. Physical fitness as a predictor of cardiovascular mortality in asymptomatic North American men. *N Engl J Med.* 1988;319:1379-1384.
71. Haskell WL. Exercise induced changes in plasma lipids and lipoproteins. *Preventive Medicine.* 1984;13:23-36.
72. Wood PD, Haskell WL, Blair SN, et al. Increased exercise level and plasma lipoprotein concentrations: a one-year randomized study in sedentary middle-aged men. *Metabolism.* 1983;32:31-39.
73. Hicky N, Mulcahy R, Bourke GJ, Graham I, Wilson-Davis K. Study of coronary risk factors relating to physical activity in 15,171 men. *BMJ.* 1975;5982:507-509.
74. Siegel WC, Blumenthal JA. The role of exercise in the prevention and treatment of hypertension. *Ann Behav Med.* 1991;13:23-30.
75. Vranic M, Wasserman D. Exercise, fitness and diabetes. In: Bouchard C, Shephard RJ, Stephens T, Sutton JR, McPherson GD, eds. *Exercise, Fitness and Health: A Concensus of Current Knowledge.* Champaign, Ill: Human Kinetics; 1990:467-490.
76. Epstein LH, Wing RR, Thompson JK, Griffin W. Attendance and fitness in aerobic exercise: the effects of contract and lottery procedures. *Behavior Modification.* 1980;4:465-479.
77. Haskell WL, Leon AS, Caspersen CJ, et al. Cardiovascular benefits and assessment of physical activity and fitness in adults. *Med Sci Sports Exer.* 1992;24:S201-S220.
78. Calabrese LH. Exercise, immunity, cancer and infection. In: Bouchard C, Shephard RJ, Stephens T, Sutton JR, McPherson GD, eds. *Exercise, Fitness and Health: A Concensus of Current Knowledge.* Champaign, Ill: Human Kinetics; 1990:567-579.
79. Stephens T. Physical activity and mental health in the United States and Canada: evidence from 4 population surveys. *Preventive Medicine.* 1988;17:35-47.
80. Glass TA, de Leon CM, Marottoli RA, Berkman LF. Population based study of social and productive activities as predictors of survival among elderly Americans. *BMJ.* 1999;319:478-483.
81. Dubos R, ed. *Mirage of Health: Utopias, Progress and Biological Change.* New York: Harper and Row; 1959.
82. McMichael T. *Human Frontiers, Environments and Disease: Past Patterns, Uncertain Futures.* Cambridge, UK: Cambridge University Press; 2001.
83. Wilcock AA, et al. Retrospective Study of Elderly Peoples' Perceptions of the Relationship Between Their Lifes' Occupations and Health. Unpublished material, University of South Australia, 1990.
84. Eisler RM. Promoting health through interpersonal skills development. In: Mattarazzo JD, Weiss SM, Herd JA, Miller NE, Weiss SM, eds. *Behavioral Health: A Handbook of Health Enhancement and Disease Prevention.* New York: John Wiley and Sons; 1984.
85. US Department of Health. Behavioral Health Services Division. Prevention Definition. <176_DOHpreventiondefinition.pdf> accessed December 2005.
86. Viner RM, Barker M. Young people's health: the need for action. *BMJ.* 2005;330:901-903.
87. Ramazzini B. *A Treatise of the Diseases of Tradesmen* (etc). London: Andre Bell et al; 1705:273.
88. Thibeault R. Occupation and the rebuilding of civic society: notes from the war zone. *Journal of Occupational Science.* 2002;9(1):38-47.
89. Hazuda H. Women's employment status and their risks for chronic disease. Colloquium presentation, University of Texas School of Public Health, Houston. In: Justice B, ed. *Who Gets Sick: Thinking and Health.* Houston, Tex: Peak Press; 1987.
90. Pelletier KR. *Mind as Healer, Mind as Slayer.* New York: Delta; 1977.
91. Klump TG. How much exercise to avoid heart attacks? *Medical Times.* 1976;4(104):64-74.
92. Arvier R, Bell A. Back injury management and prevention in the New South Wales coal mining industry. The Australian Association of Occupational Therapists 15th Federal Conference. Sydney, Australia, 1988.
93. Rudge MA. Occupational therapy in the underground mining industry. The Australian Association of Occupational Therapist's 15th Federal Conference. Sydney, Australia; 1988.
94. Schwartz RK. Cognition and learning in industrial accident injury prevention: an occupational therapy perspective. In: Johnson JA, Jaffe E, eds. Health promotive and preventive programs: models of occupational therapy practice. *Occupational Therapy in Health Care.* 1989;6(1):67-85.
95. Stout JD. Occupational therapists' involvement in safe transportation for the handicapped. In: Johnson JA, Jaffe E, eds. Health promotive and preventive programs: models of occupational therapy practice. *Occupational Therapy in Health Care.* 1989;6(1):45-56.
96. Olson L, Heanery C, Soppas-Hoffman B. Parent-child activity group treatment in preventive psychiatry. In: Johnson JA, Jaffe E, eds. Health promotive and preventive programs: models of occupational therapy practice. *Occupational Therapy in Health Care.* 1989;6(1):29-43

97. Deily J. Home safety program for older adults. In: Johnson JA, Jaffe E, eds. Health promotive and preventive programs: models of occupational therapy practice. *Occupational Therapy in Health Care*. 1989;6(1):113-124.

98. South Australian State Program. Falls Prevention Program for the Elderly. Noarlunga Community Health Service, South Australia. 1992.

99. Reducing Falls: Examples of local and national collaborative falls prevention strategies. *Occupational Therapy News*. October 2005;13(10):22-25.

100. Dubos R. Changing patterns of disease. In: Brown RG, Whyte HM, eds. Medical Practice and the Community: Proceedings of a Conference Convened by the Australian National University, Canberra. Canberra: Australian National University Press; 1968:59.

101. Maslow A. *The Farther Reaches of Human Nature*. Viking Press; 1971.

Suggested Reading

Cromwell FS. Our challenges in the seventies. Occupational therapy today—tomorrow. Proceedings of the 5th International Congress. Zurich, 1970:232-238.

Fidler GS, Fidler JW. Doing and becoming: purposeful action and self actualization. *Am J Occup Ther*. 1978;32:305-310.

Finn GL. Update of Eleanor Clarke Slagle Lecture: the occupational therapist in prevention programs. *Am J Occup Ther*. 1977;31(10):658-659.

Grossman J. Preventive health care and community programming. *Am J Occup Ther*. 1977;31(6):351-354.

Laukaran VH. Toward a model of occupational therapy for community health. *Am J Occup Ther*. 1977;31:71.

West W. The growing importance of prevention. *Am J Occup Ther*. 1969;23:223-231.

West W. The emerging health model of occupational therapy practice. Proceedings of the 5th International Congress of the WFOT, Zurich, 1970.

World Health Organization. *Global Strategy on Diet, Physical Activity and Health. Chronic Disease Information Sheets*. World Health Organization Documents and Publications: 2004.

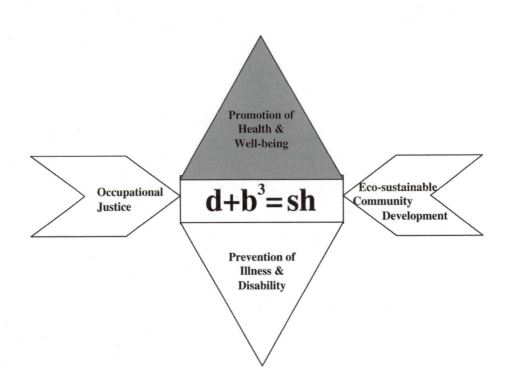

OCCUPATION-FOCUSED APPROACH TO THE PROMOTION OF HEALTH AND WELL-BEING

Theme 10:

"Health is a positive concept emphasizing social and personal resources, as well as physical capacities. Therefore, health promotion is not just the responsibility of the health sector, but goes beyond healthy life-styles to well-being."
WHO, *Ottawa Charter for Health Promotion*, 1986.

The chapter addresses:
* The concepts of health promotion and well-being
  * Health promotion
  * Well-being
* What is an occupation-focused approach to health promotion and well-being?
* Why an occupation-focused approach to health promotion and well-being is necessary
* Action-research: occupation-focused approach to health promotion and well-being
  * Well doing, being, becoming, and belonging
  * Working toward WHO "health for all" objectives across the globe

The sum of this text has been gathering momentum to this last chapter in which consideration is given to an occupation-focused approach to the promotion of health and well-being. The first chapter introduced the topic of health and well-being and set the direction for the exploration that followed of how occupation is an integral aspect. Health has been considered as a natural phenomenon and people as a species within ecosystems. In these terms, it was recognized that until fairly recent times, what humans did naturally to survive and maintain their health was concerned with what are now referred to as the prerequisites of health. As populations grew and occupation patterns changed, the experience of health and illness also changed. Rules were established that were based on observation of the differing natures of people, where and how they lived, what they did and felt about what they did, and how they experienced life. Because the physiological bases for such rules were found to be wrong when modern medicine evolved, the ancient rules were largely disregarded without due consideration of their worth. A period of limbo while medical science grew apace led to a lack of direction about how to prevent illness and promote health. The establishment of the WHO began to alter that loss of direction, and for over half a decade, has provided the modern world with guidance to improve the experience of health and to reduce illness and early mortality. Some of that guidance has been directed to political administrations throughout the world who failed to respond expediently because of factors such as pressure from multinational corporations or technologically-driven economic policies that ignored the ecological nature of the health of the world and its peoples. Ecological degradation, poverty and illness for millions, and reliance on a "live now, reverse the consequences later" cult has been the result.

Using the concepts of doing, being, and becoming to provide both directions and boundaries to what is a very diverse subject, the ancient rules of health and the directives of the WHO were explored to test goodness of fit. The exploration has, time after time, touched on the twinned notions of health and well-being from an occupational focus, and so it is fitting that the final chapter should entwine the ideas just as the WHO did when it provided the definition of health in its constitution in the 1940s. The chapter will follow much the same format as the previous 3 and will start by reviewing the concepts, including those that have come to light throughout the book.

The Concepts of Health Promotion and Well-Being

The concepts of health promotion and well-being bring together the concepts of the first 3 approaches and adds to them. In Chapter 7, it is clear that the WHO calls for health promotion initiatives that encourage people "to take care of each other, our communities and our natural environment," and regard both ecological sustainability and community development as fundamental to their health and well-being.[1] It also brings into the frame the notion of belonging that integrates the concepts of occupation with people's social needs as a basic and integrated requirement. Chapter 8, which considered an occupational justice approach, points out that there are global inequities in the experience of health and well-being, in part, because of a lack of awareness or policies that enable people to participate in doing, being, or striving to become according to their needs, capacities, and potential. It is, as the WHO has recognized in the OCHP, necessary for all people "to satisfy needs" and to "identify and realize aspirations."[1] Chapter 9 considered the prevention of illness from an occupational perspective, and it is clear that many of those approaches will also enable people to experience improved health and well-being, as well as preventing illness. Public health embraces both preventive and health-promoting approaches despite some ideological difference between them, particularly with regard to the largely medical disease orientation of the first and a basic rejection of that in the second, health promotion, instead, following a holistic approach that incorporates social well-being.[2]

HEALTH PROMOTION

The WHO included in its seminal OCHP ideas that are clearly compatible with those of doing, being, and becoming as the themes of the chapters discussing those concepts reveal. The OCHP addressed as primary the need for all people to meet the basic requirements of life. This is clearly achieved through what people do, the sociopolitical and economic constraints and liberties of their situation that enable or control what they do, the opportunities available to them, and the environmental factors that impact on what they can do. It almost goes without saying that health promotion and well-being cannot be achieved without those requirements being met or being facilitated by global and national agendas. That this is not always the case is almost beyond belief and points to obvious advocacy approaches that are required. The *Jakarta Declaration* priorities for health promotion in the 21st century include the pursuit of:

> *... policies and practices that: avoid harming the health of individuals; protect the environment and ensure sustainable use of resources; restrict production of and trade in inherently harmful goods and substances such as tobacco and armaments, as well as discourage unhealthy marketing practices; safeguard both the citizen in the marketplace and the individual in the workplace; and include equity-focused health impact assessments as an integral part of policy development.*[3]

"The need to respond to each individual's spiritual quest for meaning, purpose and belonging"[3] that appeared in the WHO theme of the chapter addressing the concept of "being" identifies the importance of how people experience and feel about what they do as an integral part of health promotion and well-being. So, too, does the theme of the next chapter on "becoming" indicate that "an individual or group must be able to identify and to realize aspirations"[1] as part of health promotion and well-being. Both "being" and "becoming" notions can be identified in other WHO/UN papers such as those addressing active aging,[4] mental health promotion,[5] and children's rights.[6]

There are those that castigate the OCHP for being too general, resulting, it is thought, in it being meaningless.[7] Reflecting that criticism, Cribb and Duncan claim its purpose is vague and elusive with significant ethical dilemmas.[8] However, they are clear that promoting health is a political activity.[8] In a similar mode, Tones maintains that promoting health is public health's radical, militant component.[9] However, it is clearly more than that, with some of the OCHP's generality being the result of the fact that it speaks to many different disciplines. As this was part of its intent, that is a particular advantage but only if the WHO and public health leaders are open to the input and contribution of different health and public spheres. That means more equal acceptance of the different ways of viewing the issues health promotion theorists and subsequent approaches seek to address, such as:

* Medicine and public health Epidemiology and disease prevention[10]
* Social sciences Social determinants and empowerment[11,12]
* Environmental sciences Ecological sustainability and global health
* Political Economic equity and development
* Occupational science Occupational determinants and enablement

While the term *health promotion* was coined in the 1970s,[13] its emergence has been linked with ideologies such as health education, preventive medicine, social medicine and social health, the women's movement, community development, and other public health participatory approaches.[2,14-16] Its ideology is, however, of much earlier origins. Readers will, perhaps, not be surprised that Owen, for one, espoused the promotion of health and well-being in the early 19th century that took an occupation-focused approach in social health terms that was inclusive of physical and mental health. Owen recognized that the interaction between occupation and health relates to the development and expression of people's capacities and potentials and to physical exercise. Examples of his explanations are in the scroll.

When society shall be based on true principles, it will not permit any of its members to be thus made small and imperfect parts of what man might be more easily made to become. It will perceive the great importance of training infants from birth, to become full-formed men or women, having every portion of their nature duly cultivated and regularly exercised.

It will discover that man has not been created to attain the full excellence and happiness of his nature, until all his faculties, senses and propensities, shall be well cultivated, and society shall be so constructed that all of them, in each individual, shall be temperately exercised, and their powers continued and increased by such exercise, until arrested by natural old age.

Owen R. Works of Robert Owen: Volume 3: Book of the New Moral World. (Pickering Masters Series). *London: Pickering & Chatto (Publishers Ltd.); 1993:156.*

It is in the highest interest of all the human race, to which there cannot be a single exception;

1st. That the entire faculties, senses and propensities, should be well cultivated, and at all times duly or temperately exercised, according to the physical and mental strength and capacity of the individual; in order that whatever may be done by each, should be performed in the best manner for the general advantage of all.

Owen R. Works of Robert Owen: Volume 3: Book of the New Moral World. (Pickering Masters Series). *London: Pickering & Chatto (Publishers Ltd.); 1993:156.*

Is it not in your interest, that each of these individuals should be placed, through life, within those external arrangements that will ensure the most happiness, physically, mentally, and morally, to the individual; and the greatest practical benefit to the whole of society?

Owen R. Twenty questions to the human race: Dedicated to the Governments of Great Britain, Austria, Russia, France, Prussia and the United States of America. *London; 1841. (New Lanark Conservation)*

Thomas Southwood-Smith, mentioned earlier for the part he played in the genesis of public health, knew and respected Owen's work. A physician, his creed was similar to Owen's and to quite a number of others of like mind in the 19th century. The name he gave to this was the "promotion of human longevity and happiness" a nomenclature similar, indeed, to "health promotion." Arguing that "there is a close connection between happiness and longevity ... to add enjoyment, is to lengthen life,"[17] Southwood-Smith suggested "it is, in fact, THE PLEASURABLE CONSCIOUSNESS WHICH CONSTITUTES THE FEELING OF HEALTH" (his emphasis).[17] He considered the development of capacities through doing both a source of pleasure and a means of prolonging life.[17,18]

... pleasure resulting from action of the organs is conducive to their com-plete development, and thereby to the increase of capacity for affording enjoy-ment; ... but also ... to the perpetuation of their action, and consequently to the maintenance of life; it follows not only that enjoyment is the end of life, but that it is the means by which life is prolonged.

Southwood-Smith T. The Philosophy of Health; or an Exposition of the Physical and Mental Constitution of Man, With a View to the Promotion of Human Longevity and Happiness. *Vol 1. London: Charles Knight; 1836:75.*

... It is interwoven with the thread of existence; it is secured in and by the actions that build up and that support the very frame-work, the material instru-ment of our being."

Southwood-Smith T. The Philosophy of Health. *Vol 1. London: Charles Knight; 1836:81-82.*

Organs of sense, intellectual faculties, social affections, moral powers, are superadded endowments of a successively higher order: at the same time they are the instruments of enjoyment of a nature progressively more and more exquisite.

Southwood-Smith T. The Philosophy of Health. *Vol 1. London: Charles Knight; 1836:85.*

Any attempt to exalt the animal life beyond what is compatible with the healthy state of the organic, instead of accomplishing that end, only produces bodily disease. Any attempt to extend the selfish principle beyond what is compatible with the perfection of the selfish, instead of accomplishing the end in view, only produces mental disease...

Southwood-Smith T. The Philosophy of Health. *Vol 1. London: Charles Knight; 1836:92.*

The ideas that were advanced by Owen, Southwood-Smith, and others in the 19th century were related to the "Utilitarian" doctrine of "happiness" attributed to Jeremy Bentham. Philosophers of that ilk also speak of "ill-being" as well as "unhappiness" to capture the negative aspects of individuals' lives.[19] Bentham proposed "nature has placed mankind under the governance of two sovereign masters, pain and pleasure. It is for them alone to point out what we ought to do."[20] Pain and pleasure could be measured accord-ing to duration and intensity.[19] Owen and Southwood-Smith's views also resulted from dismay of the health horrors experienced because of the socio-occupational changes that industrialization brought. At that time, they compared the life of the rich industrialists with the desperate lives of the laboring poor. They would be shocked anew if they were to return to many parts of the world today and saw equally horrific consequences of the present times. In developing countries, they could observe people starving, with no way to meet their basic requirements, partially because of the greed of multinational corpora-tions, self-seeking economic policies, and environmental mismanagement. The names of the players are different but the picture is similar. Or they might look on at the health effects on the people of war-torn countries and following acts of terrorism. They could observe those too in affluent postindustrial nations along with riots of all kinds, children and youths living in the streets, violence and substance abuse rife along with lethargy and over-indulgence. The lean and the fat living side by side, the blitzed and the bored, the alienated and the complacent all experiencing less than optimal health because of many factors, one of which is a lack of appreciation of the health-promoting effects of occupation. The concept of a balance of occupations across the sleep-wake continuum and a variety throughout days and weeks to exercise a range of capacities; to meet the basic requirements for health; to provide meaning purpose, satisfaction, and belonging; and to encourage potentialities is not yet understood by the majority. It is apparent in the directives of the WHO. This organization, despite the critiques of the general nature of its health promotion directives, appears to appreciate that people have a need for more than income through what they do and that this is an important aspect of health and well-being. Health promotion, like illness prevention, offers different levels of approach.[2,21] There are 4 of these:

1. Promoting health, well-being, and quality of life for the general population and prevent health-damaging behavior and illness.

2. Promoting health, well-being, and quality of life for people who have already experienced health damage to effect behavior change or retard progression.

3. Promoting health, well-being, and quality of life for people with chronic diseases or disability.

4. Promoting health, well-being, and quality of life for the terminally ill.

WELL-BEING

The WHO defined well-being in the 2000 prefinal draft of the ICCIDH-2 that was superseded by the ICF in 2002.[22] The earlier document provides the following description that may assist readers to understand how well-being is deemed to be beyond healthy lifestyles:

> Well-being is a general term encompassing the total universe of human life domains including physical, mental and social aspects (Education, Employment, Environment, Etc.), that make up what can be called a 'good life'. Health domains are a subset of domains (Seeing, Speaking, Remembering, Etc.) that make up the total universe of human life.[23]

This interesting description appears to imply a very limited view of health in line with medicine's orientation to body and mind while recognizing the affinity and connectedness to other aspects of life. It is, perhaps, surprising in an organization that gave the world such a broad definition of health 60 years ago that it remains current and controversial despite rapidly changing times. The definition, like the OCHP, has been critiqued for lack of specificity and so too has the concept of "well-being." All are useful, but especially for the fact that they have wide potential, attract debate, and are applicable across all domains of interest thus encouraging multidisciplinary and intersectoral endeavor to improve health and well-being. The WHO possibly increased the debatable nature of the definition by including social as well as physical and mental well-being, but the inclusion has enabled a valuable social model of health to emerge, although sadly, it is separated from the other 2 in most cases of health research and care. However, just as was the case in the 19th century with the genesis of public health, at the present time it is the social health problem of poverty that is the most critical in terms of global population health and requires the most attention if physical, mental, and social well-being are to be improved across the globe.

It is useful in some ways to separate physical, mental, and social well-being as in Chapter 1 in order to investigate them thoroughly, but it is also necessary to recognize that they work in unison. That became apparent in the discussion in the last chapter when the WHO initiatives toward physical activity were explored. Indeed, it can be claimed that physical well-being is recognized as a feeling or mental state. It is experienced as pleasure in the exercise of body parts while "doing something" and in the relaxing after-effects of activity. This is particularly so when function is challenged beyond the norm and the challenge is met, and for many people this is enhanced if the doing is shared with others. The extent of pleasure elicited can vary accounting, to some extent, for different interest levels in physical exercise. Maslow claimed that muscular people have to use their muscles to "feel good and to achieve the subjective feeling of harmonious, successful, uninhibited functioning."[24] The apparent rise of interest in feeling well, along with defeating disease, has led to an apparent fascination in all manner of sport and has also been associated with a growth of alternative health services such as acupuncture, reflexology, herbalism, homeopathy, naturopathy, massage, aromatherapy, and relaxation therapy for those unhappy with the extent of solutions provided by conventional medicine. The more holistic notions of traditional Asian philosophies have been influential. This has increased acknowledgment that well-being is related to spiritual, social, and behavioral factors, such as where and how people live and what they believe in, as well as physical factors such as self-care practices, the amounts and types of activity they pursue, and balance between rest, relaxation, and work.[25-27]

In America, the idea of "wellness" began an upward trek from the mid 20th century. Halbert Dunn, a physician, conceptualized and defined wellness in 1954 as "an integrated method of functioning which is oriented toward maximizing the potential of which the individual is capable within the environment where he is functioning[28] According to Dossey, the wellness health model assumes that every individual has innate capacities for healing, nurture, self-reflection, taking risks, and for making change toward wellness; that all people are searching for answers about the life process, meaning, and purpose; and that health is also about individuals being able to live according to their beliefs.[29] Wellness embraces a multidimensional concept of balance, referring to work, play, and rest; to nutritional balance; to balance between use of physical, psychological, intellectual, and spiritual capacities; as well as within self, environment, and culture.[30]

This occupation-focused concept begs the question of whether well-being is possible despite incapacity or imminent death. One obvious answer is that it depends upon how the incapacity or impending death is perceived and whether or not it prevents meeting doing, being, becoming, and belonging requirements according to current need. Another answer: because no 2 individuals will possess the same range of capacities nor have the same experiences that impact upon their development or their life course, in a sense, anyone can be seen as incapacitated to some extent, and even death can be as imminent even if most people conveniently forget that point. Some people can sing, others are tone deaf; some are athletic, others are clumsy; some are shy, others are outgoing. Such capacities, often endowed from birth, or the lack of them are generally accepted as within the normal range of human differences, yet when these relate to a fundamental capacity, such as bipedalism, vision, intellect, or fluid movement, or when such capacity is lost after birth, those so afflicted are described by others as disabled and are frequently classified as unhealthy or unwell whether or not the person so incapacitated sees it that way. At a 1991 seminar on stroke, opinions about the potential for people to experience health and well-being following stroke were canvassed. Most of those who had a stroke and their relatives and caregivers believed it possible for them to experience health and well-being despite loss of capacity, but not all health workers agreed. In fact, one physician expressed very vehemently his opinion that any person with hemiplegia could not be considered healthy.[31] Such attitudes appear prevalent in societies in which physical perfection, career success, and individual goals and needs have assumed dominance over communal living despite antidiscriminatory legislation.

It is also in such societies that people commonly talk, with some degree of regret, about loss of community spirit. Even so, many still seek to change other cultures that hold fast to long-held community and extended family values into becoming more "Western." Indeed, people from postindustrial societies are so imbued with the values of material, technological, and economic growth and have given such "prominence to our separate nature that we have become alienated from the most fundamental truth of our nature, our spiritual oneness with the living universe," and our dependence on maintaining its physical health.[32,33]

The concept behind this occupation-focused approach to health promotion and well-being encompasses the relationship between all life from cellular to global factors, from biological to sociocultural, and microscopic to macroscopic levels. What people do, be, or strive to become affects health and well-being on an individual basis through the integrative systems of the organism; on a social level through shared activity, the continuous growth of occupational technology and sociopolitical activity; and on a global level through occupational development affecting the natural resources and ecosystems. Any or all of these can have negative or positive effects on health, and all are inextricably linked. This implies that practitioners focusing on promoting the health-giving relationship of occupation have to consider or explore all levels by focusing on what and how it can improve physical, mental, social, spiritual, and environmental well-being.

What Is an Occupation-Focused Approach to Health Promotion and Well-Being?

I accept as definition of an occupation-focused approach to the promotion of health and well-being the one provided by the WHO and part of which provides the chapter theme:

> Health promotion is the process of enabling people to increase control over, and to improve, their health. To reach a state of complete physical, mental and social well-being, an individual or group must be able to identify and realize aspirations, to satisfy needs, and to change or cope with the environment. Health is, therefore, seen as a resource for everyday life, not the objective of living. Health is a positive concept emphasizing social and personal resources, as well as physical capacities. Therefore, health promotion is not just the responsibility of the health sector, but goes beyond healthy lifestyles to well-being.[1]

In the first edition of this book, I proffered the definition provided by Hettler, from the University of Wisconsin, of wellness as "an active process through which individuals become aware of and make choices toward a more successful existence."[34] That remains valuable; however, I have chosen, in this edition, to instead focus on the definition of health promotion provided in the OCHP. I have done so because parts of it have provided chapter themes throughout the book, so this last chapter, in its entirety, will help readers to bring the ideas to a workable state of closure. I have also chosen to use this definition because it is recognizably occupation focused and because it provides a way to clearly identify important issues to promote population health that are widely acknowledged. The term *well-being* has been chosen rather than *wellness* because it, too, is used repeatedly by the WHO. It also appears to be in more common usage than *wellness* in many countries, where if the latter is used it is more often applied to popular, fashionable, or naturopathic aspects of health than main-stream approaches. The ideas about wellness that were introduced in the first edition remain pertinent and useful and still appear within the chapter.

This approach is applicable to populations and communities as well as individuals and is aimed at promoting physical, mental, social, and occupational health and well-being for all people across the globe, as well as those in need of medical or mainstream health practitioner intervention. An integrated, multiprofessional, holistic approach utilizing overlapping strategies to functional health and well-being,[35] the approach is complementary to, and informed by, medical science but is based to a greater extent on behavioral, social, and environmental sciences. These encompass health education, community development, empowerment and justice, prevention, and economics and politics.[36,37] Also relevant is the emerging science of occupation, which accepts that people influence the state of their health through what they do and how, why, and where they do it.[38,39] People can improve their health and lengthen life through what they do when it is oriented toward maximizing potential within many environments; enhances feelings of satisfaction; provides meaning, purpose, and belonging; and meets basic health needs.[40,41] These mechanisms have been explored within the text as natural means to maintain and improve health and well-being, while also implying that health is not the objective of living but a resource to use while people go about doing what is required or enjoyable in everyday life in many different and interactive ways.

The approach holds as its central belief that people are occupational beings and that occupation should be a source of health as nature intended. If that is so and continues to be the case, it is possible to improve physical, mental, social, and occupational health and well-being by maximizing opportunities and maintaining or developing environments with diverse possibilities to meet the differing and equally valuable capacities of all people. Support for research to such ends and information that is widely and effectively dispersed is required. This should promote holistic understanding of occupation for well-being. People need information and assistance about what they should do toward reaching such a state because promotion of health goes beyond lifestyles based on known "health behaviors." Physical, mental, social, and occupational well-being across the globe should be a primary focus of governments, health professions, and others.

The principles of this approach hold that health promotion is the process of enabling people to increase control over, and to improve, their health and that this can be attained through doing. Because, at present, there is only limited attention given to how socio-economic-political decisions affect the promotion of health and well-being through what people do, it is held that understanding at the highest level needs to be increased. Individuals, community groups, and total populations must be enabled to satisfy needs, identify and realize aspirations, and adapt what they do according to environmental factors. To enable understanding of the place of doing, being, and becoming to promote health and increase well-being, wide dispersion of WHO directives and what they mean is required to assist achievement of health for all in the 21st century. Action across a wide variety of public sectors and fields will assist policies and action to promote health and well-being. Promotion of health and well-being is not just the responsibility of the health sector (Table 10-1).

The OCHP definition provides guidelines for this approach:

* Health promotion is the process of enabling people to increase control over, and to improve, their health.

Table 10-1

Foundations of an Occupation-Focused Approach to Health Promotion and Well-Being

Basis of Approach	Underlying Beliefs	Underlying Principles
Applicable to populations, communities, and individuals	Humans are occupational beings, and occupation should be a source of health	Natural health can be attained, maintained, and improved through doing
Aimed at promoting physical, mental, social, and occupational health and well-being	Physical, mental, social, and occupational health and well-being can be improved for all people	Health promotion is the process of enabling people to increase control over, and to improve, their health
An integrated method of functioning based on behavioral, social, environmental, and occupational science	Research and information about the promotion of physical, mental, social, and occupational well-being should be inclusive and holistic	Socioeconomic-political decisions affect the promotion of health and well-being through what people do
People can improve the state of their health through what they do when it is oriented toward maximizing potential within many environments	Health is a positive concept emphasizing social and personal resources, as well as physical capacities	Individuals or groups must be able to identify and realize aspirations, to satisfy needs, and to change or cope with the environment
Health is a resource for everyday life, not the objective of living	People need information and assistance about what they should do to reach a state of physical, mental, and social well-being	Wide dispersion of WHO directives will assist achievement of health for all in the 21st century
Is holistic and diverse, addressing many different and interactive ways to promote health and well-being	Promotion of health goes beyond healthy lifestyles to physical, mental, social, and occupational well-being across the globe and should be a primary focus of governments, health professions, and others	Promotion of health and well-being is not just the responsibility of the health sector. Action from various fields will assist policies and action to promote health and well-being

Three methods—enabling, advocacy, and mediation—were introduced in Chapter 1 as those deemed by the WHO as most suited to affect the promotion of health and well-being through the efforts of all people.[1] With recommendation of those methods comes recognition that it is what arises from within each person and community that has the most impact on people's motivation and behavior. Public health and health promotion practitioners have linked the 3 methods by using the term *empowerment*, which is claimed by them to be the "key philosophical tenet" and "guiding principle" of health promotion.[2,36]

Empowerment is seen as the link between participatory and client- or community-centered rhetoric and action because it facilitates the acquisition of choice thereby increasing control over ways to improve health.[42] Professional groups such as the UK "Society for Health Education and Promotion Specialists" advocate that participation and empowerment of people are the foremost objectives of health promotion approaches.[43] Occupational therapists have also embraced participatory,[44,45] client-centered[46] approaches during the last decades but, on the whole, have adopted "enablement" as a key principle of their practice.[47,48] Empowerment is a recently favored term in occupational therapy literature, but it sits somewhat uncomfortably within the rhetoric of a profession largely dominated by medical values and, on the whole, keen to maintain a nonpolitical stance.[49,50] Despite this, there have been moves in the direction of participation and empowerment by occupational therapy associations, educators, and some practitioners.[51-53] Thibeault and Hebert, for example, link issues of partnership, community decision making, and goal setting in their community development and health promotion model,[54] while Townsend and Landry claim "awareness of the need to shape environments to enhance occupational performance locates occupational therapists' practice implicitly and sometimes explicitly in the work of enabling empowerment and justice."[55]

* Health is a resource for everyday life, not the objective of living.

Following an occupation-focused health promotion approach to well-being embraces a belief that the potential range of what people do, be, and strive to become is the primary concern and that health is a byproduct. A varied and full occupational lifestyle will coincidentally maintain and improve health and well-being if it enables people to be creative and adventurous physically, mentally, and socially; if without undue disruption life needs are met, and appropriate exploration of self-need and environmental adaptation is attainable; if the experience of all human emotions is possible; if meaningful and supportive relationships enable a sense of belonging; and if sufficient physical, intellectual, spiritual, and social challenges to stimulate neuronal physiology are balanced by timely relaxation. For people to experience timelessness and "higher-order meaning," regular or high-powered "doing" and "feeling" requires interweaving with time for simply "being" or reflection on "becoming."[56,57] A lifestyle with such ingredients will not prevent all illness, disability, or untimely death, but coupled with modern medical approaches, there has been sufficient evidence of positive trends in the latter part of the 20th century to be able to claim such potential health results.

Engagement in occupations needs not have health outcomes in mind but meet other life needs. This text has illustrated that the total range of an individual's purposeful, meaningful, and fulfilling occupations can maintain homeostasis and keep body parts and mind functioning efficiently and so sustain health because this was the case in much of early times. Occupations can maintain and enhance joint stability and range, muscle tone, body size, cardiovascular fitness, respiratory capacity, interest and meaning, social interaction and needs for belonging, and balance between challenges and relaxation. Sufficient rest and relaxation as part of regular schedules prevents overuse and allows time for repair. Integral to engagement in life's occupations physically, mentally, and socially, healthy people who are not under- or overstressed are able to meet reasonable demands, accept responsibility, plan ahead, respond to problems, and establish realistic goals. People experience occupational well-being when they are able to carry out activities they need or wish to do without undue consideration of their physical, mental, and social capacities or status and when the environment in which they live allows such activity. In agreement with how the National Mental Health Association of America describes the mentally well, occupationally healthy people might experience fear, anger, love, jealousy, guilt, joy, and all of the human emotions but would not be overwhelmed by them. Rather they would feel comfortable about themselves and be able to accept disappointments as part of life. They would be comfortable with and interested in other people, able to give and receive love, and have satisfying and lasting relationships.[58]

The exploration in this text supports the proposition that people need to actively make use of their physical, mental, and social capacities to enjoy well-being naturally and links this with social needs for belonging.[59] It is further verified by how the number of older people who lead active lives following a wide range of occupations tend to feel better, to require less medical attention, and to live longer than those who are isolated and sedentary.[40,60,61]

* Health is a positive concept emphasizing social and personal resources, as well as physical capacities.

It has become clear throughout the text that the WHO definition of health recognized the connection between social well-being and that of a physical or mental nature long ago. It is in the field of public health that the truth of this is recognized most. Yet, social well-being is left, predominantly, in the hands of sociopolitical engineers. The predominance of medical personnel heading public health has led to a preponderance of physically related health issues being addressed. Despite the bias, this has been useful because of the interactive nature of the brain; social well-being is dependent on feeling good in the other domains.

In terms of this approach, social well-being is seen as the result of satisfying and stimulating social relationships between family members and within communities through a range of shared, supporting, or complementary occupations and roles. Occupations that have most obvious beneficial effects on health are those that people feel good about or that they know make others feel good; those that perhaps endow them with some kind of social status; those that enable them the freedom to effectively use personal capacities in combination with activities that are socially sanctioned, approved, and valued, even if only by a subculture.[62] It is this social health need that causes people to embrace causes and occupations that may be unhealthy in other ways. Rioting and war-making are obvious current examples.

* Health promotion is not just the responsibility of the health sector, but goes beyond healthy lifestyles to well-being.

In many ways, occupational therapy straddles the gap between medical and community health care. This is one reason why it has experienced a "poorness of fit" with the medical model. In common with the medical model, occupational therapy has taken a mainly individual perspective that could be applicable to population approaches as well. Because of their mixed interest, it is not surprising that some occupational therapy definitions of health from the mid 1970s on feature ideas that go beyond the health sector and include well-being. The American Occupational Therapy Association definition of 1976 is a case in point, describing health as:

> An individual state of biological, social, and emotional well-being whereby an individual is capable and able to perform those tasks or activities which are important or necessary to him to promote or maintain a sense of well-being. The individual state of health is influenced by forces such as heredity, behavior, physical environment, and the economic and social system in which he lives.[63]

Occupational therapists' interest may also reflect the wider attention to health promotion that has occurred alongside similar beliefs and approaches about life in the wider community. The wellness movement that emerged in the early 1960s is one of these.[64,65] Definitions of wellness include some ideas that resonate with those in this text, such as holism, meaning, purpose, philosophy of living, and a state of being[29,66] that hold appeal to people outside the medical profession and so have the potential for empowering and enabling others. Descriptions also embrace occupation-focused values such as:

* "An optimal or ideal condition toward which to strive."[67]
* "A context for living."[68]
* "A lifestyle ... to reach optimal potential."[69]
* "A state of mental and physical balance and fitness."[70]

Additionally, because the wellness model tends to follow the humanist tradition of growth ideologies, it is an approach suited to all people, including those who are physically, mentally, socially, or occupationally disadvantaged and usually aimed at personal growth and well-being, self-esteem, performance, roles, and quality-of-life skills.

Outside the medical field, in America particularly, a "wellness" approach has been adopted on many industrial, business, and corporate work sites[71-74]; is used as a marketing tool[75]; and has become a business offering in its own right,[76] with courses available on becoming a "wellness trainer."[77] In this corporate context, Opatz has defined health promotion in wellness terms as "systematic efforts by an organization to enhance the wellness of its members through education, behavior change, and cultural support."[78]

Quality of life is another accepted term used within and outside the medical fraternity to consider well-being. Its use in the latter will have been noted in earlier chapters, and it appears to feature often in the social and behavioral sciences. The Quality of Life Research Unit at the University of Toronto identifies quality of life as the degree to which a person enjoys life's possibilities in 3 major domains that touch on those addressed in this text.[79] They are being, belonging, and becoming. The "being domain" is inclusive of personal identity and personal physical, psychological, and spiritual factors. The "belonging domain" includes personal fit within the physical, social, and community environment. The "becoming domain" includes engagement in purposeful activities to meet personal needs and goals, including those of a practical, leisure, and growth nature.[79] The Ontario Social Development Council describes quality of life as the "product of interplay among social, health, economic and environmental conditions which affect human and social development."[80] The council claims the purpose of quality of life indexes is to monitor people's living and working conditions to focus attention on community action to improve health.[80] Quality of life has been addressed in many occupational therapy publications addressing such issues as living circumstances, empowerment, hope, motivation, meaning, satisfaction, happiness, socializing, expanding horizons, and promoting health.[47,81-83] These issues point to the need to develop partnerships with wide-ranging groups in an ongoing process, to be reflective and creative in seeking participation, and to be supportive and proactive of initiatives that have the potential to promote health and increase well-being in many differing spheres. For example, it may be that support of union-initiated structural and legislative changes to work-site health issues would be an effective means to promote improved health. According to a 1990s survey of 11,000 new members of 12 trade unions in the United Kingdom, along with better pay, improved health and safety, equity, and social justice were most often reported by members as what they wanted from union membership.[84]

Both wellness and quality of life approaches can be applied to both individual and population approaches as we have seen. Both favor development of self-responsibility and the achievement of happiness or personal goals, as does this occupation-focused approach. However, there is a fine line between self-responsibility and environmental influence. Too much emphasis on self-responsibility can lead to victim blaming, which may be unfounded in the light of epidemiological data that point to environmental and social conditions as major contributors to illness. As Antonovsky argues:

... It is disingenuous to, however, talk about getting enough sleep while disregarding the economic pressures on tens of millions of people, which compel them to moonlight or work extra shifts; to talk about eating well but say nothing of the powerful advertising industry; to talk of not smoking and drinking moderately yet be blind to the manifold social stressors that lead people to use smoking and drinking as maladaptive coping responses.[85]

Additionally, considering "achievement of one's goals" as the only criterion for health can be as narrow as a biomechanical approach to health that only considers physical factors.[86] This occupation-focused approach encompasses more than the achievement of individual goals. Instead, it points to a need for greater understanding of all people's occupational needs from the attaining of the prerequisites of life itself to the opportunities within populations around the global stage for realizing both individual and community aspirations that exercise body, mind, spirit, and social capacities inherent in everyone in a way that is healthy for the earth itself.

* An individual or group must be able to identify and realize aspirations, to satisfy needs, and to change or cope with the environment.

The chapters addressing doing, being, and becoming as aspects of occupation for health explored this last theme in many ways. It is possible to conclude, at this point, that the WHO appears correct in associating what people do and need to do are important aspects of health and can be instrumental in promoting health and well-being. Satisfying needs, coping with the environment, and realizing aspirations are integral to the first 3 approaches as well as this final one.

Why an Occupation-Focused Approach to Health Promotion and Well-Being Is Necessary

If we take the WHO premise that health is not the objective of living and that "good health is a major resource for social, economic and personal development and an important dimension of quality of life,"[1] then an approach to promote health so that living can be enjoyed by as many people as possible makes remarkably good sense. Reliance on medicine to put right illness-provoking approaches to life appears counterproductive. The latter is the way things are at present. The previous chapter gave some indication of the suffering of many because of that view. Medicine to repair damage is very expensive, and technological advances keep the costs continually escalating. The cost in monetary terms and in suffering could be substantially reduced if advice about and programs aimed at health and well-being were better financed, advertised, and promoted. During the last few months in Australia, it has been heartening to see media advertising provided by government that has picked up on the WHO and public health push to encourage people to become more physically active. This will have some impact on some people, but those who need most help may require professional programs to make changes to their lives. During the same time period, public-funded advertising about ecologically sustaining practices as part of daily living at the local level has become more evident also. All professional health encounters and action-research community endeavors should reinforce such messages. If from a single source, advertising has been found to be less effective, taking many years to achieve health promoting objectives as, for example, has been the case with the cessation of cigarette smoking.

Incorporating health promotion into ordinary life is the obvious way to go if health is deemed the desirable byproduct. That points to exploration and incorporation of ways of doing, being, becoming, and belonging that are the means to both survival needs and health and well-being. The formulas that precede the last 4 chapters encapsulate the notion and could be used as a promotional device: doing, being, becoming, and belonging leads to people surviving and experiencing positive or negative health ($db^3 = p \pm sh$). The positive or negative aspects of doing, being, becoming, and belonging need to be explicated to the world at large.

A listing of particular issues for which a health-promoting approach could be effective is required, knowing that the issues will change along with change to natural, sociopolitical, physical, technological, familial, cultural, and spiritual environments. The first issue has to be poverty and the need to find ways for people everywhere to meet the requirements of survival in ways that address their other biological needs provided naturally by occupation. Ways of doing that reduce the risk of infectious diseases and NCDs are paramount also. This, of course, includes all the occupations that are related to food, to physical activity, and to the reduction of substance abuse. Occupations of a hostile nature in all parts of the world are another concern. This requires long-term peace-building strategies to be developed and instigated whether the cause is war, terrorism, rioting, or aggressive behavior. Much of the conflict could be caused or aggravated by lack of occupational satisfaction on a population as well as an individual scale, and that this should be a consideration that peacemakers need to bear in mind.

The promotion of mental health is another major thrust that is required. The WHO recognizes that "most health care resources are spent on the specialized treatment and care of the mentally ill, and to a lesser extent on community treatment and rehabilitation services. Even less funding is available for promoting mental health."[87] They explain "mental health promotion is an umbrella term that covers a variety of strategies, all aimed at having a positive effect on mental health. The encouragement of individual resources and skills and improvements in the socio-economic environment are among them."[87] Although integrated systems theories predominate today, the effects of Cartesian dualism[88] remain in practice with disorders of mind and body being treated by different medical specialists in different locations, and the alleviation of social and ecological disorders being the province of totally separate agencies.

The older dualism of body versus mind, or the modern one of body-mind versus socioenvironmental, is contrary to the holistic notion of health and occupation resulting from all parts of brain and body working in harmony within social, natural, or human made environments. Integrative notions of health have not been well integrated into mainstream health care practices.[89-93] Rehabilitation concerned with tertiary health promotion and opportunities for specially trained health professions to assist with personal skill development and maximizing potential and quality of life, which was an extension of conventional medicine for people following illness or disability, have declined over the past 20 years to token services. This factor alone points to the promotion of health being seriously neglected, even for people with special or particular needs. Life counseling is an up and coming service in more affluent areas of the world, but there is little commonality in the education and approaches of this group. Public health practitioners and occupational therapists that follow a health-promoting philosophy could be extremely successful in such a role.

Isolation and sedentary lifestyles are factors that the British Geriatrics Society worries are likely to become increasingly widespread problems.[94] Eminent US psychologist, John Cacioppo, agrees, pointing to the US Census Bureau projections that show by 2010, 31 million Americans will be living alone.[61] Loneliness is characterized by feelings of isolation, of being disconnected, and of not belonging, and he believes "the strength of social isolation as a risk factor is comparable to obesity, sedentary lifestyles and possibly even smoking."[95] With similar concerns, Stoddart, Sharp, and Harvey call for specific investigations about the determinants of social support, networks, and activities that are required to prevent dependency in old age.[96] The UN and WHO active aging policies build upon such knowledge and concerns.[4,97] The WHO accepts:

> The essence of Fries's tenets, that chronic diseases and physical decline "originate in early life, develop insidiously" and can be prevented, as well as his vision—rejecting conventional predictions of an ever more feeble older populace—now lie at the heart of today's approach to NCDs, aging and health with its focus on the life course, health promotion, and "active aging."[98]

That illness prevention and health promotion have occurred to some extent already has meant that the "compression" of morbidity predicted by Fries in 1980[99] has begun to take effect, but his acceptance of a common duration of life years has needed adjustment because its length is increasing along with extension of its quality. McMurdo argues that it is "the undreamed of improvements in average life expectancy that have thrust aging to the forefront of attention" and suggests "laying to rest the pervasive misconception that all the ills of old age are 'just old age' would represent a major breakthrough for health care of older people."[100] While more people in affluent countries are now predicted to live to over a 100 years because of lifestyle improvements, those in developing and increasingly industrial regions are following the pattern of an insidious development of NCDs.[41]

Dossey explains that facilitating "the journey toward understanding the wellness process" is particularly useful "when people are under varying degrees of stress or illness" and "lose their appreciation for life's purpose and meaning."[29] It appears important to look below surface issues because "a person can be living a process of wellness and yet be physically handicapped, aged, scared in the face of challenge, in pain, imperfect...."[29] Diseases or symptoms may, in fact, be "the body-mind's attempt to solve a problem."[101] The wellness model may be a useful adjunct to conventional medicine[102] to counteract the trend toward increasingly restricted acute care with a focus on high technology, which is expensive and expects a passive, rather than participatory, attitude from consumers.

Limitation of practice occurs even in community agencies that conform to a conventional medical model. Minimal resources for large numbers of referrals mean that occupational therapists and others in health care teams have experienced difficulty in being able to practically implement their beliefs in health rather than illness approaches. Domiciliary/home care service guidelines, for example, establish a clear focus on primary care and rehabilitation, but a study undertaken in South Australia as early as 1987 revealed that although 80% of the occupational therapists surveyed expressed a belief that domiciliary care provides an appropriate base for health promotion programs, which they were keen to offer, only 9% of occupational therapists were able to provide this type of intervention[103] (Table 10-2). A 2003 study by Flannery and Barry suggests that limited resources in terms of time staff and funding remain the major perceived barrier to occupational therapists becoming health promoters.[104]

The holistic view held by the few occupational therapists involved in the population health field demonstrates awareness of an integrative and broad-based understanding of what well-being encompasses. For example, attendees at a seminar were each asked to record immediate responses to the question, "What is the relationship between health and occupation?" Eight themes emerged when the responses were categorized and embraced mental, physical, social, function, brain/body, quality of life, the environment, and the nature of the relationship (Table 10-3). Perhaps the mismatch of their vision with the mainly restrictive nature of the work expected of them is a reason for an apparent lack of understanding of what they could offer to population health.

Table 10-2

Constraints to Providing Health Promotion in Current Work

| | | Response | |
		Number	Percentage
Satisfied with amount	No	180	72.0%
of health promotion	Yes	47	18.8%
done in job	Don't know	23	9.2%
	Total	250	100.0%
Constrained by time to develop/implement program		118	46.8%
Constrained by heavy workload		118	46.8%
Constrained by limited staff and resources		99	39.3%
Constrained by employing agency policy		37	14.7%
Constrained by fear of invading individuals' rights		15	6.0%
Other constraints		18	7.1%

Table 10-3

Occupational Therapists' View of Relationship Between Occupation and Health

Category	Frequency	Key Words (Common Responses)
Mental	28.5%	Self-esteem, motivation, meaning, satisfaction, purpose, concentration
Function	16.0%	Goal-directed, skills, talents, opportunities, competence
Physical	13.5%	Energy, strength, exercise, tone, cardiovascular fitness
Social	12.5%	Role, status, relationships, value
Brain/body	10.0%	Balance, growth, unity, capacity
Quality of life	7.0%	Quality of life, well-being, positive
Nature of relationship	6.0%	Direct, inseparable, complementary, interdependent
Environment	2.5%	Adaptation, ecological, global
Other	4.0%	Hard to define, occupational therapy

Action-Research: Occupation-Focused Approach to Health Promotion and Well-Being

Readers will recall that the *Jakarta Declaration* identified 5 health promotion priorities for the 21st century; namely, the advancement of social responsibility for health, an increase in investments for health development, an expansion of partnerships for health promotion, an increase in empowerment of individuals and communities, and the building and safeguarding of health promotion infrastructures.[3] An action-research occupation-focused approach to the promotion of health and well-being would be aimed at those priorities. It would do so by focusing on what, how, why, and with whom people

Figure 10-1. Action-research toward occupation-focused health promotion and well-being.

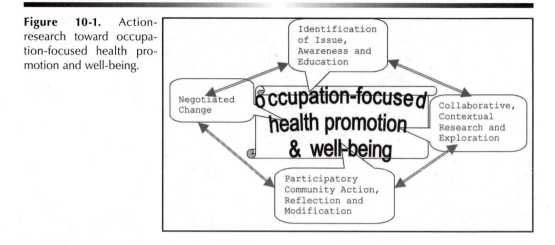

engage in the doings of ordinary life and would explore aspects of occupation within a community or population and the influence of socio-political infrastructures. It would focus debate and raise awareness about the health benefits of meeting the natural needs of people to engage in occupations that provide for their basic requirements, exercise their particular capacities, and enable them to grow and develop according to their potential and as part of a community of people with whom they feel a sense of belonging. It would do so in consultation and participation within the community to enable action for change. Action would again include mediation, advocacy, and negotiation. Outcomes would suggest further exploration, awareness raising, and action, perhaps for other communities in close proximity or far away. The process could continue, monitoring and effecting change toward promoting well-being by occupation in accord with the needs of the population (Figure 10-1).

To enable and empower people toward improvement in health and well-being can take many forms. It might include coaching, encouraging, facilitating, guiding, listening, prompting, or reflecting.[55] It might involve mass media campaigns or action to highlight issues of legislation that disempower or disenable. It might include health education campaigns aimed at occupational behavior change. Counseling or group programs might be used along with community development or self-help initiatives aimed at personal development. For this particular approach, a focus on what people do is central: how they interact with the world and with others through what they do; what they feel they need to do but cannot; what they value and would like to do now or in the future; how they understand the relationship of what they do with their health status; how they discourse about what they do; how they go about changing what they do; or feeling good about what they do. The approach would also focus on social structures, practices, and media influences on what people do or do not do. It would aim at enabling an increased awareness of how culture, the economy, or political ideologies or activities affect what can be done and how popular discourse and ideas act on notions about occupational values, skill development, and issues such as work, recreation, or power. The approach could require the learning of new skills or new ways of doing. It would also require skill building programs to empower action and to enable participants to communicate effectively, to research and explore the background to perceived problems, to make decisions, to follow through with their ideas, and to practice new ways of doing.

Because this text has used the terms *doing, being,* and *becoming* to explore the idea of an occupational perspective of health, it is appropriate to use the same terms at the conclusion to bring the ideas full circle. Added to those is the idea of "belonging" that has surfaced during the exploration as intimately connected with them and that is particularly appropriate in an action-research approach. The following section presents some current issues suitable for action-research toward promoting health and well-being.

WELL DOING, BEING, BECOMING, AND BELONGING

How people obtain the requirements for living in any part of the world could be the focus of action-research. It appears from the exploration in this text that simply providing the requirements or the wherewithal to obtain them should only be a short-term solution in cases of emergency. Over the longer term, lack of necessity to "do" can lead to social, mental, and physical illness that in turn can lead to further disorders in communities. Except in emergencies, what people do to acquire the necessities of life must meet their biological needs and exercise their particular capacities to some extent at least. That implies that people need to be more aware of their skills and capacities than is the case for most at present. The concept may appear to be common sense and current practice, but that is far from the case. Many people do not know themselves well, education may not be available or not interest them because it fails to tap into their capacities, and employment may be sought because in affluent countries it is trendy, well-paid, and carries status, and in developing countries it is the only kind available. Lack of employment creates health disasters in the developing world and, in social-welfare states, may appear more attractive than working at something outside popular parameters if self-knowledge is limited.

Social determinants and equity issues may make self-knowledge and development even harder for some people, so programs for particular groups might be necessary to increase the integration of those who are severely marginalized, such as "refugees, disaster victims, the socially alienated, the mentally disabled, the very old and infirm, abused children and women, and the poor."[5] This approach recommends increasing all people's self-awareness and understanding of the occupation and health relationship so that necessary change can be effective.

Occupational behavior develops from the earliest age. Because this is the case, the origins of physical inactivity and the development of increasingly sedentary lifestyles that are current concerns can be traced from childhood. Profiling the multidimensional occupation patterns of children requires "a broad understanding of the complex, interrelated contextual, interpersonal, intrapersonal and temporal aspects of occupational performance."[105] Poulsen and Ziviani provide input on such profiling and a conceptual framework for advice on the optimal balance between physically active and sedentary pursuits that underpins physical and mental health.[105] Access to the WHO international program to stimulate mother-infant interaction is another avenue that could be utilized to improve the emotional, social, cognitive, and physical development of children particularly for those whose living conditions are stressful and socially impoverished.[106]

Education is a primary concern. The WHO points out a direction for potential action-research in its Mental Health fact sheet when it calls for the establishment of "child friendly schools."[5] This initiative is aimed at promoting sound psychosocial environments that encourage "tolerance and equality." It recommends[5]:

* "Active involvement and cooperation."
* Avoidance of physical punishment.
* Intolerance of bullying.
* A "supportive and nurturing environment."
* "Education which responds to the reality of the children's lives."
* "Helps to establish connections between school and family life."

* "Encourages creativity as well as academic abilities."
* Promotes self-esteem and self-confidence.
* More involvement in fostering healthy social and emotional development of pupils.

Any or all of those actions could be the focus of action-research, or run in conjunction with the WHO "life skills curriculum" developed to enable the growth of sound and positive mental health, which includes "problem-solving, critical thinking, communication, interpersonal skills, empathy, and methods to cope with emotions."[5] Making use of this curriculum could be valuable. Those past school years who for some reason were deprived of the chance to learn and develop capacities are another group in need of assistance. Programs similar to those for school-aged children can be adapted and used in action-research when deemed appropriate and desirable by participants.

Practical-based programs would also be valuable for those who want to develop particular skills such as maintain a home, build shelter, store clean water, grow food, or learn to cook, for example. Scott, Verne, and Fox note that food preparation skills appear to have been lost in younger generations in affluent countries, and this appears more so in poorer populations and those ethnically challenged in an unfamiliar environment.[107,108] There are links to NCDs[109] and to social exclusion.[110] In situations such as this, action-research could address the specific needs of the group by, for example, increasing marketing skills; awareness of food types and sources within communities; group access to information about healthy eating linked to doing; and group investigation of food production sources.[111] Enlisting support of community organizations and government agencies for and in programs of this nature can be empowering, and it may be that mediating or advocating on behalf of an action-research community to such effect could be the role most suited to the health professional members.

WHO *Active Ageing* policy guidelines are fundamental to health promotion and well-being.[4] They provide direction for action to and for all older people[4]:

* Realizing physical, social, and mental potential.
* Continuing to participate in society.
* Continuing to participate in economic, cultural, spiritual, and civic affairs.
* Being assured of adequate protection, security, and care when necessary.

Because of the agist orientation of postindustrial societies, less attention is given to provision of opportunities within normal life to doing, being, becoming, and belonging for older people than to support them when their health declines. Numerous studies demonstrate the benefits of active lifestyles that provide meaning, purpose, and continued development with like-minded others.[39,40,112-115] Decline is not necessarily a part of normal aging but occurs if there is a lessening in activity and participation. In either case, it is useful to bear in mind Wilson's view of working with older people as a "privilege of recognizing, respecting and integrating the richness and individuality of a person's longer lifespan."[116] There is a great need for action-research within communities throughout the world to assist understanding of this concept and to promote continuing good health for older people by, for example, enabling and extending social support networks and leisure opportunities.[117,118] Programs in which older people empower and assist younger people in many spheres will be particularly effective for both provider and receiver.

The word *function* is used by the WHO in the ICF (earlier versions classified the effects of disability in terms of dysfunction) as an active descriptive term that encompasses the necessary doings of daily life.[119] In the first chapter of this text, Greiner, Fain, and Edelman explained, "Functioning is integral to health," recognizing its physical, mental, and social domains include activity-exercise, roles-relationships, sleep-rest,[120] cognition-perception, self-perception-self-concept, and coping-stress tolerance and that loss of function may be a sign of ill health.[121] Any or all of these integrate doing with being, becoming, and belonging and might be issues that require attention within particular communities.

Meaning, purpose, and choice are fundamental to self worth,[122] quality of life, and well-being as existential philosophers contend.[123] Control also appears to be important.[124,125] All are inherent in people's doing, being, becoming, and belonging, but that can be either positive or negative in health terms.[47] The action-research process needs to ensure that the negative is recognized and discarded and the positive is experienced. It is a sad indictment of the affluent world that the negative effects of what, how, and why people get to "do" must be partly to blame for the increased incidence of depression that has reached what is described as epidemic proportions.[126] That also implies, as is clear from the exploration reported in this text, that economic, material, and educational advantages alone are insufficient to ensure health and well-being. Research indicates that when people "are given an opportunity to gain personal meaning from everyday activities, when their sense of optimism is renewed, and where they believe that there is choice and control in their lives" it is possible to avert depression.[125-127] This suggests that action-research could be centered on population understanding of the notions of doing, being, becoming, and belonging in association with health and well-being outcomes. There is support from a range of studies,[128-131] not least to counteract deficit-based services, a lack of voice, and communication barriers.[132] A capabilities framework developed by Amartya Sen and others in tune with the social model of disability might be useful here. Common themes include the relationship between social barriers and individual limitations, the importance of autonomy, the value of freedom, and dissatisfaction with income as a measure of well-being.[133]

Tertiary and quaternary approaches toward health promotion and quality of life for people with chronic diseases, disability, or terminal illness could fit into current occupational therapy in either medical or social care-based services. Extended programs in the community to embrace action-research in terms of physical activity and diet toward control of NCDs or eating disorders,[134] for example, would not only be timely, they could elicit support and resources additional to the norm. It is timely to progress in this way because of overwhelming acceptance at present of the significance of physical activity and diet in medical, economic, and humanitarian terms. In many places, occupational therapists are involved in discharge planning and assessments that would provide an avenue to extend services into health-promoting physical activity programs, to offer people more than coping skills, the provision of aids to daily living, and helping with the organization of assistance. Atwal suggests "in order to promote healthy discharge planning the occupational therapy profession needs to ensure that educational establishments provide appropriate training on the aging process, health promotion and discharge procedures."[135] Part of that process entails putting in place support mechanisms to provide people with opportunities to make choices, to enable them to set their own goals and to make life more meaningful.[136,137] Enabling terminally ill people to self-actualize or to accomplish long-held dreams is another health-promoting initiative that may stimulate community-based action-research and elicit community support. Focusing on health promotion rather than independence will provide benefits for the latter, for as Geller and Warren maintain, "both rehabilitation and healing are meant to enhance all aspects of well-being, restore integrity to a person, and facilitate the creation of meaning."[138] Enabling people to make responsible and healthy life-style choices calls for attention to behavioral, social, political, and environmental issues and to a matching of personalities, capacities, needs, meaning, and challenge with environmental factors.[139-142]

Environmental issues could be a focus of action-research toward well-being. An essential yet often forgotten aspect of health initiatives is the benefit derived through interaction with natural environments. The most celebrated early hospitals for the treatment of tuberculosis were situated in beautiful and isolated natural environments, and patients often lived and slept in outdoor rooms. There are current moves to reincorporate the natural world into the design of settings where medicine is practiced. Theories, hypotheses, and experimental evidence demonstrate positive effects on human health such as a lessening of the physiological effects of stress on the autonomic nervous system.[143] The built environment, too, can lessen or aggravate feelings of disease to the extent that a phenomenon known as "sick building syndrome" is acknowledged in public health. Many people experience the same environment throughout a lifetime that may significantly impact on their experience of health. Others constantly change where and how they live, yet the impact of moving house is well recognized as a major life stressor. New-age architecture is being responsive to health and quality of life needs by beginning to develop "lifetime homes" that are flexible to meet people's changing needs throughout the lifespan and "smart homes" that incorporate assistive technology.[144] Action-research that focuses on occupation-health related environmental issues is long overdue.

As part of a program to provide occupational science and therapy students at Deakin University in Australia with the skills required to set up action-research programs, they are required to explore a community health issue from an occupational perspective. One such group of first year students in 2005 explored "occupational environments." Recognizing that environments can inhibit or enhance people's engagement and performance in occupation, they understood they are also determinants of individual, population, and ecological health. Taking one example, they chose to focus on the difficulties experienced by Sudanese immigrants in an Australian city in accessing occupations of need and choice. The students proposed and developed an 8-week program that incorporated practical learning experiences. The key objective was to develop Sudanese immigrants' skills in the community and particularly in the use of public transport[145] (Figure 10-2). Small-scale action-research projects such as this can take multiple issues and enable and empower communities to act toward attaining increased health and well-being.

Working Toward World Health Organization "Health for All" Objectives Across the Globe

It has been heartening to find that the health-promoting and well-being directions recognized within WHO policies over the last 30 years have, increasingly, espoused the importance of what people do, how they experience and feel about what they do, that doing should encompass potential and meaning as well as the prerequisites of survival, and that the interactive nature of doing and belonging can be health giving. Making clear to WHO and other health, political, and economic organizations the congruence of an occupational perspective of health with those ideas is critical. To create a new profession to engage in action-research toward occupation-focused policies and initiatives would be a waste. It is time to act now.

As this text was being written, the sixth global conference on health promotion was taking place in Bangkok, its theme centering on the health issues emanating from a globalized world. The Charter calls for making the promotion of health central to the global development agenda, a core responsibility for all governments, a key focus of communities and civil society, and a requirement for good corporate practice. It urges[146]:

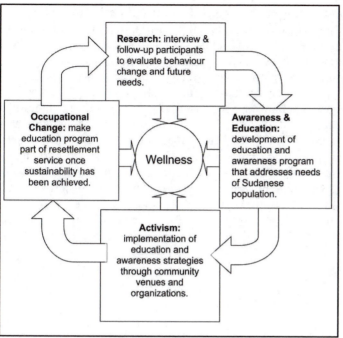

Research: interview & follow-up participants to evaluate behaviour change and future needs.

Occupational Change: make education program part of resettlement service once sustainability has been achieved.

Wellness

Awareness & Education: development of education and awareness program that addresses needs of Sudanese population.

Activism: implementation of education and awareness strategies through community venues and organizations.

Figure 10-2. Student initiated small-scale action-research project to develop Sudanese immigrants' skills in the community and particularly in the use of public transport.

* Advocacy "for health based on human rights and solidarity."

* Investment "in sustainable policies, actions and infrastructure to address the determinants of health."

* Capacity building "for policy development, leadership, health promotion practice, knowledge transfer and research, and health literacy."

* Regulation and legislation toward "a high level of protection from harm" and the enabling of "equal opportunity for health and well-being for all people."

* Building alliances and partnerships with "public, private, nongovernmental and international organizations and civil society to create sustainable action.

Public health practitioners have based their health promotion work on the WHO directives since the New Public Health emerged some 3 decades ago. However, their interest in occupation has been largely bounded by popular use of the word limiting it to paid employment. Taking up an occupation focus would not require a change of allegiance on their part, just a broader appreciation of occupation in line with many of the WHO directives as outlined in this text. For occupational therapists, the major change from current practice would be consideration of, and action toward, underlying sociopolitical and ecological issues and emphasis on all the population, not only sick or disabled individuals. Additionally, they would need to be open to the negative as well as positive health outcomes of occupation. Both disciplines would be required to understand and accept social illness such as war, under or over-employment, and poverty as domains of concern of equal importance to physical and mental illness as defined by medical science. It remains debatable whether either discipline will make such changes, although both have the philosophical persuasion and the potential to contribute to a wide-ranging and holistic occupation-focused approach to health promotion and well-being in line with WHO directives.

Failure to recognize the underlying factors that influence the relationship between occupation and health and failure to accept responsibility for research and action in this domain would be negligent. However, there is a major problem for occupational therapists. The profession continues to be largely unrecognized as a scientific discipline with a distinctive and important contribution to make to public health, and for it to articulate and follow a direction different from dominant paradigms implies that the profession has "to stick its neck out." A leading Australian social commentator suggests that although in current society there is a "need to encourage new ideas, dissident views, debates, and critics," those who argue have had "to speak the same language and work from similar sets of assumptions to those in power."[147] In the case of the WHO health promotion rhetoric, health is inextricably bound up with people's doing, being, becoming, and belonging, but it has been interpreted within public health from its own dominant paradigms, and the occupational elements have been largely disregarded. This leaves a major question as to whether public health will welcome, or even recognize, the potential contributions of occupational therapy's distinct and different viewpoint, or accept a different focus for its own discipline.

References

1. World Health Organization, Health and Welfare Canada, Canadian Public Health Association. *Ottawa Charter for Health Promotion*. Ottawa, Canada: Author; 1986:3.
2. Scriven A, ed. *Health Promoting Practice: The Contribution of Nurses and Allied Health Professionals*. Basingstoke, UK: Palgrave Macmillan; 2005.
3. World Health Organization. *Jakarta Declaration on Leading Health Promotion into the 21st Century*. Geneva: Author; 1998.
4. World Health Organization. *Active Ageing*. Geneva: Author.
5. World Health Organization. *Mental Health: Strengthening Mental Health Promotion. Fact Sheet N°220*. Geneva: Author; 2005.
6. World Health Organization. *Childrens Rights*. Office of the High Commissioner for Human Rights. Fact sheet No 10 (Rev.1) The Rights of the Child. Geneva. 1989. Available at: http://www.unhohr.ch/html/menu6/2/fs/0.htm. Accessed April 20, 2006.
7. Seedhouse D. *Health Promotion: Philosophy, Prejudice and Practice*. 2nd ed. Chichester, UK: Wiley; 2004:28-32.
8. Cribb A, Duncan P. *Health Promotion and Professional Ethics*. Oxford, UK: Blackwell Science; 2002.
9. Tones K. Health promotion: the empowerment imperative. In: Scriven A, Orme J, eds. *Health Promotion: Professional Perspective*. Basingstoke, UK: Palgrave Macmillan; 2001.
10. Department of Health. *The Report of the Chief Medical Officer's Project to Strengthen the Public Health Function*. London: The Stationers Office; 2001.
11. Mittelmark M. Global health promotion: challenges and opportunities. In: Scriven A, Garman S, eds. *Promoting Health: Global Issues and Perspectives*. Basingstoke, UK: Palgrave Macmillan; 2005.
12. Laverack G. *Health Promotion Practice: Power and Empowerment*. London: Sage; 2004.
13. Lalonde M. *A New Perspective on the Health of Canadians*. Ottawa: Information Canada; 1974.
14. Green LW, Frankish JC. Health promotion, health education and disease prevention. In: Koop CE, Pearson CE, Schwarz MR, eds. *Critical Issues in Global Health*. San Francisco, Calif: Jossey Bass; 2002.
15. Nutbeam D. Foreword. In: Bunton R, MacDonald G, eds. *Health Promotion: Disciplines, Diversity and Development*. 2nd ed. London: Routledge; 2002,
16. Scriven A, Garman S, eds. *Promoting Health: Global Issues and Perspectives*. Basingstoke, UK: Palgrave Macmillan; 2005.
17. Southwood-Smith T. *The Philosophy of Health; or an Exposition of the Physical and Mental Constitution of Man, with a view to the Promotion of Human Longevity and Happiness*. Vol 1. London: Charles Knight; 1836:101.
18. Wilcock AA. *Occupation for Health. Volume 1. A Journey from Self Health to Prescription*. London: British College of Occupational Therapists; 2001.
19. Crisp R. *Well-being. Stanford Dictionary of Philosophy*. 2001. Accessed January 2006.

20. Bentham J. *An introduction to the principles of morals and legislation.* Burns J, Hart HLA, eds. Oxford, UK: Clarendon Press; 1996:1.
21. Ewles L, Simnett I. *Promoting Health: A Practical Guide.* Edinburgh, UK: Bailliere Tindall; 2003:29.
22. World Health Organization. *International Classification of Functioning, Disability and Health.* Geneva: Author; 2000.
23. World Health Organization. *International Classification of Functioning, Disability and Health. Prefinal Draft.* Geneva: Author; 2002.
24. Maslow AH. *Toward a Psychology of Being.* 2nd ed. New York: D Van Nostrand Co; 1968:201.
25. Hetzel BS, McMichael T. *L S Factor: Lifesyle and Health.* Ringwood, Victoria: Penguin; 1987.
26. Iwami M. Occupation as a cross-cultural construct. In: Whiteford GE, Wright-St Clair V, eds. *Occupation and Practice in Context.* Sydney: Elsevier/Churchill Livingstone; 2005.
27. Iwami M. Situated meaning: an issue of culture, inclusion, and occupational therapy. In: Kronenberg F, Simo Algado S, Pollard N. *Occupational Therapy Without Borders: Learning From the Spirit of Survivors.* London: Elsevier Ltd; 2005
28. Dunn H. *High Level Wellness.* Arlington, Va: RW Beatty; 1954.
29. Dossey BM, Guzzetta CE. Wellness, values clarification and motivation. In: Dossey BM, Keegan L, Kolkmier LG, Guzzetta CE. *Holistic Health Promotion. A Guide for Practice.* Rockville, Md: Aspen Publishers; 1989:69-70.
30. Howard RB. Wellness: obtainable goal or impossible dream. *Post Graduate Medicine.* 1983;73(1):15-19.
31. Wilcock AA. Workshop: Holistic Health Care, Occupational Therapy and Stroke. Seminar on Stroke, National Heart Foundation, Auckland, New Zealand, November 1991.
32. The Asian NGO Coalition, IRED Asia, The people centred development forum. Economy, Ecology and Spirituality: Toward a Theory and Practice of Sustainablity. 1993.
33. Potter VR. Bioethics, the science of survival. *Biology and Medicine.* 1970;14:127-153.
34. Hettler W. Wellness—the lifetime goal of a university experience. In: Matarazzo JD, et al, eds. *Behavioral Health. A Handbook of Health Enhancement and Disease Prevention.* New York: John Wiley and Sons; 1990:1117.
35. Tannahill A. What is health promotion. *Health Education Journal.* 1985;44:167-168.
36. Jones L. Promoting health: everybody's business? In: Katz J, Peberdy A, Douglas J, eds. *Promoting Health: Knowledge and Practice.* Basingstoke, UK: Macmillan; 2000.
37. Katz J, Peberdy A, Douglas J, eds. *Promoting Health: Knowledge and Practice.* Basingstoke, UK: Macmillan; 2000.
38. Wilcock A. The occupational brain: a theory of human nature. *Journal of Occupational Science: Australia.* 1995;2(1):68-73.
39. Clark F, Azen SP, Zemke R, et al. Occupational therapy for independent older adults: A randomized controlled trial. *JAMA.* 1997;Oct 22/29:1321-1326.
40. Glass TA, de Leon CM, Marottoli RA, Berkman LF. Population based study of social and productive activities as predictors of survival among elderly Americans. *BMJ.* 1999;319:478-483.
41. Kalache A, Aboderin I, Hoskins I. Compression of morbidity and active aging: key priorities for public health policy in the 21st century. Bulletin of the World Health Organization. Geneva: World Health Organization; Accessed 2005. <Bull World Health Organvol.80no.3Genebra2002>
42. Labonte R. Foreword. In: Laverick G, ed. *Health Promoting Practice: Power and Empowerment.* London: Sage; 2004.
43. Society of Health Education and Promotion Specialists. Health promotion in Transition, Paper 5: Principles and Philosophy. Birmingham, UK: SHEPS; 2002. In: Scriven A, ed. *Health Promoting Practice: The Contribution of Nurses and Allied Health Professionals.* Basingstoke, UK: Palgrave Macmillan; 2005.
44. Law M. Distinguished Scholar Lecture: Participation in the occupations of everyday life. *Am J Occup Ther.* 2002;56:640-649.
45. Law M, Baum CM, Baptiste S. *Occupation Based Practice: Fostering Performance and Participation.* Thorofare, NJ: SLACK Incorporated; 2002.
46. Sumsion T. Promoting health through client centred occupational therapy practice. In: Scriven A, ed. *Health Promoting Practice: The Contribution of Nurses and Allied Health Professionals.* Basingstoke, UK: Palgrave Macmillan; 2005.
47. Canadian Association of Occupational Therapists. *Enabling Occupation: An Occupational Therapy Perspective.* Ottawa: CAOT Publications; 2002.
48. Letts L, Rigby P, Stewart D, eds. *Using Environments to Enable Occupational Performance.* Thorofare, NJ: SLACK Incorporated; 2003.
49. Corring D, Cook J. Client-centred care means that I am a valued human being. *Can J Occup Ther.* 1999; 66(2):71-82.

50. Honey A. Empowerment versus power: consumer participation in mental health services. *Occupational Therapy International.* 1999;6(4):257-276.

51. College of Occupational Therapists. *COT Strategy: From Interface to Integration.* London: Author; 2002.

52. Madill H, Townsend E, Schultz P. Implementing a health promotion strategy in occupational therapy and practice. *Can J Occup Ther.* 1989;56(2):67-72.

53. Letts L, Fraser B, Finlayson M, Walls J. *For the Health of It! Occupational Therapy Within a Health Promotion Framework.* Toronto, Ontario: CAOT Publications; 1996.

54. Thibeault R, Hebert M. A congruent model for health promotion in occupational therapy. *Occupational Therapy International.* 1997;4(4):271-293.

55. Townsend E, Landry J. Interventions in a societal context: Enabling participation. In: Christiansen CH, Baum CM, eds. *Occupational Therapy Performance, Participation, and Well-Being.* Thorofare, NJ: SLACK Incorporated; 2005:507.

56. do Rozario L. Ritual, meaning and transcendence: the role of occupation in modern life. *Journal of Occupational Science: Australia.* 1994;1(3):46-53

57. Rappaport R. *Ecology, Meaning, and Religion.* Richmond, Va: North Atlantic Books; 1979.

58. Payne WA, Hahn DB. *Understanding Your Health.* 4th ed. St. Louis, Mo: Mosby; 1995:26.

59. Wilcock AA, et al. Retrospective Study of Elderly Peoples' Perceptions of the Relationship Between Their Lifes' Occupations and Health. Unpublished material, University of South Australia, 1990.

60. Ciechanowski P, Wagner E, Schmaling K, et al. Community-integrated home-based depression treatment in older adults: a randomized controlled trial. *JAMA.* 2004;291:1569-1577.

61. Cacioppo J. Biological costs of social stress in the elderly. Paper given at the American Psychological Association. Washington, D.C. 2000. (Reported in: The University of Chicago Chronicle. Vol 19. No.20. Aug 17 2000).

62. Maguire G. An exploratory study of the relationship of valued activities to the life satisfaction of elderly persons. *Occupational Therapy Journal of Research.* 1983;3:164-171.

63. American Occupational Therapy Association. Glossary: essentials for an approved program for the occupational therapy assistant. *Am J Occup Ther.* 1976;30:262.

64. Neville R. *Play Power.* London: Cape; 1970.

65. Roszak T. *The Making of a Counter Culture.* New York: Doubleday; 1969.

66. Johnson J. Wellness and occupational therapy. *Am J Occup Ther.* 1986;40(11):753-758.

67. Reed KL, Sanderson SN. *Concepts of Occupational Therapy.* Baltimore: Williams & Wilkins; 1980:92.

68. Johnson JA. Wellness: Its myths, realities and potential for occupational therapy. *Occupational Therapy in Health Care.* 1985;2(2):117-138.

69. White VK. Promoting health and wellness: a theme for the eighties. *Am J Occup Ther.* 1986;40(11):743-748.

70. Thomas TL, ed. *Taber's Cyclopedic Medical Dictionary.* 18th ed. Philadelphia: F.A. Davis; 1997:2110.

71. Zechetmayr M. Wellness programs and employee assistance programs in industry. *Arena Review.* 1986;10(1):28-42.

72. Conrad P. Wellness in the workplace: potentials and pitfalls of worksite health promotion. *Milbank Quarterly.* 1987;65(2):255-275.

73. Conrad P, Walsh DC. The new corporate health ethic: lifestyle and the social control of work. *International Journal of Health Services.* 1992;22(1):89-111.

74. Walsh DC, Jennings SE, Mangione T, Merrigan DM. Health promotion versus health protection? Employees' perceptions and concerns. *Journal of Public Health Policy.* 1991;12(2):148-164.

75. Melaleuca: The Wellness Company. Experience the New Product Store. Accessed 2006.

76. National Exercise and Sports Trainers Association. Corporate Fitness and Trainers Programs. 2006.

77. Spencer University of Southern California. Executive Certification in Health Promotion and Corporate Wellness. Available at: http://vw.spenceruniversity.org/ - 18k. Accessed April 2006.

78. Opatz JP. *A Primer of Health Promotion: Creating Healthy Organizational Cultures.* Washington, DC: Oryn Publications; 1985:7.

79. Quality of Life Research Unit. University of Toronto. Notes on "Quality of Life". Accessed. November 2005.

80. Ontario Social Development Council, 1997. Notes on "Quality of Life." Accessed November 2005.

81. Christiansen CH, Baum C, eds. *Occupational Therapy: Enabling Function and Well-Being.* 2nd ed. Thorofare, NJ: SLACK Incorporated: 1997.

82. Punwar AJ, Peloquin SM, eds. *Occupational Therapy: Principles and Practice.* 3rd ed. Philadelphia: Lippincott Williiams and Wilkins; 2000

83. Stein F, Roose B. *Pocket Guide to Treatment in Occupational Therapy.* San Diego, Calif: Singular Publishing Co; 2000.

84. Whitston C, Waddington J. Why join a union? *New Statesman and Society.* 1994;7(329):36-38.

85. Antonovsky A. The sense of coherence as a determinant of health. In: Matarazzo JD, et al, eds. *Behavioral Health. A Handbook of Health Enhancement and Disease Prevention.* New York: John Wiley and Sons; 1990:124.

86. Boddy J, ed. *Health: Perspectives and Practices.* New Zealand: The Dunmore Press; 1985:48.

87. World Health Organization. *Mental Health Promotion.* Accessed November 2005.

88. Descartes R. *Discourse on the Method of Rightly Conducting the Reason, IV.* New York: The Liberal Arts Press; 1954.

89. Rosi EL. *The Psychobiology of Mind-Body Healing.* New York: WW Norton and Co, Inc; 1986.

90. Pert C. The wisdom of receptors: neuropeptides, the emotions, and bodymind. *Advances.* 1986;3(3):8-16.

91. Dossey B. The psychophysiology of bodymind healing. In: Dossey B, et al. *Holistic Health Promotion: A Guide for Practice.* Rockville, Md: Aspen Publishers; 1989.

92. Emeth EV, Greenhut JH. *The Wholeness Handbook: Care of Body, Mind and Spirit for Optimal Health.* New York: The Continuum Publishing Co; 1991.

93. Pelletier KR. *Sound Mind, Sound Body.* New York: Simon and Schuster; 1994.

94. British Geriatrics Society. Health Promotion and Preventive Care. (reviewed 2005). BGS Compendium Document 4. Accessed January 2006.

95. Harms B. (News Office). New research reveals how loneliness can undermine health. The University of Chicago Chronicle. Vol 19. No.20. Aug 17 2000.

96. Stoddart H, Sharp D, Harvey I. Letters: social networks are important in preventing dependency in old age. *BMJ.* 2000;320:1277.

97. United Nations. 2nd UN World Assembly on Ageing. Madrid, Spain: 2002.

98. World Health Organization. Health and aging: A discussion paper. Geneva: World Health Organization; 2001. Unpublished document WHO/NMH/HPS/01.1. In: Kalache A, Aboderin I, Hoskins I. Compression of morbidity and active aging: key priorities for public health policy in the 21st century. Bulletin of the World Health Organization. Geneva: World Health Organization; Accessed 2005. <Bull World Health Organvol.8 0no.3Genebra2002>

99. Fries JF. Aging, natural death, and the compression of morbidity. *N Engl J Med.* 1980;303:130-5.

100. McMurdo MET. A healthy old age: realistic or futile goal? *BMJ.* 2000;321:1149-1151.

101. Ryan RS, Travis JW. *The Wellness Workbook.* Berkley, Calif: Ten Speed Press; 1981:xv.

102. Levenstein S. Wellness, health, Antonovsky. *Advances.* 1994;10(3):26-29.

103. Wilcock AA. Domiciliary care, occupational therapists and health promotion. The Proceedings of the Australian Association of Occupational Therapists 15th Federal Conference. Sydney, Australia, 1988.

104. Flannery G, Barry M. An exploration of occupational therapist' perceptions of health promotion. *Irish J Occup Ther.* 2003;33-41.

105. Poulsen AA, Ziviani, JM. Health enhancing physical activity: factors influencing engagement patterns in children. *Australian Occupational Therapy Journal.* 2004;51(2):69-79.

106. World Health Organization. International program to stimulate mother-infant interaction. Accessed 2005.

107. Scott P, Verne J, Fox C. Promoting better nutrition: the role of dieticians. In: Scriven A, ed. *Health Promoting Practice: The Contribution of Nurses and Allied Health Professionals.* Basingstoke, UK: Palgrave Macmillan; 2005.

108. Lang T, Raynor G, eds. *Why Health is the Key to the Future of Food and Farming.* London: UK Public Health Association, Chartered Institute of Environmental Health, Faculty of Public Health Medicine, National Heart Forum and Health Development Agency; 2002.

109. James WPT, Nelson M, Ralph A, Leather S. Socioeconomic determinants of health: the contribution of nutrition to inequalities in health. *BMJ.* 1997;314:1545-1548.

110. Leather S. *The Making of Modern Malnutrition: An Overview of Food Poverty in the UK.* London: Caroline Walker Society; 1996.

111. Department of Health. Towards a Food and Health Action Plan: Discussion Paper. London: Department of Health; 2004.

112. Yaffe K, Barnes D, Nevitt M, Lui L, Covinsky R. A prospective study of physical activity and cognitive decline in elderly women. *Arch Intern Med.* 2001;161(14):1703-1708.

113. McIntyre A, Bryant W. Activity and participation. In: McIntyre A, Atwal A, eds. *Occupational Therapy for Older People.* Oxford, UK: Blackwell Publishing; 2005.

114. Mather AS, Rodriguez C, Guthrie MF, McHarg AM, Reid IC, McMurdo MET. Effects of exercise on depressive symptoms in older adults with poorly responsive depressive disorder. *Br J Psychiatry.* 2002;180:411-415.

115. Manson JE, Greenland P, La Croix AZ, et al. Walking compared with vigorous exercise for the prevention of cardiovascular events in women. *N Engl J Med.* 2002;347(10):716-725.

116. Wilson L. Activity and participation: part 2. In: McIntyre A, Atwal A, eds. *Occupational Therapy for Older People.* Oxford, UK: Blackwell Publishing; 2005.

117. Mayers CA. The Casson Memorial Lecture 2000: Reflect on the past to shape the future. *Br J Occup Ther.* 2000;63(8):358-366.

118. Reynolds F, Kee Hean Lim. The social context of older people. In: McIntyre A, Atwal A, eds. *Occupational Therapy for Older People.* Oxford, UK: Blackwell Publishing; 2005.

119. World Health Organization. *International Classification of Functioning, Disability and Health*. Geneva: World Health Organization; 2001.

120. Labyak S. Sleep and circadian schedule disorders. *Nurs-clin;North Am*. 2002;37(4):599-610.

121. Greiner PA, Fain JA, Edelman CL. Health defined: objectives for promotion and prevention. In: Edelman CL, Mandle CL, eds. *Health Promotion Throughout the Lifespan*. 5th ed. St Louis, Mo: Mosby; 2002:6.

122. Somner KL, Baumeister RF. The construction of meaning from life events. In: Wong PT, Fry PS, eds. *The Human Quest for Meaning*. Mahwah, NJ: Erlbaum; 1998.

123. Plahuta JM, McCulloch BJ, Kasarshis EJ, Ross MA, Walter RA, McDonald ER. Amyotrophic lateral sclerosis and hopelessness: psychosocial factors. *Soc Sci Med*. 2002;55:2131-2140.

124. Hammell KW. Using qualitative evidence to inform theories of occupation. In: Hammell KW, Carpenter C, eds. *Qualitative Research in Evidence-Based Rehabilitation*. Edinburgh: Churchill Livingstone; 2004.

125. Hammell KW. Dimensions of meaning in the occupations of daily life. *Can J Occup Ther*. 2004;71:5:296-305.

126. Murray CJL, Lopez AD. *The Global Burden of Disease*. Geneva: WHO; 1996.

127. Christiansen C. Defining lives: Occupation as identity: an essay on competence, coherence, and the creation of meaning. Eleanor Clarke Slagle lecture. *Am J Occup Ther*. 1999;53:547-558.

128. Rask K, Astedt-Kurki P, Paavilainen E, Laippala P. Adolescent subjective well-being and family dynamics. *Scandinavian J of Caring Science*. 2003;17(2):129-138.

129. Gunnarsdottir S, Bjornsdottir K. Health promotion in the workplace: the perspective of unskilled workers in a hospital setting. *Scandinavian Journal of Caring Science*. 2003;17(1):66-73.

130. Guinn B, Vincent V. Select physical activity determinants in independent-living elderly. *Activity, Adaptation, Ageing*. 2002;26(4):17-26.

131. Messias DK, De-Jong MK, Mcloughlin K. Being Involved and making a difference: Empowerment and well-being among women living in poverty. *Journal of Holistic Nursing*. 2005;239(1):70-88.

132. Sheehy K, Nind M, Emotional well-being for all: mental health and people with profound and multiple learning disabilities. *British Journal of Learning Disabilities*. 2005;33(1):34-38.

133. Burchardt T. Capabilities and disability; the capabilities framework and the social model of disability. *Disability in Society*. 2004;19(7):735-751.

134. Harris P. Health promotion in eating disorders: The contribution of occupational therapists. In: Scriven A, ed. *Health Promoting Practice: The Contribution of Nurses and Allied Health Professionals*. Basingstoke, UK: Palgrave Macmillan; 2005.

135. Atwal A. Healthy discharges for older persons: a health promotion role for occupational therapists in acute health care. In: Scriven A, ed. *Health Promoting Practice: The Contribution of Nurses and Allied Health Professionals*. Basingstoke, UK: Palgrave Macmillan; 2005.

136. Menon S. Toward a model of psychological health empowerment: implications for health care in multicultural communities. *Nurse Education Today*. 2002;22:28-39.

137. Sinclair K. World connected: The international context of professional practice. In: Whiteford GE, Wright-St Clair V, eds. *Occupation and Practice in Context*. Sydney: Elsevier/Churchill Livingstone; 2005.

138. Geller G, Warren LR. Toward an optimal healing environment in pediatric rehabilitation. *J Alternat Complement Med*. 2004;10(Supp1):S179-S192.

139. Christiansen CH, Townsend EA. *Occupation: The Art and Science of Living*. Upper Saddle River, NJ: Prentice Hall; 2004.

140. Callahan D. *False Hope*. New York: Simon & Schuster. 1998.

141. Csiksentmihalyi M. *Flow: The Psychology of Optimal Experience*. New York: Harper and Row; 1990.

142. Christiansen CH, Little BR, Backman C. Personal projects: a useful approach to the study of occupation. *Am J Occup Ther*. 1998; 52(6):439-446.

143. Irvine KN, Warber SL. Greening healthcare: practicing as if the natural environment really mattered. *Alternative Ther Health Med*. 2002;8(5):76-83.

144. Atwel A, Farrow A, Sivell-Muller M. Environmental impacts, products and technology. In: McIntyre A, Atwal A, eds. *Occupational Therapy for Older People*. Oxford, UK: Blackwell Publishing; 2005.

145. Boromeo B, Burgess N, Deutscher B, Fox C, McArthur J, O'Donnell L, Quick L. 'They've got a ticket to ride': Addressing the public transport needs of Sudanese re-settlers in Melbourne. Deakin University Occupational Science and Therapy: 1st year student project; 2005.

146. World health Organization. Bangkok Charter for Health promotion in a Globalized World. 6th Global Conference on Health Promotion. Bangkok: 2005. Available at: http://www.who.int/health promotion/conference/6gchp/bangkok_charter/en/index.html>

147. Cox E. A truly civil society: lecture 1: broadening the views. The 1995 Boyer Lectures. Australia: Radio National Transcripts; 1995:Nov 7.

Suggested Reading

Clark F, Azen SP, Zemke R, et al. Occupational therapy for independent older adults: A randomized controlled trial. *JAMA.* 1997;Oct 22/29:1321-1326.

Fries JF. Aging, natural death, and the compression of morbidity. *N Engl J Med.* 1980;303:130-135.

Hammell KW. Dimensions of meaning in the occupations of daily life. *Can J Occup Ther.* 2004;71:5:296-305.

Iwami M. Occupation as a cross-cultural construct. In: Whiteford GE, Wright-St Clair V, eds. *Occupation and Practice in Context.* Sydney: Elsevier/Churchill Livingstone; 2005.

Johnson JA. Wellness: its myths, realities and potential for occupational therapy. *Occupational Therapy in Health Care.* 1985;2(2):117-138.

Jones L. Promoting health: everybody's business? In: Katz J, Peberdy A, Douglas J, eds. *Promoting Health: Knowledge and Practice.* Basingstoke, UK: Macmillan; 2000.

Kalache A, Aboderin I, Hoskins I. Compression of morbidity and active aging: key priorities for public health policy in the 21st century. *Bulletin of the World Health Organization.* Geneva: World Health Organization; 2002.

Laverack G. *Health Promotion Practice: Power and Empowerment.* London: Sage; 2004.

Murray CJL, Lopez AD. *The Global Burden of Disease.* Geneva: WHO; 1996.

Poulsen AA, Ziviani, JM. Health enhancing physical activity: Factors influencing engagement patterns in children. *Australian Occupational Therapy Journal.* 2004;51(2):69-79.

Scriven A, ed. *Health Promoting Practice: The Contribution of Nurses and Allied Health Professionals.* Basingstoke, UK: Palgrave Macmillan; 2005.

Southwood-Smith T. *The Philosophy of Health; or an Exposition of the Physical and Mental Constitution of Man, with a view to the Promotion of Human Longevity and Happiness.* Volume 1. London: Charles Knight; 1836.

Epilogue: Summation and Challenge

Within the confines of my research, it was possible to explore only some of the more obvious connections and philosophical associations implied by the theory of human nature I proposed in Chapter 2. The exploration has, however, tested it in many directions and, in the main, supported its contentions. A theory of human nature must consider the biological characteristics that all humans share. Additionally, because I was relating the theory to health and survival, it appeared wise to subject it to other notions about health and survival of a biological nature that have been subjected to rigorous study by scientists of many disciplines. For this reason, I explored ideas held by evolutionary scientists and geneticists and considered the theory in terms of neuroscientific understanding of human behavior. This furthered my belief that physiological systems support and promote occupation to such an extent that the need "to do" is so natural, so much a part of being, that humans have failed to recognize it as an entity. It is the means to survive and to achieve health. Instead, people have reduced the holistic concept of occupation by dividing it and then made it more complex by endowing specific aspects with particular value.

The value and the division of occupation has altered with its evolution and because of cultural diversity. It has also altered because humans' occupational nature has immense variability, so that no 2 people have the same occupational capacities, potential, or needs, and these are susceptible to and developed according to environmental demands. Despite the variability, it was possible to tease out 6 major functions of occupation, which form a 3-way link with survival and health. These functions enable:

1. The attainment of the prerequisites of survival and health such as sustenance, self-care, and shelter.

2. Safety from and apparent superiority over predators and the environment.

3. Balanced exercise of personal, physical, mental, and social capacities.

4. The finding of meaning, purpose, choice, and satisfaction through doing.

5. Development so that each person and the species will flourish.

6. A sense of belonging through shared occupations that cannot be achieved satisfactorily by an individual.

The variability between people and cultures over time made it important to subject economic evolution to an occupational perspective; this reinforced a view held by many that human action (occupation) shapes culture and is, in turn, shaped by culture. People's potential for new and different pursuits, for exploring ways of making their lives easier, and giving themselves time for chosen occupations has led to a situation in which the products and results of doing appear to have assumed a greater importance than "natural" human need or the health and survival of the ecosystem on which humans depend.

An exploration of the history of ideas that surround health, well-being, and illness uncovered underlying determinants that have resulted from humans' occupational natures, from the economic base of societies, the ways of structuring them, and the values that emanate from them. The institutions and activities resulting from these foundations and their effect upon the occupational experience of individuals and communities can lead to positive or negative health outcomes. Research and action are required to promote the positive or inhibit the negative from an occupational perspective. I am convinced that the study of health, from this perspective, requires serious and immediate consideration, research, and action at individual, community, and environmental levels. Action-research is an obvious choice of methodology, alongside epidemiology, to explore the underlying determinants of health and ill health from an occupational perspective.

The 4 approaches discussed in this section of the book were chosen, in part, because different aspects of public health are demonstrated and, in part, because together they represent a holistic paradigm of occupation within population health practice. They also, in large measure, summarize the outcomes of the exploration undertaken in this history of ideas.

An ecologically sustainable community development approach seeks population health based on the development of self-sustaining occupational infrastructures. This broad perspective concentrates on encouraging local community action that will enhance well-being through changes to sociopolitical institutions and activities at global, national, or local levels. Linked with ecological sustainability, the approach strives toward the transformation of economic, political, and sociocultural structures so that the world and its interdependent life systems and organisms will survive healthily in the long term. As the occupational nature of people is, in large part, to blame for the underlying factors that have led to the present unacceptable state of the ecology and nation-centered economic policies, the transformation of occupational behaviors, that meet both human and ecological needs, is essential.

An occupational justice approach aspires to a more equitable experience of health and access to occupations conducive to well-being, conditions that are health giving for affluent and developing nations alike, and access to appropriate medical and preventive services for all people. Occupational inequities and injustices prevail universally, affecting health outcomes negatively; action-research toward identifying and eradicating both inequities and injustice is required urgently.

An occupation-focused preventive approach to illness and disability is concerned with preventing people from experiencing negative health outcomes because of a poor appreciation of the links between health, illness, and people's doing, being, and strivings to become. It is about limiting occupation-based risk factors of illness and disability such as poverty, urbanization, substance abuse, and physical inactivity for individuals and populations. Prevention of individual and community occupations and occupational institutions that erode health and lead to disability, disease, or premature death are central to that approach.

This occupation-focused health promotion approach is aimed at improvement in health and well-being for all people across the globe. It takes into account biological needs and physiological factors such as homeostasis that are part of natural health mechanisms. It draws on the WHO prerequisites for health and directives for increased physical activity and mental and spiritual growth toward potential and self-actualization. It encourages occupation-focused social action-research toward sociopolitical understanding of people's occupational health needs. Patterns of occupation, occupational balance, satisfaction, creativity, choice, and opportunity to meet unique capacities, meanings, and potential are important.

Five specific issues have been addressed in this second edition:
1. Health as a natural state that is dependent on occupation as the means to maintain and enhance it.
2. A theory of the place of occupation in human life, health, and survival.

3. Occupation, defined as doing, being, and becoming, as a positive and negative influence on health.

4. The potential contribution of occupation-focused approaches to population health based on current WHO directives.

5. Possible occupation-focused action-research for occupational therapists or public health practitioners to improve ecosustainable community development, occupational justice, health, and well-being world-wide, and to prevent illness, disability, and premature death.

In a 19th century paper, *Dedicated to the Governments of Great Britain, Austria, Russia, France, Prussia and the United States of America*, Robert Owen posed 20 questions to the human race. Among them were:

"Is it not in the interest of the human race that everyone should be so taught, and placed, that he would find his highest enjoyment to arise from the continued practice of doing all in his power to promote the well-being, and happiness, of every man, woman, and child, without regard to their class, sect, party, country or colour?"

Owen R. Paper: Dedicated to the Governments of Great Britain, Austria, Russia, France, Prussia and the United States of America. *London: New Lanark Conservation; 1841.*

GLOSSARY

action-research: Research aimed at social change through self-reflective inquiry undertaken by participants within any shared situation to increase understanding of the ideologies and practices of their particular situation and to empower and improve them through action. It is usually described as a dynamic, spiraling process with ongoing observation, reflection, planning, and action and is aligned with critical research.

agrarian: A way of life centered on an agricultural economy.

alienation: A state in which through historically created human possibilities a person, community, or society is estranged to an activity or its results or products, the nature in which it lives, other human beings, and to self.

artifact: A purposefully formed object; any object used, modified, or made by humans.

Arts and Crafts movement: A 19th century English social and aesthetic movement, largely antimachines. Founded by William Morris and his Pre-Raphaelite associates.

atomistic societies: Societies such as many in the "West" that are based on individualism, external connections, causal and reductionistic explanations, rule orientation, and artificial frameworks.

biotope: The smallest subdivision of a habitat characterized by a high degree of uniformity in its environmental conditions, plants, and animal life.

Broca's area: Part of the human cerebral cortex involved in speech production. It is situated in the left frontal lobe and named after Paul Broca, a French surgeon.

capacities: Innate and sometimes undeveloped potential, aptitude, ability, talent, trait, or power of individuals for anything in particular.

Cartesian dualism: Separation of mind and soul from body and brain. The former can exist without the latter and withstand its corruption and death (term based on the work of René Descartes, see Descartian).

coercion: Constrain into obedience.

community development: Community consultation, deliberation, and action to promote individual, family, and community responsibility for self-sustaining development and well-being.

copying-fidelity: Reproduction of exact copies.

critical research: A research approach oriented toward advocacy and criticism in order to unmask the ideological roots in self-understanding that constrain equity and support hegemony, and to empower individuals/groups toward greater autonomy, social justice, and emancipation. It is openly ideological, political, and socially analytical.

critical social science: An interpretive critique of society, especially of the theoretical bases of its organization.

cytoarchitectonic maps: Maps of the brain in terms of the structure and function of cells.

delayed return economies: Time investment in the future is part of daily life.

Descartian (link with Cartesian dualism): René Descartes (1596–1650), French philosopher and mathematician. After a Jesuit education and military service, he settled in Holland. Descartes' *Discourse on Method* (1637) introduced themes that he developed in his greatest work, *The Meditations* (1641). Asking "How and what do I know?" he arrived at his famous statement "Cogito ergo sum" ("I think, therefore I am"). From this he proved to his own satisfaction God's existence (he was a Roman Catholic) and hence the existence of everything else. He believed that the world consisted of 2 different substances—mind and matter (the doctrine of Cartesian dualism).

division of labor: The separation of tasks. It may take several forms such as social division of labor according to the economics of different societies and communities; division of labor by gender, which is a basic structural element in human social organizations that originates from differences in human physiology; and division of labor between workers who perform only a partial operation in production and what is produced is a social product of the collective workers.

DNA (deoxyribonucleic acid): The chief ingredient of chromosomes, DNA is necessary for the organization and functioning of living cells.

ecological sustainability: To uphold and support the ecology and ecosystems by practices that maintain, and continue to maintain, the natural environment and the relationships of different species.

ecology: The scientific study of organisms in their natural environment, including the relationships of different species with each other and the environment.

ecosystem: A biological community and the physical environment associated with it.

electrophoresis: A technique for the analysis and separation of colloids; used extensively in studying mixtures of proteins, nucleic acids, carbohydrates, enzymes, etc. In clinical medicine it is used for determining the protein content of body fluids.

epidemiology: The basic science of public health and preventive medicine. Originally, the study of epidemic diseases and their control.

epigenesis: The development of an organism from an undifferentiated cell, consisting in the successive formation and development of organs and parts that do not pre-exist in the fertilized egg.

ethology: The study of animal and human behavior. Central to the ethologist's approach is the principle that animal behavior (like physical characteristics) is subject to evolution through natural selection, through the development of the individual, and, in humans, in cultural history.

existentialism: A philosophical movement that rejects the metaphysical and centers on an individual person as a being in the world. It has as a major tenet that every person is unique, and cannot be explained in reductionist physiological terms. It aims toward a comprehensive concept of human existence and uses phenomenological methods to grasp the "essence" of peoples' consciousness, feelings, moods, experiences, and relationships.

fecundity: The fertility of an organism. Normally all organisms, assuming they reach reproductive age, are sufficiently fecund to replace themselves several times over. Darwin noted this, together with the fact that population numbers nevertheless tended to remain fairly constant. These observations led him to formulate his theory of evolution by natural selection.

feminism: A doctrine and movement advocating the granting of the same social, political, and economic rights to women as the ones granted to men.

flow: A state of consciousness when people are so involved in an activity that nothing else seems to matter; of optimal experience, transcendence, and enjoyment when individuals are challenged but engaged within the scope of their abilities.

founder effect: The genetic consequences of founding a new population with few individuals. The founder population will most likely differ genetically from its parent population because it will contain only a fraction of the total genetic variation. Any recessive gene will increase in frequency.

gene: A unit of heredity composed of DNA. In classical genetics, a gene is visualized as a discrete particle, forming part of a chromosome, that determines a particular characteristic.

gene flow: The exchange of genes among populations either directly by migration or by diffusion of genes over many generations.

general systems theory: A theory put forward by von Bertalanffy that, in the broadest sense, refers to a collection of general concepts, principles, tools, problems, and methods associated with all kinds of systems.

genetic drift: The random change of gene frequencies over time that happens in all populations but can take place rapidly in small populations.

genome: The complete set of genetic information in every living organism. Human genome consists of 3000 million matching pairs of nucleotides.

hegemony: Domination or leadership, especially the predominant influence of one state over another.

high longevity: Long life.

history of ideas: Discipline that studies the history and development of ideas and theories in terms of their origins and influences.

holism: Philosophical theory that wholes are greater than the sum of their parts. In health care, treating of the whole person rather than the symptoms of a disease. First used in modern times by JC Smuts in 1928.

hominid: Of the primate family including humans and their fossil ancestors (Latin *Homo homin* = man).

Homo: The genus of primates that includes modern humans (modern *Homo sapiens* sometimes known as *Homo sapien sapiens*, the only living representative) and various extinct species, of which 4 or 5 are usually recognized although the number is uncertain.

  * *H. habilis*: the earliest species (small and large forms, probably 2 species).

  * *H. erectus*: descended from *H. habilis*.

  * *H. sapiens*: descended from *H. erectus*.

  * Neanderthal man (*H. sapiens Neanderthalensis* or *H. Neanderthalensis*).

Homo erectus: A direct ancestor of modern man who appeared about 1.5 million years ago and lived to 300,000 years ago. Fossils of *H. erectus*, which are sometimes called Pithecanthropus (ape man), are similar to present-day man except that there was a prominent ridge above the eyes and no forehead or chin. They had crude stone tools and used fire.

Homo habilis: Probably the earliest *Homo*. Fossils of *H. habilis* were first found at Olduvai Gorge in Tanzania. Estimated to have lived at least 2.3 to 1.5 million years ago. Gracile and delicate-boned toolmaker.

Hormic School of Psychology: An early psychological school of thought centered on vital or purposeful energy, and related to Jung's view of the importance of an individual's search for meaning in life.

humanism: A nonreligious philosophy based on belief in potential of human nature rather than in religious or transcendental values.

humoral theory: An earlier and long living physiological theory in which health was contingent upon a balance between 4 humours: blood, phlegm, black bile, and yellow bile. It formed the basis of rules for health that served preventive and curative purposes and population health maintenance and promotion. Based, largely, on acute observations of the natural world.

immediate return economies: Hand-to-mouth subsistence existence.

individualism: A social theory that emphasizes the importance of the individual.

kin selection: Natural selection of genes that tends to cause the individuals bearing them to be altruistic to close relatives. These relatives have a higher probability of bearing identical copies of those same genes than do other members of the population. Thus, kin selection for a gene that tends to cause an animal to share food with a close relative will result in the gene being spread through the population because it (unconsciously) benefits itself. The more closely two animals are related, the higher the probability that they share some identical genes and therefore the more closely their interests coincide. Parental care is a special case of kin selection.

!Kung San: Hunter-gatherer peoples who live on the northern fringe of the Kalahari Desert. Their language has a characteristic clicking sound that is represented by ! prefixing Kung.

long distance exchange: The exchange of objects as currency a long distance from where the objects are found or made. Seashells found hundreds of miles inland are a particularly good example.

Marxist structuralism: A philosophy of science or method of inquiry that has affinities with Realism. It investigates "systems" in terms of totality, self-regulation, and transformation.

Mendelian genetics: The theory of heredity that forms the basis of classical genetics, proposed by Gregor Mendel (1822–1884) in 1866. Mendel suggested that individual characteristics were determined by inherited "factors."

moral treatment: The first systematic treatment that commenced in the last decade of the 18th century providing responsible care for an appreciable number of people with mental illness. "Moral" was used in this early context as the equivalent of "emotional" or "psychological" (from the same root as morale) and also has to do with custom, conduct, way of life, and inner meaning.

mutation: Genetic change that, when transmitted to offspring, gives rise to heritable variations (Latin muto = change).

neo-Darwinism: *See* synthetic Darwinism.

neophilia: Love for, great interest in what is new; novelty.

nepotism: Favoritism shown to relatives, especially in conferring offices.

neural Darwinism: Gerald Edelman's theory of the biological development of the brain within an individual's lifespan, rooted in Darwinian notions of natural selection. See also neuronal group selection.

neuronal group selection: The central theory of Edelman's neural Darwinism. It has 3 major tenets: a dynamic selection process that sets up the neuroanatomical characteristics of individuals during development; patterns of responses selected from this anatomy during experience; and physiology and psychology that give rise to behavior through re-entry, a process of signaling between brain maps. *See also* re-entrant signaling.

new public health: Global Public Health initiatives of recent years based on the *Declaration of Alma Ata* and the *Ottawa Charter for Health Promotion*. Emphasis is on primary health care, illness prevention, and health promotion.

Occident: Europe and America as distinct from the Orient (Latin occidens -entis = setting, sunset, west).

occupation: All that people need, want, or are obliged to do; what it means to them; and its ever-present potential as an agent of change. It encapsulates doing, being, and becoming.

occupational alienation: Sense of isolation, powerlessness, frustration, loss of control, and estrangement from society or self as a result of engagement in occupation that does not satisfy inner needs.

occupational balance: A balance of engagement in occupation that leads to well-being. For example, the balance may be among physical, mental, and social occupations; between chosen and obligatory occupations; between strenuous and restful occupations; or between doing and being.

occupational deprivation: Deprivation of occupational choice and diversity because of circumstances beyond the control of individuals or communities.

occupational imbalance: A lack of balance or disproportion of occupation resulting in decreased well-being.

occupational justice: The promotion of social and economic change to increase individual, community, and political awareness, resources, and equitable opportunities for diverse occupational opportunities that enable people to meet their potential and experience well-being.

occupational potential: Future capability to engage in occupation toward needs, goals, and dreams for health, material requirement, happiness, and well-being.

occupational science: The rigorous study of humans as occupational beings.

occupational technology: Means and tools by which material things are produced in a particular civilization that change ways of "doing."

occupational therapy: "Promoting health and well being through occupation. The primary goal of occupational therapy is to enable people to participate successfully in the activities of everyday life. Occupational therapists achieve this outcome by enabling people to do things that will enhance their ability to live meaningful lives or by modifying the environment to better support participation."[1]

ontogeny: The development of an individual from egg to adult throughout the lifespan.

organic communities: Societies in which natural functions, role perspectives, mutual interdependence, and intrinsic relationships are paramount.

phylogeny: The evolutionary history of species.

physiological neophilia: Everything new is attractive in puberty.

polymorphism: Diversity occurring within biological populations.

pragmatism: A philosophy of the late 19th and 20th centuries that interprets truth in terms of practical effects. "Meaning" can best be understood by examining its consequences on human activity.

praxis: Doing, acting, action, practice; free, universal, creative, and self-creative activity. Can be any kind of activity, but often used for business or political activity, accepted practice or custom, and as a descriptor in action-research.

prerequisites of health: Peace, shelter, education, food, income, a stable eco-system, sustainable resources, social justice, and equity.[2]

preventive medicine: The application of Western medical and social science to prevent disease, prolong life, and promote health in the community through intercepting disease processes.

proto humans: Early members of the hominidae family such as Australopithecus (Greek protos, proto = first).

public health: Public health addresses the health of the population as a whole by "fulfilling society's interest in assuring conditions in which people can be healthy."[3]

radiator theory: A theory proposed by Dean Falk, an anthropologist, that the evolution of increased brain size was dependent on adequate cooling through heat dispersal. This theory is based on the differences in cranial vessels and drainage patterns (foramen in the skull) between australopithecines and early *Homo* brains. These patterns become increasingly elaborate over evolutionary time.

reciprocity: Mutual action, exchange, practice of give and take.

reductionism: A philosophical stance associated with empiricism and scientific "disciplines" in which understanding is achieved through the study of parts and their effects on each other.

re-entrant signaling: A term used by Edelman in his theory of neural Darwinism. Brains contain multiple maps that automatically adapt their boundaries to changing signals to categorize and make sense of perceptions. The maps are connected by parallel and reciprocal connections. Re-entrant signaling occurs along these connections. This means that, as groups of neurons are selected in a map, other groups in different maps may also be selected at the same time. Re-entrant signaling is the process by which correlation and coordination of such selection events are achieved.[4]

Regimen Sanitatis: Rules of health. The name given to a medico-literary phenomenon originating at the ancient University of Salerno in Southern Italy providing 6 major rules for living known as the "non-naturals." Based on Hippocrates.

self-actualization: People becoming what they have the potential to become. Full humanness. The development of the inner nature and needs and biological potential of people. People becoming what they have the potential to become.

sexual dimorphism: The male and female of a species are distinctly different (eg, in size or shape).

social Darwinism: A largely discredited doctrine of the late 19th and early 20th centuries that applied (mostly erroneously) Darwin's theory of biological evolution to societies.

social justice: The promotion of social and economic change to increase individual, community, and political awareness, resources, and opportunity for health and well-being.

sociobiology: The study of animal behavior, especially social behavior, from the perspective of evolution by natural selection.

synthetic Darwinism: A modern synthesis of Charles Darwin's arguments of natural selection with Gregor Mendel's mechanisms of heredity. This was accomplished in the 1940s by a group of evolutionists and geneticists and accounts for the origin of genetic variation as mutations in DNA as well as rearrangement of genetic structures in a process known as recombination. Also known as neo-Darwinism.

temporality: Of time (Latin tempus -por = time).

topobiology: A term used by Edelman in his theories about brain evolution because many transactions leading to shape are place dependent (topo = place).

Utopia: An imagined perfect place, perfect society, or state of things. The term emerged during the Renaissance in the 14th through 16th centuries, being coined by Sir Thomas More as the name he gave to his ideal city-state.

Wernicke's area: A region of the human brain in the left parietotemporal region involved in the comprehension of speech. Named after neurologist Carl Wernicke (1848-1905).

References

1. World Federation of Occupational Therapists. Definition: 2004. Available at: www.wfot.org.au/officefiles/final%20definitionCM20042.pdf. Accessed April 25, 2006.
2. World Health Organization, Health and Welfare Canada, Canadian Public Health Association. *Ottawa Charter for Health Promotion*. Ottawa, Canada: WHO; 1986.
3. Institute of Medicine, Committee for the Study of the Future of Public Health, Division of Health Care Services. *The Future of Public Health*. Washington, DC: National Academy Press; 1988.
4. Edelman G. *Bright Air, Brilliant Fire: On the Matter of the Mind*. London: Penguin Books; 1992.

INDEX

WAIT

...*There's More!*

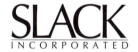